T0229541

ADDITIONAL VOLUMES IN PREPARATION

Cutaneous Infection and Therapy

edited by
Raza Aly
Karl R. Beutner
Howard Maibach
University of California School of Medicine
San Francisco, California

informa
healthcare

New York London

First published in 1997 by Marcel Dekker.

This edition published in 2011 by Informa Healthcare, Telephone House, 69-77 Paul Street, London EC2A 4LQ, UK.

Simultaneously published in the USA by Informa Healthcare, 52 Vanderbilt Avenue, 7th Floor, New York, NY 10017, USA.

Informa Healthcare is a trading division of Informa UK Ltd. Registered Office: 37–41 Mortimer Street, London W1T 3JH, UK. Registered in England and Wales number 1072954.

A CIP record for this book is available from the British Library.

Library of Congress Cataloging-in-Publication Data available on application

ISBN-13: 9780824798260

Orders may be sent to: Informa Healthcare, Sheepen Place, Colchester, Essex CO3 3LP, UK
Telephone: +44 (0)20 7017 5540
Email: CSDhealthcarebooks@informa.com
Website: http://informahealthcarebooks.com/

For corporate sales please contact: CorporateBooksIHC@informa.com
For foreign rights please contact: RightsIHC@informa.com
For reprint permissions please contact: PermissionsIHC@informa.com

Series Introduction

During the past decade there has been a vast explosion in new information relating to the art and science of dermatology as well as fundamental cutaneous biology. Furthermore, this information is no longer of interest only to the small but growing specialty of dermatology. Scientists from a wide variety of disciplines have come to recognize both the importance of skin in fundamental biological processes and the broad implications of understanding the pathogenesis of skin disease. As a result there is now a multidisciplinary and worldwide interest in the progress of dermatology.

With these factors in mind, we have undertaken a series of books specifically oriented to dermatology. The series has been purposely broad in focus and has ranged from pure basic science to practical, applied clinical dermatology. Thus, while there is something for everyone, all editions in the series should ultimately prove to be valuable additions to the dermatologist's library.

The latest addition to the series by Raza Aly, Karl R. Beutner, and Howard Maibach is both timely and pertinent. The authors are well known authorities in the fields of cutaneous microbiology and clinical skin infections. We trust that this volume will be of broad interest to scientists and clinicians alike.

Alan R. Shalita
SUNY Health Science Center
Brooklyn, New York

Preface

Cutaneous Infection and Therapy reviews the latest developments in the field and summarizes current knowledge, hypotheses, and opinions. The most recent advances in treating cutaneous fungal, bacterial, and viral infections are examined. Cutaneous infections are among the most common afflictions in humans. Emphasis is on the clinical perspective rather than laboratory microbiology, although enough of the latter is included to place the clinical aspect in proper context. This volume is a source of information for dermatologists, as well as for clinicians and clinical scientists with interests in cutaneous infections.

The skin, being our exposed or external organ, is readily accessible to a vast number of microbial organisms. We are exposed to these organisms on a nearly continuous basis during many of our normal daily activities. While the skin and our natural host and immunological defenses are well adapted to protecting us from this onslaught, skin infections remain a major cause of human morbidity. Virtually everyone will have one or more cutaneous infections, at least episodically. One might wonder why everyone is not continuously afflicted with multiple infections. Given the rate of exposure versus the number of symptomatic individuals, one would say we are doing quite well.

The spectrum of cutaneous infection is broad in terms of the pathogenic organisms, which include fungi, yeast, bacteria, and viruses, as well as a variety of hosts, which include infants, children, and adults— both immunocompetent and immunocompromised—as well as diffuse natural history ranging from acute self-limited infections to chronic and recurrent infections. Expression of these infections can be brought on by preexisting factors such as local mechanical trauma or one's immunological status, sexual habits, occupation, or skin care. These conditions are diagnosed and treated by a variety of clinicians, from generalists to specialists. As illustrated by the diverse background of the authors in this volume, research on these infections is an active area for scientists and clinicians, including microbiologists, medicinal chemists, dermatologists, infectious disease specialists, gynecologists, pediatricians, and orobiologists. These efforts are directed at diagnosis, better understanding of epidemiology and natural history, and a constant search for new therapies and therapeutic approaches. This volume represents a snapshot of the state of cutaneous infections in the mid-1990s. Research may rapidly make this an old snapshot, and the more rapidly this happens, the better all our patients will be.

The authors who have contributed to this book represent a cross-section of authorities in the many specialized areas that characterize our knowledge of skin infection and therapy. They include investigators in microbiology, dermatology, infectious diseases, orobiology, and various areas of pharmaceutical industry. We are grateful for their efforts in preparing such well-written material. Significant efforts have been made to minimize repetition and overlap. In some cases, however, information is deliberately repeated to provide a necessary frame of reference.

This volume will be valuable to the variety of clinicians and scientists who share our interests and enthusiasm about cutaneous infections.

Raza Aly
Karl R. Beutner
Howard Maibach

Contents

I. BACTERIAL INFECTIONS

Contents ix

Contributors

Raza Aly, Ph.D. Department of Dermatology, University of California School of Medicine, San Francisco, California

Dennis E. Babel, Ph.D. Department of Microbiology, Michigan State University, East Lansing, Michigan

Robert L. Baran, M.D. Nail Disease Center, Cannes, France

Robert G. Bartolo, Ph.D. Department of Personal Cleansing Product Development, The Procter & Gamble Company, Cincinnati, Ohio

Cynthia A. Berge, M.T., ASCP Department of Clinical Research and Biometrics, The Procter & Gamble Company, Cincinnati, Ohio

David I. Bernstein, M.D. Division of Infectious Diseases, Children's Hospital Medical Center, Cincinnati, Ohio

Karl R. Beutner, M.D., Ph.D. Department of Dermatology, University of California School of Medicine, San Francisco, California

Woubalem Birmachu 3M Pharmaceuticals, St. Paul, Minnesota

Jacalyn L. Bryan, R.N., M.S., C.I.C. Association of State and Territorial Health Officials, Washington, D.C.

Marvin T. Case 3M Pharmaceuticals, St. Paul, Minnesota

Komal Chopra, M.D. Department of Microbiology/Immunology, University of Texas Medical Branch, Galveston, Texas

Peggy Clarke, MPH American Social Health Association, Research Triangle Park, North Carolina

Jackie Cohran, R.N., M.S., C.I.C. Department of Infection Control Epidemiology, Prince George's Hospital Center, Cheverly, Maryland

Marcus A. Conant, M.D. Department of Dermatology, University of California School of Medicine, San Francisco, California

Graham Darby, B.Sc., M.A., Ph.D. Department of Therapeutic Research, Glaxo Wellcome, Stevenage, England

Gray Davis, Ph.D. Department of International OTC Antiviral Development, Glaxo Wellcome, Research Triangle Park, North Carolina

Piet De Doncker, Ph.D. Departments of Clinical Research/Dermatology and Infectious Diseases, Janssen Research Foundation, Beerse, Belgium

Charles Ebel, B.A. *Sexual Health Magazine*, Durham, and Herpes Advice Center, Research Triangle Park, North Carolina

Jan Faergemann, M.D., Ph.D. Department of Dermatology, Sahlgrenska University Hospital, Gothenburg, Sweden

David S. Feingold, M.D. Department of Dermatology, Tufts University School of Medicine, Boston, Massachusetts

Grace Forde, M.D. Departments of Neurology and Anesthesia, University of California School of Medicine, San Francisco, California

Ilona J. Frieden, M.D. Departments of Dermatology and Pediatrics, University of California School of Medicine, San Francisco, California

John F. Gerster, Ph.D. Drug Discovery Department, 3M Pharmaceuticals, St. Paul, Minnesota

Sheila J. Gibson 3M Pharmaceuticals, St. Paul Minnesota

Angella Glidden, M.D. Department of Microbiology/Immunology, University of Texas Medical Branch, Galveston, Texas

John R. Graybill, M.D. Department of Medicine, University of Texas Health Science Center at San Antonio and Audie Murphy Veterans Hospital, San Antonio, Texas

Deborah Greenspan, B.D.S., D.Sc., hon FDS RCS Edin. Department of Stomatology, University of California School of Medicine, San Francisco, California

Christopher J. Harrison, M.D. Department of Pediatrics, Creighton University and University of Nebraska Medical Center, Omaha, Nebraska

Edgar L. Hill, M.S.P.H. Department of Virology, Glaxo Wellcome, Research Triangle Park, North Carolina

David U. Himmelberger, M.S. Health Outcomes Group, Palo Alto, California

Jerry J. Hutchinson, B.Sc., Ph.D. Department of Advanced Tissue Repair Research and Development, ConvaTec, Ltd., Deeside, Clwyd, Wales

Linda M. Imbertson 3M Pharmaceuticals, St. Paul, Minnesota

H. S. Jaffe, M.D. Department of Clinical Affairs, Gilead Sciences, Inc., Foster City, California

Russell C. Johnson, Ph.D. Department of Microbiology, University of Minnesota Medical School, Minneapolis, Minnesota

Bruce H. Keswick, Ph.D. Clinical Research and Biometrics Department, The Procter & Gamble Company, Cincinnati, Ohio

Edna K. Kretzer, R.N., M.S., CFNP Department of Medicine, Johns Hopkins Bayview Medical Center, Baltimore, Maryland

Elaine L. Larson, R.N., Ph.D., FAAN Georgetown University School of Nursing, Washington, D.C.

Patricia Lee, M.D. Department of Microbiology/Immunology, University of Texas Medical Branch, Galveston, Texas

Eva Lydick, Ph.D. Department of Epidemiology, Merck Research Laboratories, West Point, Pennsylvania

Howard Maibach, M.D. Department of Dermatology, University of California School of Medicine, San Francisco, California

Michael R. McGinnis Department of Pathology, University of Texas Medical Branch, Galveston, Texas

Brian William McGuire, Ph.D. Department of Clinical Research, Gilead Sciences, Inc., Foster City, California

Richard L. Miller, Ph.D. Department of Pharmacology, 3M Pharmaceuticals, St. Paul, Minnesota

William Charles Noble, Ph.D., D.Sc., FRC Path. Institute of Dermatology, St. Thomas' Hospital, London, England

Charles G. Prober, M.D. Department of Pediatrics, Stanford University Medical Center, Stanford California

Azer Rashid, M.D., Ph.D. Department of Dermatology, Khyber Medical College, Peshawar, Pakistan

James E. Rasmussen Department of Dermatology, University of Michigan Medical Center, Ann Arbor, Michigan

Michael V. Reitano, M.D. National Advice Centers, *Sexual Health Magazine*, and New York University Hospital, New York, New York

Michael J. Reiter 3M Pharmaceuticals, St. Paul, Minnesota

M. D. Richardson University of Glasgow, Glasgow, Scotland

David T. Roberts Southern General Hospital, Glasgow, Scotland

Michael C. Rowbotham, M.D. Departments of Neurology and Anesthesia, University of California School of Medicine, San Francisco, California

Theodore C. Spaulding, Ph.D. International OTC Antiviral Development, Glaxo Wellcome, Research Triangle Park, North Carolina

Spotswood L. Spruance, M.D. Department of Internal Medicine, University of Utah School of Medicine, Salt Lake City, Utah

Jerry O. Stern, M.D. National Advice Centers and New York University Hospital, New York, New York

Mark A. Tomai, Ph.D. Drug Discovery Department, 3M Pharmaceuticals, St. Paul, Minnesota

Stephen K. Tyring, M.D., Ph.D. Departments of Dermatology, Microbiology/Immunology, and Internal Medicine, University of Texas Medical Branch, Galveston, Texas

Geo von Krogh, M.D., Ph.D. Department of Dermatology and Venereology, Karolinska Hospital, Stockholm, Sweden

Tamara L. Wagner 3M Pharmaceuticals, St. Paul, Minnesota

Thomas J. Walsh, M.D. Pediatric Branch, National Cancer Institute, Bethesda, Maryland

Deborah D. Watson, B.S. Personal Cleansing Product Development, The Procter & Gamble Company, Cincinnati, Ohio

Richard J. Whitley, M.D. Departments of Pediatrics, Microbiology, and Medicine, The University of Alabama at Birmingham, Birmingham, Alabama

1

Factors Modulating Cutaneous Flora

Raza Aly and Howard Maibach
University of California School of Medicine, San Francisco, California

INTRODUCTION

Various cutaneous factors control the survival of pathogenic microorganisms on human skin and the development of infection. The ability to eliminate or control exogenous bacterial life has been ascribed to both physical and chemical factors. Purely physical factors cause dehydration and desiccation of microorganisms. Chemical factors include antimicrobial substances derived from bacteria, keratinocytes, and pilosebaceous and eccrine gland secretions. Several of these factors operate selectively to eliminate different organisms from skin. Adherence factors present on bacterial cell walls and on the cell surface of epithelia recently have been implicated in bacterial colonization. There is a remarkable specificity involved in the adherence of various bacteria to different skin sites. Although these factors probably operate cooperatively, their relative importance or necessity is undetermined.

The specific identity of the chemical agents is particularly wanting. In general, intact skin and mucous membranes provide barriers to the invading microorganisms. Once barriers have been breached, phagocytosis and intracellular processing of bacteria become the primary functions of the host to eradicate the infecting organisms. This chapter discusses, for the most part, those factors that are primarily related to the skin.

BACTERIAL FACTORS

Microbial antagonisms regulating the resident flora on the skin, although mechanistically complex, play an important role in host susceptibility to infection. Berntsen and McDermott (1) noted that hospitalized patients treated with tetracycline acquired nasal staphylococci more frequently than appropriate controls. They postulated that the use of antibiotics resulted in increased transmissibility of staphylococci. Antibiotics markedly changed the indigenous microbial flora, and this may have provided the setting in which resistant organisms multiplied and become the predominant flora.

Probably the most interesting example of a complex succession of microorganisms in a skin lesion is in tinea pedis (2). Here the toe web becomes infected with a dermatophyte, which may be assisted by its production of antibacterial antibiotics such as penicillins and amino-glycosides. These antibiotic-producing fungi can eliminate the susceptible normal microflora, aided perhaps by chemotaxis, and the release of nutrients from killed bacteria (3,4). The fungal antibiotics also encourage secondary overgrowth by resistant "large colony coryneforms"—mainly *Brevibacterium epidermidis*—and to a lesser extent by *Staphylococcus aureus* and gram-negative bacilli. This mixed infection corresponds to the dermatophytosis complex stage of athlete's foot, in which the original dermatophyte infection has been mainly or entirely replaced by a secondary coryneform infection, resistant to antifungal and many antibacterial agents.

Sprunt et al. (5) demonstrated that viridans streptococci, which predominate in the oropharynx flora of most individuals, can inhibit the growth of enteric gram-negative bacilli. The overgrowth of enteric bacteria at these sites follows therapy with massive doses of penicillin. They proposed that the suppression of streptococci by antibiotics results in the loss of inhibitory action on gram-negative bacteria, thereby permitting multiplication of the previously inhibited (or newly introduced) bacilli. Patients carrying streptococci resistant to the antibiotic did not experience overgrowth of enterics when the same antibiotic was given. These patients had recently received penicillin. Such exposure to the antibiotic favored the selection of resistant strains of streptococci in the oropharynx.

We observed that certain strains of viridans streptococci from the nose of normal subjects inhibit *S. aureus* and *Staphylococcus pyogenes* when grown together on trypticase soy agar. Also, prior intraallontoic infection of chicken embryos with viridans streptococci protected them from the challenge of virulent strains of *S. aureus* (6).

The phenomenon of bacterial interference has been utilized to control cross-infection of the skin and nasal mucosa by staphylococci. *S. aureus* 502A, obtained from a nurse and infants in hospital nurseries who were free from staphylococcal disease, was capable of colonizing nasal mucosa and umbilicus when artificially applied. This aspect of bacterial interference has been utilized as a therapeutic tool in patients with recurrent furunculosis (6a). Viable *S. aureus* 502A is required to demonstrate this bacterial interference phenomenon. Patients with extensive burns or neoplastic conditions, or those who are chronically ill or immunosuppressed would be potential beneficiaries from such ecological approaches. In these patients, administration of antibiotics often leads to the overgrowth of more dangerous microbial flora.

The opposite effect, satellitism (i.e., the growth enhancement of one organism by another), is a little understood phenomenon of the microbial ecology of skin. It is not known whether the bacteria involved in this phenomenon exert their effects by production of essential growth factors or destruction of toxic substances. The role of satellitism in the ecology of skin requires systemic study.

The incidence of systemic infection caused by gram-negative organisms has recently increased. The widespread use of antibiotics effective predominantly against gram-positive organisms has been incriminated as the most likely cause for this shift. Of particular interest is the gram-negative folliculitis seen in patients receiving long-term antibiotics for the treatment of acne vulgaris (7). Marples et al. (8) reported a higher rate of colonization of the anterior nares of acne patients following prolonged use of antibiotics. The incidence rate was 73% in these patients. The pustular lesions are grouped around the nose and fan out on the cheeks. The intensive use of soap containing hexachlorophene is bacteriostatic against gram-positive bacteria (9,10). The combined action of prolonged use of antibiotics and antibacterial soaps that suppress gram-positive bacteria creates an ecological vacuum for proliferation of gram-negative bacteria.

CUTANEOUS FACTORS

Eccrine Sweat

Eccrine sweat contains factors that inhibit the growth of *Microsporum gypseum* and *Epidermophyton inguinale* (11). This fungicidal property was attributed to acetic, propionic, caprylic, and lactic acids, leading to the early development of fatty acid topical therapy of superficial cutaneous fungus infections.

Surface Lipids

Lipids of both pilosebaceous and keratinocyte origin are called surface lipids. Distinction as to origin is not made. Burtenshaw (12) prepared crude ether extracts of skin and tested them against common bacterial pathogens. *Streptococcus pyogenes,* viridans streptococci, *Corynebacterium diphtheriae,* and certain strains of *S. aureus* were sensitive to these extracts. Ricketts et al. (13) used acetone to obtain lipids from the skin surface and demonstrated that true fatty acids comprised 35 to 45% of skin lipids. *S. aureus* and *S. pyogenes,* when exposed to various concentrations of these fatty acids, were more sensitive to unsaturated than to saturated fatty acids.

Nicholaides (14) demonstrated that surface skin lipids contain more fatty free acids than either sebaceous glands or epithelial cells alone. When free fatty acid levels on skin are high, triglyceride levels are low, and vice versa. The relative proportion of free fatty acids to total lipids is variable. One reason for this variability is that lipid deposited on the human skin surface undergoes lipolysis by lypolytic enzymes derived from skin bacteria and fungi, and possibly by lipases of cutaneous origin.

Endogenous (Keratinocyte) Versus Exogenous (Pilosebaceous) Lipids

Lipids primarily of keratinocytic origin are termed *endogenous lipids,* while those of pilosebaceous origin are known as *exogenous lipids.* Histochemical and chemical analyses demonstrate that sebum in sebaceous cysts contains no free fatty acids (15,16). It is only after sebum leaves the sebaceous glands and is exposed to the external environment that fatty acids are formed. Sebum on the skin surface comprised approximately 25% of odd chain length and branched fatty acids, while the epidermal layer had only 6%. Kligman (17) showed that sebum smeared on filter paper discs was not inhibitory to staphylococci and streptococci on brain heart infusion blood agar. Blood and albumin neutralize the antimicrobial effectiveness of fatty acids; thus the in vitro system utilizing blood agar plates selected by Kligman to study the antibacterial effect of sebum may not be appropriate. Further, the chemical composition of sebum and epidermal lipids is qualitatively and quantitatively different. However, no study has compared directly the antimicrobial effects of lipids collected from the forehead (largely sebum) versus those collected from the palm and forearm, which are mostly epidermal in origin. A comparison of the bactericidal effect of lipids derived from different areas would be useful.

We substantiated earlier studies demonstrating that when *S. pyogenes, S. aureus,* or *Candida albicans* were deposited on normal skin and occluded for 5 hours, their numbers were reduced significantly (18). In contrast, forearms washed with acetone allowed greater persistence of deposited bacteria. Further observations demonstrated that (a) antimicrobial activity returned after 5 hours or upon replacement of acetone extracts of the skin and (b) the phenomenon was not due to bacterial interference. The ability to inhibit growth of *S. aureus* on skin was not uniform. Many individuals had the capacity to destroy greatly reduce artificially applied *S. aureus,* while in others, this organism persisted or multiplied (19). This relationship was not noted with *S. pyogenes.* However, subjects demonstrating *S. aureus* persistence also demonstrated persistence of *C. albicans,* and those subjects not showing *S. aureus* persistence on their skin also resisted *C. albicans* multiplication. Subjects allowing multiplication of bacteria on their skin were designated *persisters* and those inhibiting growth of bacteria were called *inhibitors*: Persisters had higher counts of normal flora (average 9.2×10^3/cm^2) than inhibitors (7.4×10^2).

There was a direct correlation between the quantitative reduction of experimentally inoculated *S. aureus* on skin and the degree of inhibition shown in vitro by acetone extracts of the skin surface material (19). Bacteria recovered from samples containing skin extracts were divided by the counts from samples containing acetone and were expressed as percent recovery. The percentage of *S. aureus* or *C. albicans* recovered was higher (79% and 55%, respectively) in persisters than in the inhibitors (47% and 28%, respectively). This difference noted for *S. aureus* was not found with *S. pyogenes.* The percentage of *S. pyogenes* recovered was 30% whether skin extracts were from low-count or high-count populations. *S. pyogenes* is most sensitive to skin lipids and, probably because of its extreme sensitivity to lipids, is seldom present on normal skin. A direct correlation between the quantitative reduction of experimental inoculation of bacteria on skin and the degree of their inhibition in vitro by acetone extracts taken from the skin surface was established (18,19).

After establishing that skin surface lipids kill certain pathogenic bacteria and *C. albicans* but not other microflora, the antifungal effects of lipid extracts were tested against *Trichophyton mentagrophytes.* The methods used were the same as for *S. aureus,* except that spores of *T. mentagrophytes* were substituted for bacteria. Fifteen subjects (nine persisters and six inhibitors) were selected. The antifungal activity between the two populations was not significantly different, but lipids did demonstrate antifungal activity. For some skin bacteria, cutaneous surface lipids may have a stimulatory rather than inhibitory role. Puhvel and Reisner (20) found that although saturated fatty acids (C8, C16) inhibited the growth of two strains of *Propionibacterium acnes*, oleic acid (unsaturated C8) promoted their growth. Oleic acid also promotes growth of cutaneous aerobic diptheroids in vitro (21).

It has been established that as compared with those of adults, the more varied flora of infants and children could be due to a relatively low level of free fatty acids on the skin. Streptococci that are very sensitive to antimicrobial effects of fatty acids are rarely found on adult skin, but occur on infant's skin (22).

In our work involving the stratum corneum lipids of humans and especially essential fatty acid–deficient mice, we discovered that the phospholipid and sphingolipid fractions of thin-layer chromatography showed strong antimicrobial activity (23,24). Pursuing this lead, we developed an in vitro assay to screen an assortment of commercial phospholipids and sphingolipids (25). The sphingosines and, to a lesser degree, stearlamine were clearly effective against *S. aureus* (4 log reduction at 6.25 μg/ml). The sphingosines were similarly active against *S. pyogenes*, *Micrococcus luteus*, *P. acnes*, *B. epidermis*, and *C. albicans*. Sphingosine and sphinganine, free phospholipids of the stratum corneum, demonstrated strong inhibitory activity for both bacteria and fungi. These results point toward new chemical approaches in antimicrobial therapy. Sphingolipids have been suggested as antiinflammatory agents because of their wide spectrum of regulatory functions in mammalian cells (26). The idea of drugs having both antimicrobial and antiinflammatory activity is exciting. The prophylactic effect of sphingosine on the survival of microorganisms subsequently applied to human skin was investigated. Strong statistically significant differences between use of the lipid and its vehicle alone were noted (27). Similar results were obtained when sphingosine was applied to an expanded normal flora of the skin.

We previously determined that sphingosine and sphinganine kill staphylococci in part by damaging their cell wall (28). We ascertained that these lipids are even stronger inhibitors than penicillin and chloramphenicol perhaps because of a more direct and rapid bactericidal effect of the cell membrane (unpublished data). Adherence of bacteria to epithelial cells would thereby be reduced as previously reported (29).

Secretory Antibodies

A wide spectrum of antibacterial antibodies occur in external secretions of the normal host. These antibodies might play an important role in host susceptibility to infections. The role of secretory antibody against bacterial infection has not been studied. Today, variation in local immunity, specifically the secretory IgA response, is the leading prospect for solving this puzzle. The mechanism by which secretory IgA mediates its antibacterial activity on mucous surfaces remains speculative. Theoretically, antibodies in secretions may react with bacteria while they are multiplying on the mucosal surfaces; hence, when the organisms become dislodged, they would have a reduced ability to reattach.

IgA antibodies found in parotid saliva can inhibit the attachment of oral streptococci to epithelial cells (30). It is expected that this property would inhibit streptococcal colonization without the involvement of phagocytes or the complement system. Such mechanisms may explain, at least in part, how IgA antibodies provide protection on mucosal surfaces.

Secretory IgA and IgG in human genital secretions inhibit the adherence of *Neisseria gonorrhoea* (31). Studies on the prevention of adhesion of *Escherichia coli* to urinary tract–epithelial cells showed that IgG and secretory IgA from the urine of a patient with acute pyelonephritis were inhibitory, as were other secretions such as breast milk or commercial globulin (32).

In naturally acquired immunity against pathogenic bacteria, the role of secretory antibodies is important in controlling bacterial colonization. A deficiency in the mechanisms of production of secretory antibodies may render the host susceptible to certain infections.

BACTERIAL ADHERENCE

Among the various known ecological factors that determines host–parasite relationships is the specific binding of microorganisms to cells and tissues. This important process is called adherence; the microbe-borne molecule that connects with a host receptor is an adhesin. Like those tenacious microorganisms inhabiting streams and other marine environments, the flora indigenous to skin and mucosa has the selective advantage of being able to stick to substrates, resisting the abrasive forces of air and fluid currents that would otherwise wash it away (33). Furthermore, like the attachment of viruses to their target cells, microbial adherence is a significant, if not crucial, step in infectivity and in subsequent infectious disease (34). Indeed, the molecular principles previously established for specific viral attachment have been found appropriate for bacteria and fungi as well.

Bacteria vary in their ability to attach to epithelial cells. *Streptococcus salivarius* and *Streptococcus sanguis*, found abundantly on the oral epithelial surface, demonstrate great affinity for these cells (35). In contrast, *Streptococcus mutans*, which are found in small numbers on oral epithelial surfaces, exhibit feeble adherence. *S. mutans* prefer instead the tooth surface. In addition to the investigations on oral streptococci, studies have been carried out on streptococci associated with pyoderma. Group A streptococci are the predominant skin pathogen. The Group A streptococci isolated from skin adhered in greater numbers to human skin epithelial cells than to buccal mucosa, whereas streptococci isolated from the throat adhered better to buccal epithelia (33). Similar host factors may be involved in people with rheumatic heart disease, because fever–associated strains of streptococci adhere more to pharyngeal cells of rheumatic fever patients than to cells of control subjects (36).

Lipoteichoic acid was among the first adhesins identified on gram-positive bacteria. It is the adhesin by which *S. pyogenes* attaches to oral mucosa cells (37). Neither M protein nor C carbohydrate had appreciable blocking ability. Furthermore, antilipoteichoic acid antiserum interfered with adherence, and purified lipoteichoic acid could attach to the outer membranes of erythrocytes and oral epithelial cells. Alkan et al. (33) later found through inhibition studies that this wall substance is also involved in streptococcal adherence to human stratum corneum cells. The oral epithelial cells of newborn infants carry less than half the receptors for *S. pyogenes* of adults; however, within 3 days, adherence counts for reach adult levels (38). Adult buccal cells constituted some 5×10^9 binding sites for lipoteichoic acid (39).

C. albicans is not normally considered part of the skin microflora, but may be isolated from the mucous membranes of the alimentary tract and vagina (40). Infection may occur at these sites of colonization especially after antibiotic or steroid treatment; for example, widespread use of the contraceptive pill is related to an increase in vaginal candidosis. In cases of immunosuppression, however, life-threatening disease due to this organism is also encountered. Adherence of *C. albicans* to buccal and cutaneous cells is probably related to a glycoprotein receptor. Pretreatment of the yeast with various polysaccharides inhibited adherence. While several carbohydrates were effective in buccal cell assays, only galactosamine, glucosamine, and mannosamine gave significant reductions with corneocytes (41).

Bacterial Adherence to Adult Nasal Epithelial Cells

We developed methods by which bacterial adherence to human nasal mucosal cells was demonstrated (42). We selected epithelial cells because for many bacteria, particularly *S. aureus*, the nose is a site for multiplication and dissemination. Vulvar skin is another reservoir for *S. aureus* (43).

We demonstrated the selective ability of bacteria to adhere to nasal mucosal cells. Significant adherence occurred with *Pseudomonas aeruginosa, S. epidermidis, S. aureus, S. pyogenes, and coryneforms, but less with S. mutans,* and *Klebsiella pneumoniae.* Staphylococci, which constitute the major flora of the anterior nares, possess a distinct advantage over *Streptococcus mitis* and *S. mutans.* They are the predominant flora of the buccal mucosa and teeth. The persistent nasal carrier status of *S. aureus* was investigated. The adherence of *S. aureus* was significantly greater (P <0.005) for the carriers of *S. aureus* than that for the noncarriers (i.e., 132 + 82 for carriers and 67 + 70 for noncarriers). This finding suggested that the greater affinity of bacteria to mucosal cells of staphylococcal carriers might be a property of the mucosal cells or host environment rather than the bacteria because *S. aureus* was a common denominator in both carriers and noncarriers. By utilizing this model, we may gain further insight in determining why some people become staphylococcal carriers and others do not.

Bacterial Adherence in Dermatitic Skin

S. aureus colonization is extremely high in patients with atopic dermatitis. The high prevalence of *S. aureus* is noted not only in eczematous skin but also in the noninvolved skin of the adjacent area and the anterior nares (44). High *S. aureus* counts occur in psoriatic plaques, although these counts are not as high as in atopics. *S. aureus* rarely becomes part of the resident flora on normal skin.

We examined epithelial cells of patients with eczema or psoriasis for their binding capacity to *S. aureus.* The adherence of *S. aureus* to the epithelial cells of atopic subjects was significantly greater when compared with normal subjects. However the difference in adherence between psoriatic epithelial cells and normal epithelial cells was not significant. The greater affinity of *S. aureus* to epithelial cells obtained from eczema patients correlates with the high density of *S. aureus* on the skin of these patients. Whereas psoriasis is primarily a skin disease of unknown origin, atopic dermatitis has been related to aberrant, hyperactive immunological conditions and hence may be merely one symptom of a systemic disorder that probably also affects the nasal mucosa and regions of the respiratory tracts (45). It also seems that the enhanced binding of staphylococci to atopic epithelial cells may be due to some inherent cellular alteration unrelated to immunological aberrations associated with the disease.

Role of Teichoic Acid and Keratinized Cells in Adherence

While working with S. aureus, we obtained suggestive evidence that multiple adhesins and receptors are involved in microbe–keratinocyte interactions. Teichoic acid is apparently one adhesin of S. aureus for nasal, labial, and vaginal cells (46–48). On investigating its inhibition of staphylococcal adherence on spinous, granular, and fully keratinized cells, we observed that teichoic acid is effective only on the keratinocytes; the number of attached bacteria on cells from the lower, less differential layers remained the same.

In conclusion, the recent recognition and investigation of microbial adherence have been a major advance in our understanding of the ecological principles leading to the establishment of a normal flora and the onset of infectious disease. This field is still fresh, particularly in dermatobiology, and much more research is needed to determine the molecular composition and arrangement of adhesins and cell receptors, their respective production and distribution, and the physicochemical aspects of the interaction. New discoveries will almost certainly ensure the development of new ecologically based forms of therapy or prophylaxis.

EFFECTS OF OCCLUSION

Bacteria survive and multiply better under occlusion. Resident flora is denser in the moist regions than on the dry areas of the skin (49,50). Most of the water on skin is derived from eccrine sweat and transepidermal water loss. In the axillary region, there is also an intermittent contribution from apocrine sweat. Occlusion and the subsequent increase of humidity, among other changes, are significant ecological forces.

Henning et al. (51) studied the bacterial flora of the skin in experimentally produced miliaria. Extensive miliaria were noted in all subjects. After 48 hours of occlusion, the bacterial population was examined to determine whether any increased density could be related to the severity of the induced miliaria. These investigations found a nine times greater increase of aerobic bacteria per square centimeter in subjects with severe miliaria than in those with a less severe disease.

Lyons et al. (52) measured the incidence of miliaria in a controlled population living under standard climatic work and hygienic conditions. They reported that miliaria rubra is primarily a staphylococcal infection of the sweat pore and that the infection occurs as a result of damage produced by heat and humidity.

Hennig et al. (51) reported that although they could not exclude the possibility that bacteria play a role in the pathogenesis of miliaria rubra, they still believed that miliaria is not related to bacterial multiplying in the sweat glands or pores following occlusion.

Kligman and Leyden (53) applied polyethylene wrap to the feet of persons with fungus-positive asymptomatic dermatophytosis. The interspaces became macerated, whitish, itchy, and foul-smelling in about a week. With removal of occlusions, rapid return to the original state was not achieved, and symptoms persisted for weeks. Occlusion of normal, fungus-free interspaces produced only asymptomatic, whitish maceration (superhydration). The feet returned to normal within several days when they were allowed to dry. With occlusion, fungus-infected interspaces showed clinical worsening, which was correlated with the overgrowth of bacteria (53).

Approaches such as the removal of shoes and separation of interspaces with soft pads lead to a decrease in the amount of moisture and bacteria and a correspondence with clinical improvement. Similarly, treatments that simultaneously suppress bacteria and fungi as well as local drying are expected to be the most effective. Aluminum chloride, a dehydrating agent, will produce considerable clinical improvement in a symptomatic wet athlete's foot in a short period.

The effects of increased hydration have been studied by occluding the skin with plastic film for several days (54). The occlusion of skin not only results in hydration, but also alters other ecological factors. For example, pH of the skin, which is acidic (4.38) before occlusion, shifts to neutral (7.05) on day 4 of occlusion. Surface levels of carbon dioxide, which promote microbial growth and alter metabolism, also increased. Other factors such as nutrients, bacterial metabolites, bacterial antagonism, skin surface lipids and salt concentration can also change upon occlusion, thus exerting a cumulative pressure on the skin microbial flora.

We suspect that the effects of occlusion are complex. Great strides have been made in understanding the factors that modulate skin flora in health and disease, although we are at the beginning of understanding the heterogeneous factors involved.

REFERENCES

1. Bernstein CA, McDermott W. Increased transmissibility of staphylococci to patients receiving an antimicrobial drug. N Engl J Med 1960; 262: 637–642.
2. Leyden JJ, Kligman AM. Interdigital athlete's foot. Arch Dermatol 1978; 114: 1466–1473.
3. Bibel DJ, Smiljanic RJ. Interaction of *Trichophyton mentagrophytes* and micrococci on skin culture. J Invest Dermatol 1979; 72: 133–137.
4. Virtanen O. Observation on the symbiosis of some fungi and bacteria. Ann Med Exp Biol Fenn 1959; 29: 352–358.
5. Sprunt K, Leidy G, Redman W. Prevention of bacterial overgrowth. J Infect Dis 1971; 123: 1–9.
6. Aly R, Maibach HI, Shinefield HR. Protection of chick embryos by viridian streptococci against the lethal effect of *S. aureus*. Infect Immun 1974; 9: 559–563.
6a. Aly R, Shinefield H, Maibach HI. Bacterial interference among *Staphylococcus aureus* strains. In: Aly R, Shinefield H (eds.). Bacterial Interference. Boca Raton, Florida: CRC Press, 1982: 13–23.
7. Fulton JE, McGinley K, Leydon JJ, Marples R. Gram-negative folliculitis in acne vulgaris. Arch Dermatol 1968; 98: 349–352.
8. Marples RR, Fulton JE, Leyden J, McGinley KJ. Effect of antibiotic in the nasal flora in acne patients. Arch Dermatol 1969; 99: 647–650.
9. Forfar JO, Gould JC, MacCabe AF. Effect of hexachloraphene on incidence of staphylococcal and gram-negative infections in the newborn. Lancet 1968; 2: 177–180.
10. Stetler H, Martin E, Plotkin S, Katz M. Neonatal mastitis due to *E. coli*. J Pediatr 1970; 76: 611–614.
11. Peck S, Rosenfeld H, Leifer W, Bierman W. Role of sweat as a fungicide. Arch Dermatol Syph 1939; 39: 126–148.
12. Burtenshaw JM. The mechanism of disinfection of the human skin and its appendages. J Hyg (Lond) 1942; 42: 184–210.
13. Ricketts CR, Squire JR, Topley E. Human skin lipids with particular reference to the self-sterilizing power of the skin. Clin Sci 1951; 1: 89–111.
14. Nicholaides N. Skin lipids, II. Lipid class composition of samples from various species and anatomical sites. J Am Oil Chem Soc 1965; 45: 691–702.
15. Nicholaides N, Wells GC. On the biogenesis of free fatty acids in human skin surface fat. J Invest Dermatol 1957; 29: 432–437.
16. Kellum RE. Human sebaceous gland lipids. Arch Dermatol 1967; 95: 218–224.
17. Kligman AM, The use of sebum. Br J Dermatol 196; 75: 307–319.
18. Aly R, Maibach HI, Strauss WG, Shinefield HR. Survival of pathogenic microorganisms on human skin. J Invest Dermatol 1972; 58: 205–210.

19. Aly R, Maibach HI, Rahman R, et al. Correlation of human in vitro and in vivo cutaneous antimicrobial factors. J Infect Dis 1975; 131: 579–583.
20. Puhvel M. Reisner RM. Effect of fatty acids on the growth of *Corynebacterium acne* in vitro. J Invest Dermatol 1970; 54: 40–52.
21. Pollack MR, Wainwright SD, Mansion ED. The presence of oleic acid-requiring diphtheroids on human skin. J Pathol Bacteriol 1949; 61: 274–276.
22. Somerville DA. The normal flora of the skin in different age groups. Br J Dermatol 1969; 81: 249–253.
23. Miller SJ, Aly R, Shinefield HR, Elias PM. In vitro and in vivo anti-staphylococcal activity of human stratum corneum lipids. Arch Dermatol 1988; 124: 209–215.
24. Bible DJ, Miller SJ, Brown BE, et al. Antimicrobial activity of stratum corneum lipids from normal and essential fatty acid-deficient mice. J Invest Dermatol 1989; 92: 632–638.
25. Bibel DJ, Aly R, Shinefield HR. Antimicrobial activity of sphingosines. J Invest Dermatol 1992; 98: 269–273.
26. Gupta AK, Fisher GJ, Elder JT, et al. Sphingosine inhibits phorbal ester-induced inflammation, ornithine decarboxylase activity, and activation of protein kinase C in mouse skin. J Invest Dermatol 1988; 91: 486–491.
27. Bibel DJ, Aly R, Shinefield HR. Topical sphingolipids in antisepsis and anti-fungal therapy. Clin Exp Dermatol 1995; 20: 395–400.
28. Bibel DJ, Aly R, Shah S, Shinefield HR. Sphingosines: antimicrobial barriers of the skin. Acta Derm Venereol 1993; 73: 407–411.
29. Bibel DJ, Aly R, Shinefield HR. Inhibition of microbial adherence by sphingosine. Can J Microbiol 1992; 38: 383–385.
30. Williams RC, Bibbons RJ. Inhibition of bacterial adherence by secretory immunoglobulin A: a mechanism of antigen disposal. Science 1972; 177: 697–699.
31. Tramont EC. An inhibition of adherence of *Neisseria gonorrhoea* by human genital secretions. J Clin Invest 1977; 59: 117–124.
32. Svanborg-Eden C, Svennerholm AM. Secretory immunoglobulin A and G antibodies prevent adhesion of *E. coli* to human tract epithelial cells. Infect Immun 1978; 22: 790–797.
33. Alkan M, Ofec I, Beachey E. Adherence of pharyngeal and skin stains of group A streptococci to human skin and oral epithelial cells. Infect Immun 1977; 18: 555–557.
34. Ofek I, Beachey EH. General concepts and principles of bacterial adherence in animals and man. In: Beachy EH, ed. Bacterial Adherence. London: Chapman and Hall; 1980: 19–44.
35. Gibbons RJ, Van Houte J. Bacterial adherence in oral microbial ecology. Annu Rev Microbiol 1975; 29: 19–44.
36. Selinger DS, Julie N, Reed WP, Williams RC. Adherence of group A streptococci to pharyngeal cells: a rile in the pathogenesis of rheumatic fever. Science 1978; 210: 455–457.
37. Ofec I, Beachey EH, Jefferson W, Cambell GL. Cell membrane binding properties of group A streptococcal lipoteichoic acid. J Exp Med 1985; 141: 900–1003.

38. Ofek I, Beachey EH, Eyal F, Morrison JC. Postnatal development of binding of streptococci and lipoteichoic acid by oral mucosal cells of humans. J Infect Dis 1977; 135: 267–274.
39. Simpson WA, Ofek I, Sarasohn C, et al. Characteristics of the binding of streptococcal lipoteichoic acid to human oral epithelial cells. J Infect Dis 1980; 141: 457–464.
40. Odds FC. Candida and Candidosis. Leicester: Leicester University Press, 1979.
41. Collins-Lech C. Kalbfleisch JH, Franson TR, Sohnle PG. Inhibition by sugars of *Candida albicans* adherence to human buccal mucosal cells and corneocytes in vitro. Infect Immun 1984; 46: 831–834.
42. Aly R, Shinefield HR, Strauss WG, Maibach HI. Bacterial adherence to nasal mucosal walls. Infect Immun 1977; 17: 546–549.
43. Aly R, Britz M, Maibach HI. Quantitative microbiology of human vulva. Br J Dermatol 1979; 101: 445–448.
44. Aly R, Maibach HI, Shinefield HR. Microbial flora of atopic dermatitis. Arch Dermatol 1977; 113: 780–782.
45. Rook AJ (ed.). Wilkinson DS, Ebling FJG. Textbook of Dermatology. 3d ed. Oxford: Blackwell Scientific, 1992.
46. Bibel DJ, Aly R, Shinefield HR, et al. Importance of the keratinized epithelial cells in bacterial adherence. J Invest Dermatol 1982; 79: 250–253.
47. Aly R, Shinefield HR, Litz C, Maibach HI. Role of teichoic acid in the binding of *Staphylococcus aureus* to nasal epithelial cells. J Infect Dis 1980; 141: 463–465.
48. Bibel DJ, Aly R, Lahti L, et al. Microbial adherence to vulvar epithelial cells. J Med Microbiol 1987; 23: 75–82.
49. Marples RR. The effect of hydration on the bacterial role of the skin. In: Maibach HI, Hildick-Smith G (eds.). Skin Bacteria and Their Role in Infection. New York: McGraw-Hill, 1965: 33–41.
50. Aly R, Maibach HI. Aerobic microbial flora of intertrigenous skin. Appl Environ Microbiol 1977; 33: 97–100.
51. Henning RD, Greffin TB, Maibach HI. Studies on changes in skin surface bacteria in induced malaria and associated hypohidrosis. Acta Derm Venereol 1972; 52: 371–375.
52. Lyons ER, Levine R, Auld D. Miliaria rubra: a manifestation of staphylococcal disease. Arch Dermatol 1962; 76: 282–286.
53. Kligman A, Leyden JJ. The interaction of fungi and bacteria in the pathogenesis of athlete's foot. In: Maibach HI, Aly R (eds.). Skin Microbiology: Relevance to Infection. New York: Springer-Verlag, 1981.
54. Aly R, Shirley C, Cunico B, et al. Effect of prolonged occlusion on the microbial flora, pH, CO_2 and transepidermal water loss on human skin. J Invest Dermatol 1978; 71: 378–381.

2

The Changing Spectrum of Streptococcal and Staphylococcal Infections

David S. Feingold

Tufts University School of Medicine, Boston, Massachusetts

History is replete with the periodic ebb and flow of infectious diseases. New diseases appear and well-described infections wax or wane for a variety of reasons including changes in the virulence of the organisms, changes in the susceptibility of the hosts, or changes in the interaction of humans with specific organisms causing new epidemiological patterns. There is grave concern expressed in the medical (1–3) and lay literature that we are in the midst of a very active phase of dangerous new and reemerging infectious diseases. AIDS is the paradigm.

This chapter explores recent changes in the spectrum of diseases caused by the major gram-positive pathogens, *Staphylococcus aureus* and *Streptococcus pyogenes* (GAS), and, more important, the lessons learned from these changes.

STAPHYLOCOCCUS AUREUS

About 30% of the normal population is colonized by *S. aureus* in the anterior nares; this percentage is possibly higher in persons with diabetes and other impaired hosts of various types (4). It is unusual for normal skin to be colonized, but diseased skin, such as skin involved with atopic dermatitis, is almost always colonized with *S. aureus*. From these loci the organisms spread to cause infection, often where there is a break in the skin, or to colonize other people or fomites (4).

The spectrum of *S. aureus* infections seems to be quite stable. The organism causes impetigo, furuncles, and wound infections in the skin. A major cause of generalized and focal systemic infections including endocarditis, pneumonia, osteomyelitis, septicemia, and a variety of other serious infections, *S. aureus* is one of the principal human pathogens in both normal and impaired hosts.

The most compelling recent concern about *S. aureus* is the emergence of antibiotic-resistant strains. Methicillin resistance and other multidrug antibiotic resistance is occurring with alarming frequency, raising the dreadful spectre of untreatable organisms in the near future (5). Fortunately, this possibility has happened only in rare instances, but it is an all too possible scenario, and if realized, will have a major impact on the spectrum of staphylococcal disease. The most important practical approach to prevent the development of antibiotic resistance is to insist on proper antibiotic usage, a difficult task indeed. Alternatively, the search for new antibiotic agents and novel methods of treatment must be pursued aggressively.

One dramatic change in the spectrum of staphylococcal infections in the last two decades illustrates strikingly how precariously the host–parasite relationship is balanced. Although clearly not a new disease, staphylococcal toxic shock syndrome (TSS) was not defined formally until 1978 (6). In the usual clinical picture, patients with focal staphylococcal infections suddenly develop fever, severe myalgias, and hypotension accompanied by a scarlatiniform rash and organ failure. One to two weeks into the course, if the patient survives the acute phase, generalized cutaneous desquamation occurs, most prominently on the hands and feet.

In 1980, attention focused on staphylococcal TSS in association with tampon use in menstruating women (7), and the reported disease incidence skyrocketed. Over the next several years, the pathophysiology of staphylococcal TSS was worked out, and the cause of the increased frequency was discovered. This knowledge led to action that decreased the incidence of the disease to its original level (8).

Some *S. aureus* strains make a toxin, TSST-1, which is one of the most significant mediators responsible for the signs and symptoms seen in staphylococcal TSS, especially in menstrual-associated disease (9). This toxin is one of the several gram-positive bacterial exotoxins, now identified as superantigens, that can effect release of cytokines from large numbers of both helper T-cells and antigen-presenting cells by a mechanism not involving the usual antigen-binding groove. The burst of superantigen-mediated cytokines including tumor necrosis factor may be responsible for much of the clinical picture of staphylococcal TSS (8,9).

The superabsorbant tampon was the other villain in the piece. When left in place too long, these tampons created a milieu in which *S. aureus* grew luxuriantly and produced large amounts of toxin (7). Removal of the superabsorbant tampon from the market eliminated this epidemic form of the disease, leaving a much lower incidence of staphylococcal TSS secondary to other focal *S. aureus* infections with toxin-producing organisms in patients susceptible to the toxin (10–13). The beneficial side effect that resulted from the study of staphylococcal TSS was recognition of this previously not understood pathologic process. It is now recognized that many other gram-positive bacterial exotoxins are superantigens that can cause disease by similar mechanisms, as we shall see with *Streptococcus*.

STREPTOCOCCUS PYOGENES

Group A beta-hemolytic streptococci or *Streptococcus pyogenes* (GAS) is the other gram-positive organism, which, along with *S. aureus*, is responsible for the majority of skin infections. Normal human skin is inhospitable to GAS, but the organism can thrive on abnormal skin surfaces such as areas of dermatitis (14). From these cutaneous sites, from the nasopharynx that is frequently colonized with GAS, and by transfer from other individuals infected or colonized with GAS, the organism initiates infection, usually in skin that has been injured by trauma or disease (15). The common GAS infections on skin and mucous membranes include the soft-tissue infections (impetigo, ecthyma, erysipelas, cellulitis) and pharyngitis. Scarlet fever, necrotizing fasciitis, GAS sepsis, and the nonsuppurative sequelae of GAS, namely glomerulonephritis and rheumatic fever, occur far less frequently.

GAS is one of the few pathogenic organisms that has had a profound influence on history. Serious epidemics of scarlet fever with mortality rates as high as 30% in children were common (16). Early in this century, scarlet fever was so feared that household quarantine was practiced by health departments, persisting in some locales into the 1950s (17). In the days before antibiotics, GAS wound infections, both civilian and military, and puerperal sepsis were often lethal (18). Rheumatic fever and to a lesser extent glomerulonephritis were important concerns, especially during World War II (18).

Even before antibiotic usage became widespread, however, the severity and incidence of invasive GAS infections declined dramatically

(18). By the 1980s, Stollerman (17) pointed out that scarlet fever was then only a "dermatologic oddity." The possible causes for the decline, in addition to an antibiotic effect, include improved socioeconomic conditions, changes in the immune status of the population, and/or a decrease in the virulence of GAS strains. Life-threatening GAS infections were still seen. For example in southern New England a severe GAS epidemic was reported in 1958–1959 (19), but for many decades, severe, neither invasive GAS infections nor the nonsuppurative sequelae were common. Unfortunately, because GAS infections were not generally reportable, few reliable incidence figures were available.

Within this context, in the 1980s and early 1990s a cluster of reports appeared in the medical literature suggesting a reemergence of severe, life-threatening GAS infections (20–25). This concern was sensationalized and exaggerated in the lay press with the description of "flesh-eating" bacterial infections (necrotizing fasciitis) and the widely publicized death of puppeteer Jim Henson with overwhelming GAS infection. Because strict case definition of severe, invasive GAS has been lacking in many reports, and incidence figures were not reliable, it has been hard to discern the truth.

Although several clusters of severe GAS infections were described in the late 1980s, most authors were careful to refer to an apparent increase in severe GAS infections. Martin and Hoiby (26) presented the most convincing data for an increase in incidence and severity of GAS infections. They studied a 1987–1988 epidemic from Norway, where the disease was reportable. They reported GAS infections including bacteremic cases with a 25% mortality rate and cases that usually involved young, otherwise healthy people. In addition a fairly convincing increase of invasive GAS infections was reported among native Americans in Pima County, Arizona, between 1985 and 1990, which consisted of severe disease in otherwise healthy people (27). Reports of less well-documented cases from diverse geographical areas such as the intermountain western United States (23), Canada (28), and Sweden (29) had similar sequelae, with severe, often life-threatening GAS infection occurring in otherwise healthy individuals.

These reports, taken as a whole, made a strong case for the emergence or reemergence of a type of streptococcal infection that was similar clinically in many respects to staphylococcal TSS and most appropriately called streptococcal toxic shock–like syndrome (TS-LS). For several reasons the term *streptococcal TS-LS* is preferable to *streptococcal toxic shock syndrome*, a term some authors have adopted. Staphylococcal TSS, as previously discussed, is clearly caused by a toxin produced at a localized, noninvasive, nonbacteremic site of infection. In streptococcal TS-LS, invasive, bacteremic disease is usually present (30) and is less clearly a pure toxin-caused syndrome.

M-proteins, capsular polysaccharides, extracellular enzymes, and other streptococcal virulence factors may be involved (31). It may be confusing and potentially dangerous to use the same *toxic shock syndrome* to apply to both staphylococcal and streptococcal disease because antibiotic treatment must be specific.

The syndrome of streptococcal TS-LS was first characterized by Cone et al. (22) and then Stevens et al. (23). The Working Group on Severe Streptococcal Infections under the auspices of the Centers for Disease Control, in an attempt to foster uniformity, suggested a strict definition for streptococcal TS-LS (Table 1) (32). Isolation of GAS and hypotension is always present in the syndrome. Severe soft-tissue infection, such as necrotizing fasciitis, occurs during the course of the illness in more than 50% of patients. The infection often begins with severe local pain and flulike symptoms. Despite therapy, rapid deterioration to multiorgan failure and death occurs in as many as 30% of patients (30).

It is unlikely that streptococcal TS-LS is a new infection. Most authors who write about this syndrome suggest that more virulent GAS have reappeared, causing a spectrum of severe manifestations of streptococcal disease as observed in earlier decades (30). A concomitant decrease in

Table 1 Proposed Case Definition for the Streptococcal Toxic Shock Syndrome

I. Isolation of group A *Streptococcus* (GAS)
   A. From a normally sterile site
   B. From a nonsterile site
II. Clinical signs of severity
   A. Hypotension
   B. ≤ 2 of the following signs
      1. Renal impairment
      2. Coagulopathy
      3. Liver involvement
      4. Adult respiratory distress syndrome
      5. A generalized erythematous macular rash that may desquamate
      6. Soft-tissue necrosis including necrotizing fasciitis, myositis, or gangrene

An illness fulfilling criteria IA and II (A and B) can be defined as a definite case. An illness fulfilling criteria IB and II (A and B) can be defined as a probable case if no other etiology for the illness is identified.
Source: Modified from Ref. 32.

individual and herd immunity to streptococcal virulence factors also may be responsible for an increase in the number of severe GAS infections.

The more virulent GAS pathogens usually possess one of the antiphagocytic M-proteins, such as M-1 or M-3. They also synthesize one or more of a class of streptococcal extracellular proteins called *streptococcal pyrogenic exotoxins* (SPEs), new names for the scarlet fever toxins or erythrogenic toxins previously described. Type A exotoxin or SPEA has predominated in some studies (23,33), whereas SPEB has been predominant in others (34). Organisms with these virulence factors had been observed only rarely in the decades before the 1980s. Several virulent strains of GAS have likely appeared, causing small clusters of severe disease in susceptible hosts (35). It is an overstatement to call this cluster of cases of invasive GAS infections an epidemic; however, they deserve careful study because of the dramatic severity of the infections, the need for early clinical recognition to prevent death, and the implications for improved therapy inherent in the suggested pathophysiology.

The virulent strains of GAS must have antiphagocytic properties, and most isolates produce SPEA or SPEB, exotoxins, which, like TSST-1 of *S. aureus*, have superantigen properties. These exotoxins may provoke the symptomatology of severe GAS by direct cytotoxicity or by the now well-described superantigen-mediated release of excessive cytokine mediators.

The spread of GAS strains horizontally from person to person is common, but horizontal spread of streptococcal TS-LS resulting in local epidemics of invasive disease is rare if it occurs. It is likely that few individuals are susceptible to streptococcal TS-LS because they are immune to one or more of the GAS virulence factors from previous exposure, or they lack the receptors for the SPE superantigens. The pool of individuals susceptible to streptococcal TS-LS thus is likely small to begin with.

The dramatic speed with which severe GAS infection can progress to hypotension, organ failure, and death is unsurpassed by any infectious process. Because streptococcal TS-LS often presents with nonspecific findings of pain and flulike symptoms, the diagnosis and, hence, early specific therapy rests on clinical suspicion and the rapid identification of GAS. Perhaps new rapid diagnostic techniques, such as immunofluorescence or DNA probes, which can identify GAS in hours rather than the days required for culture, can improve the treatment success rate.

Ideal treatment is prevention. Developing a vaccine against a critical streptococcal produce is an attractive but elusive goal.

With our present therapy, mortality from streptococcal TS-LS is unacceptably high. What improvements in treatment may stem from our new understanding of the pathophysiology of severe GAS infections?

1. If necrotizing fasciitis or collections of pus are present, early surgical drainage or debridement is mandatory to increase the antibiotic efficacy and to physically decrease the load of exotoxin(s).
2. Penicillin, although a wonderful drug for the treatment of GAS infections, may not be optimal antibiotic therapy for streptococcal TS-LS. Antibiotic inhibitors of protein synthesis such as clindamycin may impair protein toxin production in vivo more rapidly than beta-lactams such as penicillin. There is experimental support for this hypothesis in vitro and in animal models (36,37).
3. Neutralization of streptococcal exotoxins involved in the pathophysiological cascade of GAS TS-LS may be effective therapy, but commercial products to achieve this goal are not available. A rational but untested approach is to take advantage of specific neutralizing antibodies to streptococcal exotoxins in pooled immune gamma globulin. Pooled gamma globulins given intravenously seems to be effective for the treatment of Kawasaki syndrome, which may also involve toxins acting as superantigens (38). Two recent case reports suggest that intravenous pooled gamma globulin also may be effective for the treatment of streptococcal TS-LS (39,40). If gamma globulin is to be effective, it should be used early rather than as a last resort in patients with suspected severe, invasive GAS infection. Specific antitoxins and cytokine agonists should be developed and examined. Unfortunately the paucity of cases of GAS TS-LS will preclude controlled clinical studies. Decisions must be based on in vitro studies, animal studies, and clinical judgment.

CONCLUSIONS

Many forces result in the waxing and waning of infectious processes. Over the last few decades, there has been significant change in the spectrum of streptococcal and staphylococcal infections. Arguably the most important change has been the reemergence of more virulent GAS strains resulting in cases of streptococcal TS-LS. The mechanisms responsible for this syndrome have been defined and provide the rational basis for therapeutic suggestions.

REFERENCES

1. Murphy FA. New, emerging and reemerging infection diseases. Adv Virus Res 1994; 43: 1–52.
2. Institute of Medicine, Emerging Infections: Microbial Threats to Health in the United States. Washington, DC: National Academy Press, 1992.
3. CDC. Address emerging infectious disease threats: a prevention strategy for the United States. MMWR 1994; 43: 1–18.
4. Noble WC. Staphylococci on the skin. In: Noble WC, ed. The Skin Microflora and Microbial Skin Disease. Cambridge, England: Cambridge University Press, 1992: 135–152.
5. Cohen ML. Epidemiology of drug resistance: implication for a post-antimicrobial era. Science 1992; 257: 1050–1055.
6. Todd J, Fishaut M, Kapral R, et al. Toxic shock syndrome associated with phage-group I staphylococci. Lancet 1978; 2: 1116–1118.
7. Shands KN, Schmid BP, Dan BB, et al. Toxic shock syndrome in menstruating women: its association with tampon use and Staphylococcus aureus and the clinical features in 52 cases. N Engl J Med 1980; 303: 1436–1442.
8. Resnick SD, Elias PM. Staphylococcal toxin-mediated syndromes. In: Arndt KA et al, eds. Cutaneous Medicine and Surgery. Philadelphia: WB Saunders, 1995: 931–938.
9. Parsonnet J. Mediators in the pathogenesis of toxic shock syndrome: overview. Rev Infect Dis 1989: 2(suppl 1): S263–S269.
10. Reingold AL, Hargrett NT, Dan BB, et al. Nonmenstrual toxic shock syndrome: a review of 130 cases. Ann Intern Med 1982; 96: 87–874.
11. Tanner MH, Liljenquist JE. Toxic shock syndrome from Staphylococcus aureus infection at insulin pump infusion sites. JAMA 1988; 259: 394–395.
12. McCarthy VP, Peoples WM. Toxic shock syndromes after ear piercing. Pediatr Infect Dis J 1988; 7: 741–742.
13. Ferfuson MA, Todd J. Toxic shock syndrome associated with Staphylococcus aureus sinusitis. J Infect Dis 1990; 161: 953.
14. Barnharn M. Streptococci and the skin. In Noble WC, ed. The Skin Microflora and Microbial Skin Disease. Cambridge, England: Cambridge University Press, 1992: 135–152.
15. Hirschmann JV. Skin infections caused by staphylococci streptococci, and the resident cutaneous flora. In: Arndt KA, et al, eds. Cutaneous Medicine and Surgery. Philadelphia: WB Saunders, 1996: 919–930.
16. Quinn RW. Epidemiology of group A streptococcal infections: their changing frequency and severity. Yale J Biol Med 1982; 55: 265–270.
17. Stollerman GH. Changing group A streptococci. The reappearance of streptococcal "toxic shock." Arch Intern Med 1988; 148: 1268–1270.
18. Denny FW. A 45-year perspective on the streptococcus and rheumatic fever: the Edward H. Kass Lecture in Infectious Disease History. Clin Infect Dis 1994; 1110–1122.

19. Black PH, Swartz MN, Sharp JT, et al. Severe streptococcal disease. Observations during an epidemic occurring in southern New England 1958–1959. N Engl J Med 1961; 264: 898–903.

20. Ispahani P, Donald FE, Aveline AJD. Streptococcal pyogenes bacteremia: an old enemy subdued but not defeated. J Infect 1988; 16: 37–46.

21. Bartter T, Dascal A, Carroll K, Curely FJ. Toxic strep syndrome: a manifestation of group A infection. Arch Intern Med 1988; 148: 1421–1424.

22. Cone LA, Woodards MS, Schlievert PM, Tomory GS. Clinical and bacteriologic observations of a toxic shock-like syndrome due to *Streptococcus pyogenes*. N Engl J Med 1987; 317: 146–149.

23. Stevens DL, Tanner MH, Winship J, et al. Severe group A streptococcal infections associated with a toxic shock-like syndrome and scarlet fever toxin A. N Engl J Med 1989; 321: 1–7.

24. Wheeler MC, Roe MH, Kaplan EL, et al. Outbreak of group A streptococcal septicemia in children: clinical, epidemiologic, and microbiological correlates. JAMA 1991; 266: 533–537.

25. Belani K, Schlievert PM, Kaplan EL, Ferrieri P. Association of exotoxin-producing group A streptococci and severe disease in children. Pediatr Infect Dis J 1991; 10: 251–254.

26. Martin PR, Hoiby EA. Streptococcal serogroup A epidemic in Norway 1987-1988. Scand J Infect Dis 1990; 22: 421–429.

27. Hoge CW, Swartz B, Talkington DF, et al. The changing epidemiology of invasive group A streptococcal infections and the emergence of streptococcal toxic shock-like syndrome. JAMA 1993; 269: 384–389.

28. Demers B, Simor AE, Vellend H, et al. Severe invasive group A streptococcal infections in Ontario, Canada: 1987–1991. Clin Infect Dis 1993; 15: 792–800.

29. Holm SE, Norrby A, Bergholm AM, Norgren M. Aspects of the pathogenesis of serious group A streptococcal infections in Sweden 1988–1989. J Infect Dis 1992; 166: 31–37.

30. Stevens DL. Streptococcal toxic-shock syndrome: spectrum of disease, pathogenesis, and new concepts in treatment. Emerg Infect Dis 1995; 1: 69–79.

31. Talking DF, Schwartz B, Black CM, et al. Association of phenotypic and genotypic characteristics of invasive *Streptococcus pyogenes* isolates with clinical components of streptococcal toxic shock syndrome. Infect Immun 1993; 61: 3369–3374.

32. The Working Group on Severe Streptococcal Infections. Defining the group A streptococcal toxic shock syndrome. Rationale and consensus definition. JAMA 1993; 269: 390–391.

33. Musser JM, Hauser AR, Kim MH, et al. *Streptococcus pyogenes* causing toxic-shock-like syndrome and other invasive diseases: clonal diversity and pyrogenic exotoxin expression. Proc Natl Acad Sci 1991; 88: 2668–2672.

34. Forni AL, Kaplan EL, Schlievert PM, Roberts RB. Clinical and microbiological characteristics of severe group A streptococcus infections and streptococcal toxic shock syndrome. Clin Infect Dis 1995; 21: 333–340.

35. Cleary PP, Kaplan EL, Handley JP, et al. Clonal basis for resurgence of serious *Streptococcus pyogenes* disease in the 1980s. Lancet 1992; 339: 518–521.
36. Stevens DL, Gibbons AE, Bergstrom R, Winn V. The Eagle effect revisited: effect of clindamycin, erythromycin, and penicillin in the treatment of streptococcal myosites. J Infect Dis 1988; 158: 23–28.
37. Stevens DL, Bryant AG, Yan S. Invasive streptococcal infection: new concepts in antibiotic treatment. Int J Antimicrob Agents 1994; 4: 297–301.
38. Kawasaki T. Kawasaki disease. Acta Paediatr 1995; 84: 713–715.
39. Barry W, Hudgins L, Donta SL, Pesanti EL. Intravenous immunoglobulin therapy for toxic shock syndrome. JAMA 1992; 267: 3315–3316.
40. Young JM. Letter. Lancet 1994; 343: 1427.

3

Treatment of Nasal Carriage of Staphylococcus Aureus

James E. Rasmussen
University of Michigan Medical Center, Ann Arbor, Michigan

INTRODUCTION

Staphylococcus aureus has always been one of the most common causes of cutaneous infections. It is also a cause of serious systemic infection such as septicemia, wound infection, pneumonia, and contamination of indwelling catheters. With the emergence of methicillin-resistant *S. aureus*, the organism has become a major cause of difficult to treat, serious infections. This organism can be of importance to dermatologists because of chronic furunculosis, increased frequency of wound infections, contamination of dermatological operating suites, and spread to patients with damaged epidermis (atopic dermatitis) and immunological disorders (HIV infection).

HISTORY OF THE CURRENT PROBLEM

Penicillin was brought into practice in 1940. By 1942 resistance was first reported and resistant *S. aureus* rapidly emerged. In a study from Boston a minimum inhibitory concentration (MIC) of > 25 µg/ml was reported in 28% of coagulase-positive *S. aureus* cultures in 1948 and in 73% in 1951 (1). The resistance factor was penicillinase, which was first isolated in *Escherichia coli* in 1940. Semisynthetic penicillins produce protection of the β-lactam ring, which prevents hydrolysis by penicillinase (β-lactamase). Methicillin is considered the prototype for this group of penicillins. Other examples include nafcillin, cloxacillin, and dicloxacillin. These compounds were introduced early in 1960, with resistance being reported almost immediately in 1961. These are generally recognized and described as methicillin-resistant *S. aureus* (MRSA). Most if not all of these organisms are also resistant to a wide range of other antibiotics including erythromycin, tetracycline, sulfonamides, quinolones, and cephalosporins. Vancomycin and rifampin are among the few antibiotics that are usually successful against MRSA. These organisms were initially more commonly isolated from large hospitals, but they quickly spread to the "community" acquired infections. During 1 year (1980) at Henry Ford Hospital in Detroit, Michigan, the prevalence of MRSA infections increased from 3% to 38% (2).

The mechanism of methicillin resistance has involved elaboration of new forms of penicillinase, as well as alteration of the typical penicillin binding sites, which decreases their affinity for penicillins and cephalosporins. Prevalence rates vary remarkably from country to country and from hospital to hospital. Patient infection rates of between 2% and 50% and hospital personnel carriage rates of between 0 and 25% have been reported. With epidemics of this organism, the percentage of carriers increases.

Patients colonized with MRSA continue to carry this organism for approximately 40 months. The most common site of chronic carriage is the nares (93%); other sites have considerably less colonization (3).

CONTROL OF NASAL CARRIAGE

Systemic

Attempts to eradicate chronic nasal carriage of *S. aureus* (including MRSA) involve topical and systemic approaches. Results using systemic agents have not been completely successful. A study of novobiocin plus rifampin for irradicating MRSA nares contamination was effective in 67% of patients. A similar study of trimethoprim sulfamethoxizole plus rifampin generated an irradication rate of only 53%.

Topical

Topical approaches have included a variety of antibiotics of which only mupirocin has shown much promise (4). Six double-blind trials have compared the effect of mupirocin ointment given intranasally twice a day for 5 days and placebo. Approximately 90% of those receiving mupirocin were free of *S. aureus*, compared to only 6% of those receiving the placebo. Approximately two-thirds of those from whom nasal carriage was eradicated were free of *S. aureus* at the end of 4 weeks (5).

A long-term study of intranasal mupirocin ointment administered twice a day for 5 days was carried out for 1 year after therapy. Results at 6 months and 1 year show that approximately 75% of the mupirocin-treated group were free of *S. aureus* compared to only about 50% of the untreated group. In addition staphylococcal hand carriage was dramatically reduced in patients receiving mupirocin, even though the antibiotic was not applied directly to these sites, implying that nasal carriage is a source of hand contamination.

Problems with mupirocin resistance have not been common in any of these studies, but they have been reported. Most resistance has been documented with long-term mupirocin therapy. It is thought that this resistance was related to alterations in isoleucyl-MRNA binding sites (6).

Competitive Replacement

A third possible way to remove *S. aureus* from the nares involves replacement therapy. In a series of well-controlled experiments, Steele (7) inoculated "benign" *S. aureus* 502A nasally. He demonstrated a substantial reduction of pathological *S. aureus* and a concomitant decrease in cutaneous infections. This protection was noted for the 6 months of the study. No apparent disease resulted from the inoculation of the SA 502A. Although this form of therapy showed great promise, it has not been pursued recently. In a personal communication with Dr. Steele, he noted that strain 502A is not commercially available and he does not believe any work has been undertaken recently on this subject.

SUMMARY

Nasal carriage with *S. aureus* is a common source of infections. This nasal carriage tends to be either transient or chronic and may last as long as 40 months. Methicillin-resistant *S. aureus* is also commonly isolated from the anterior nares of carrier individuals. Attempts to remove these organisms with systemic agents are not uniformly successful and expose patients to systemic drugs. Intranasal application of mupirocin is safe and effective. Application twice a day for 5 days will produce beneficial results in 80% to 90% of patients, and approximately two-thirds of them will remain clear for approximately 1 year. Intranasal application will also decrease carriage at other sites such as the hands.

REFERENCES

1. Findland M. Changes in susceptibility of selected pathogenic bacteria to widely used antibiotics. Ann NY Acad Sci 1971; 182: 5–20.
2. Saravolatz LD, Pohlod DJ, Arking LM. Community-acquired methicillin-resistant *Staphylococcus aureus* infections: a new source for nosocomial outbreaks. Ann Intern Med 1982; 97: 325–329.
3. Sanford MD, Widmer AF, Bale MJ, et al. Efficient detection and long-term persistence of the carriage of methicillin-resistant *Staphylococcus aureus*. Clin Infect Dis 1994; 19: 1123–1128.
4. Walsh TJ, Standiford HC, Reboli AC, et al. Randomized double-blinded trial of rifampin with either novobiocin or trimethoprim-sulfamethoxazole against methicillin-resistant *Staphylococcus aureus* colonization; prevention of antimicrobial resistance and effect of host factors on outcome. Antimicrob Agents Chemother 1993; 37: 1334–1342.
5. Doebbeling BN, Breneman DL, Neu HC. Elimination of *Staphylococcus aureus* nasal carriage in health care workers: analysis of six clinical trials with calcium mupirocin ointment. 1993; 17: 466–474.
6. Kauffman CA, Terpenning MS, He X, et al. Attempts to eradicate methicillin-resistant *Staphylococcus aureus* from a long-term care facility with the use of mupirocin ointment. Am J Med 1993; 94: 371–378.
7. Steele RW. Recurrent staphylococcal infection in families. Arch Dermatol 1980; 116: 189–190.

4

Skin Infections with Gram-Negative Bacilli

William Charles Noble
St. Thomas' Hospital, London, England

The gram-negative bacilli are relatively rare on normal human skin except in the moist areas such as the axillae, groin, and toewebs and in the antecubital fossa (1). The most common skin resident is *Acinetobacter*, which has undergone taxonomic reevaluation in the last decade expanding from 2 species to more than 15. The species found on normal human skin are most likely to be *A. johnsonii, A. lwoffi,* and a number of currently unnamed genospecies (2). Skin infection with *Acinetobacter*, however, is rare. Most infection is seen in catheterized patients in urology or intensive care units and is due chiefly to *A. baumannii,* but also representatives of many other species (3). The groin, the perineum, and perianal areas are frequently colonized with gram-negative bacilli, and many of these may be derived from fecal contamination. In the elderly this may also reflect urinary tract infection (4). Organisms such as *Pseudomonas aeruginosa,* however, tend not to cause clinical infection of the skin unless the area is very wet (5).

The toewebs are the chief site of carriage and infection in the feet. In the United Kingdom, various studies by a single group of workers revealed carriage rates of 8% in normal students, 14.5% in female and 29% in male office workers, 41% in industrial workers wearing heavy boots, and 58% in coal miners (6–8). The species recovered were varied but *Acinetobacter, Enterobacter,* and *Escherichia* spp. were found in all groups. The coal miners had the most extensive flora, and much of this was probably due to environmental contamination. Quantitative studies in the United States reported gram-negative bacilli as a minority population in 10% of normal individuals and as forming 0.01% on the total flora (9). Experimentally, clinically apparent infection by gram-negative bacilli, especially *Pseudomonas aeruginosa*, occurs only where the skin in hyperhydrated (5), which no doubt accounts for foot infection in soldiers undergoing swamp training (10) and in coal miners (7). Generally both high temperatures and high humidities are necessary to elevate the numbers of bacilli on the skin (11), but these conditions are normal in coal mines or in the confines of an occlusive industrial boot. Foot infection is most commonly caused by *P. aeruginosa* and/or *Proteus mirabilis* (7).

P. *aeruginosa* may infect apparently intact skin. Recent reports include the familiar green nail syndrome (13), but other *Pseudomonas* species such as *P. cepacia (Burkholderia cepacia)* (14,15) and *P. paucimobilis* (16) infect preexisting lesions. *Aeromonas hydrophila* also infects under some conditions, and skin lesions may follow exposure to contaminated water (17–19). The role of other members of the skin flora in checking infection by gram-negative bacilli is not known, but treating dermatophyte-infected feet with antifungals eliminates the fungi but results in an increase in bacilli; the application of povidone iodine reverses the trend (8).

The hands act chiefly as vectors for gram-negative bacilli and may become, at least temporarily, colonized by bacilli in health care workers or others exposed to high concentrations of organisms (20–22). In individuals outside hospitals, the species found are chiefly derived from the gut. Effective hand washing by health care personnel keeps populations in check (23). Not all carriage can be described as transient, however, because the same species can be recovered from the hands over several weeks (24). Nurses carry *Klebsiella pneumoniae* more frequently than do others, and persons with hand dermatoses carry *P. aeruginosa* more often and may be responsible for the spread of gram-negative infections in a ward (22,25).

Skin infections may occur with almost any gram-negative bacillus. Some may be secondary such as the painful, nonpruritic, macular, erythematous rash caused by legionella in a small percentage of patients with legionellosis (26,27). Brucella skin lesions are described in brucellosis (28,29). Pathogens of animal origin such as salmonella, shigella, brucella, and yersinia are especially liable to cause infections in veterinarians (30–32). Some probably reflect the long-term use of antibiotics, especially the gram-negative folliculitis seen in acne patients (33,34).

In children, *Haemophilus influenzae*, usually type B, remains an occasional cause of cellulitis on the face of young children, especially boys (35–37). Toxin production by *Pasteurella multocida* is responsible for skin lesions associated with animal bites, especially from cats (38,39).

In recent years, two gram-negative bacilli have received special attention: *P. aeruginosa* and the marine vibrios, especially *Vibrio vulnificus*.

P. aeruginosa has long been known as a cause of folliculitis and may be a contributor to gram-negative folliculitis after therapy for acne vulgaris. About a decade ago, there was much interest in the outbreaks of "hot-tub dermatitis" or jacuzzi dermatitis (40–42). This tended to appear 2 to 3 days after the use of a jacuzzi or whirlpool tub in which the patient had spent much time in hot water. Most infections cleared up rapidly without therapy when the skin was allowed to dry out, although some recurrences in sweaty individuals were reported. Another leisure activity that can apparently result in *Pseudomonas* folliculitis is mud wrestling (43). Recent studies have added the loofah sponge to the list of fomites that can distribute *P. aeruginosa*, and it has been indicated that the sponge is a sufficient growth medium for the organism when contaminated with human cell debris and kept moist (44). A rare instance of *Pseudomonas* folliculitis following epilation has been recorded (45). Potentially more significant, brushes used for shaving before surgery may contain gram-negative bacilli, which result in local or deep infection (46). *P. aeruginosa* may also cause septicemia in patients with AIDS and may be associated with skin infections or other localized infection such as otitis (47,48). The appearance of skin lesions may be the herald of septicemia in neutropenic patients and should be taken seriously (49,50).

A full appreciation of noncholera vibrios as causes of skin and deeper infection is of comparatively recent origin, despite comprehensive descriptions in earlier literature (51,52). Recent reports have included studies on *Vibrio vulnificus* infections from Mexico (53), Taiwan (54), Korea (55), Australia (56), and Mississippi Gulf coastal waters (57). Most reports have in common exposure to an aquatic environment with contamination of skin lesions leading to a severe necrotizing cellulitis and bullae that may progress to a fatal septicemia. Skin lesions may also appear in patients with the rapid onset, frequently fatal, septicemia, which is the second form of *V. vulnificus* infection. The third form is a severe diarrhea. Tetracycline is the antibiotic of choice, although strains are also usually sensitive to ampicillin. Some other noncholera vibrios also cause similar disease, and some may require more vigorous therapy. The skin lesions may be the result of a metalloprotease activity (58). Preexisting disease such as cirrhosis may predispose to infection after ingestion of contaminated shellfish when the necrohemorrhagic bullae are secondary to septicemia (53,59).

Therapy of infections due to the gram-negative bacilli is necessarily as diverse as the bacilli themselves (60). Reported therapies range from nothing other than maintaining a dry skin for *Pseudomonas* folliculitis to the use of ofloxacin and cephalexin (61,62) for deep-seated lesions. Ticarcillin plus clavulanate (63), cefotaxime, and ciprofloxacin (64) also have been effective in a variety of infections caused by gram-negative bacilli. Laboratory help in determining sensitivity patterns may prove invaluable.

REFERENCES

1. Noble WC. Other cutaneous bacteria. In: Noble WC ed. The Skin Microflora and Microbial Skin Disease. Cambridge: Cambridge University Press, 1993: 210–231.
2. Grimont PAD, Bouvet PJM. Taxonomy of acinetobacter. In: Towner KJ, Bergogne-Berezin E, Fewson CA, eds. The Biology of the Acinetobacter. New York: Plenum Press, 1991: 25–36.
3. Tjernberg I, Ursing J. Clinical strains of acinetobacter classified by DNA-DNA hybridization. APMIS 1989; 97: 595–605.
4. Ehrenkranz NJ, Afonso BC, Eckert DG, Moskowitz LB. Proteeae species bactiuria accompanying Proteeae species groin skin carriage in geriatric patients. J Clin Microbiol 1989; 27: 1988–1991.
5. Hojyo-Tomoka MT, Marples RR, Kligman AM. Pseudomonas infection in superhydrated skin. Arch Dermatol 1973; 107: 723–727.
6. Noble WC, Hope YM, Midgley G, et al. Toewebs as a source of gram-negative bacilli. J Hosp Infect 1986; 8: 248–256.
7. Howell SA, Clayton YM, Phan QG, Noble WC. Tinea pedis: the relationship between symptoms, organisms and host characteristics. Microb Ecol Health Dis 1988; 1: 131–135.
8. Hay RJ, Clayton YM, Howell SA, Noble WC. Management of combined bacterial and fungal infections in coal miners. Mycoses 1988; 31: 316–319.
9. Aly R, Maibach HI. Aerobic microbial flora of intertriginous skin. Appl Environ Microbiol 1977; 33: 97–100.
10. Rietschel RL, Allen AM. Immersion foot: a method for studying the effects of protracted water exposure on human skin. Milit Med 1976; 141: 778–780.
11. McBride ME, Duncan WC, Knox JM. Physiological and environmental control of gram-negative bacteria on skin. Br J Dermatol 1975; 93: 191–199.
12. Suter L, Rabbat RM, Nolting S. Gramnegativer fussinfekt. Mykosen 1979; 22: 109–114.
13. Agger WA, Mardan A. *Pseudomonas aeruginosa* infection of intact skin. Clin Infect Dis 1995; 20: 302–308.
14. Taplin D, Bassett DCJ, Mertz PM. Foot lesions associated with *Pseudomonas cepacia*. Lancet 1971; 1: 568–571.
15. Mandell IN, Feiner HD, Price NM. Simberkoff M. *Pseudomonas cepacia* endocarditis and ecthyma gangrenosum. Arch Dermatol 1977; 113: 199–202.
16. Peel MM, Davis JM, Armstrong WLH, et al. *Pseudomonas paucimobilis* from a leg ulcer on a Japanese seaman. J Clin Microbiol 1979; 9: 561–564.

17. Fulghum DD, Linton WR Jr, Taplin D. Fatal *Aeromonas hydrophila* infection of the skin. Southern Med J 1978; 71: 739–741.
18. Young DF, Barr RJ. *Aeromonas hydrophila* infection of the skin. Arch Dermatol 1981; 117: 244.
19. Gold WL, Salit IE. *Aeromonas hydrophila* infections of the skin and soft tissue: report of 11 cases and review. Clin Infect Dis 1993 16: 69–74.
20. Ligtvoet EEJ, Mouton RP. Hands and nebulizers as a route of transmission of gram-negative bacilli in an intensive care unit. Antonie van Leeuwenhoek 1982; 48: 204–205.
21. Casewell M, Phillips I. Hands as a route of transmission for *Klebsiella* species. Br Med J 1977; 2: 1315–1317.
22. Parry MF, Hutchinson JH, Brown NA, et al. Gram-negative sepsis in neonates: a nursery outbreak due to hand carriage of *Citrobacter diversus*. Pediatrics 1980; 65: 1105–1109.
23. Adams BC, Marrie TJ. Hand carriage of aerobic gram-negative rods by health care personnel. J Hyg Camb 1982; 89: 3–31.
24. Adams BC, Marrie TJ. Hand carriage of aerobic gram-negative rods may not be transient. J Hyg Camb 1982; 89: 33–45.
25. Buxton AE, Anderson RL, Werdegar D, Atlas E. Nosocomial respiratory tract infection and colonization with *Acinetobacter calcoaceticus*. Am J Med 1978; 65: 507–513.
26. Helms CM, Johnson W, Donaldson MF, Corry RJ. Pretibial rash in *Legionella pneumophila* pneumonia. JAMA 1981; 245: 1758–1759.
27. Ample NM, Ruben FL, Norden CW. Cutaneous abscess caused by *Legionella micdadei* in an immunosuppressed patient. Ann Intern Med 1985; 102: 630–632.
28. Gee-Lew BM, Nicholas EA, Hirose FM et al. Unusual skin manifestation of brucellosis. Arch Dermatol 1983; 119: 56–58.
29. Ariza J, Servitje O, Pallares R, et al. Characteristic cutaneous lesions in patients with brucellosis. Arch Dermatol 1989; 125: 380–383.
30. Kurtz JB. Leg abscess caused by *Salmonella heidelberg*. Lancet 1976; 1: 200–201.
31. Stoll DM. Cutaneous shigellosis. Arch Dermatol 1986; 122: 22.
32. Neimi KM, Hannuksela M, Salo OP. Skin lesions in human yersiniosis. Br J Dermatol 1976; 94: 155–160.
33. Leyden JJ, Marples RR, Mills OH, Kligman AM. Gram-negative folliculitis—a complication of antibiotic therapy in acne vulgaris. Br J Dermatol 1973; 88: 533–538.
34. Blankenship ML. Gram-negative folliculitis: follow-up observations in 20 patients. Arch Dermatol 1984; 120: 1301–1303.
35. Rasmussen JE. *Haemophilus influenzae* cellulitis. Case presentation and review of the literature. Br J Dermatol 1973; 88: 547–550.
36. Sokal RJ, Bowden RA. An erysipelas-like scalp cellulitis due to *Haemophilus influenzae* type B. J Pediatr 1980; 96: 60–61.
37. Spencer RC, Barnham M. *Haemophilus influenzae* cellulitis. Br Med J 1975; 2: 615.

38. Elling F, Pedersen KB,. Hogh P, Foged NT. Characterization of the dermal lesions induced by a purified protein from toxigenic *Pasteurella multocida*. APMIS 1988; 96: 50–55.

39. Francis DP, Holmes MA, Brandon G. *Pasteurella multocida*: infections after animal bites and scratches. JAMA 1975; 233: 42–45.

40. Silverman AR, Nieland ML. Hot tub dermatitis: a familial outbreak of *Pseudomonas* folliculitis. J Am Acad Dermatol 1983; 8: 153–156.

41. Chandrasekar PH, Rolston KVI, Kannangara W, et al. Hot tub-associated dermatitis due to *Pseudomonas aeruginosa*. Arch Dermatol 1984; 120: 1337–1340.

42. Schleck WF III, Simonsen N, Sumarah R, Martin RS. Nosocomial outbreak of *Pseudomonas aeruginosa* associated with a physiotherapy pool. Can Med Ass J 1986; 134: 909–913.

43. Adler AI, Altman J. An outbreak of mud-wrestling-induced pustular dermatitis in college students. Dermatitis palaestrae limosae. JAMA 1993; 269: 502–504.

44. Bottone EJ, Perez AA II, Oeser JL. Loofah sponges as reservoirs and vehicles in the transmission of potentially pathogenic bacterial species to human skin. J Clin Microbiol 1994; 32: 469–472.

45. Trueb RM, Elsner P, Burg G. *Pseudomonas aeruginosa* folliculitis after epilation. Hautarzt 1993; 44: 103–105.

46. Oie S, Kamiya A. Microbial contamination of brushes used for preoperative shaving. J Hosp Infect 1992; 21: 103–110.

47. Sangeorzan JA, Bradley SF, Kauffman CA. Cutaneous manifestations of *Pseudomonas* infection in the acquired immunodeficiency syndrome. Arch Dermatol 1990; 126: 832–833.

48. Flores G, Stavola JJ, Noel GJ. Bacteremia due to *Pseudomonas aeruginosa* in children with AIDS. Clin Infect Dis 1993; 16: 706–708.

49. Bodey GP. Dermatologic manifestations of infections in neutropenic patients. Infect Dis Clin North Am 1994; 8: 655–675.

50. el Baze P, Thyss A, Vinti H, et al. A study of nineteen immunocomprised patients with extensive skin lesions caused by *Pseudomonas aeruginosa* with and without bacteremia. Acta Derm Venereol 1991; 71: 411–415.

51. West PA. The human pathogenic vibrios—a public health update with environmental perspectives. Epidemiol Infect 1989; 103: 1–34.

52. Wickboldt LG, Sanders CV. *Vibrio vulnificus* infection: case report and update since 1970. J Am Acad Dermatol 1983; 9: 243–251.

53. Porras-Cortes G, Viana JJ, Chavez-Mazari B, Sieera-Madero J. *Vibrio vulnificus* in Mexico: a case report and review of the literature. Rev Invest Clin 1994; 46: 495–498.

54. Chuang YC, Yuan CY, Liu CY et al. *Vibrio vulnificus* infection in Taiwan: report of 28 cases and review of clinical manifestations and treatment. Clin Infect Dis 1992; 15: 271–276.

55. Park SD, Shon HS, Joh NJ. *Vibrio vulnificus* in Korea: clinical and epidemiologic findings in seventy patients. J Am Acad Dermatol 1991; 24: 397–403.

56. Maxwell EL, Mayall BC, Pearson SR, Stanley PA. A case of *Vibrio vulnificus* septicaemia acquired in Victoria. Med J Aust 1991; 154: 214–215.

57. Penman AD, Lanier DC Jr, Avara WT III, et al. *Vibrio vulnificus* wound infections from the Mississippi Gulf coastal waters. South Med J 1995; 88: 531–533.
58. Miyoshi S, Hirata Y, Tomochika K, Shinoda S. *Vibrio vulnificus* may produce a metalloprotease causing an edematous skin lesion in vivo. FEMS Microbiol Lett 1994; 121: 321–325.
59. Hally RJ, Rubin RA, Fraimow HS, Hoffman-Terry ML. Fatal *Vibrio parahemolyticus* septicemia in a patient with cirrhosis. A case report and review of the literature. Dig Dis Sci 1995; 40: 1257–1260.
60. Noble WC. Gram-negative bacterial skin infections. Semin Dermatol 1993; 12: 336–341.
61. Gentry LO, Rodriguesz-Gomez G. Ofloxacin treatment of difficult infections of the skin and skin structure. Cutis 1993; 51: 55–58.
62. Powers RD, Schwartz R, Snow RM, Yarborough DR III. Ofloxacin versus cephalexin in the treatment of skin, skin structure, and soft tissue infections in adults. Clin Ther 1991; 13: 727–736.
63. File TM, Tan JS. Ticarcillin-clavulanate therapy for bacterial skin and soft tissue infections. Rev Infect Dis 1991; 13(suppl 9): S733–S736.
64. Gentry LO, Ramirez-Ronda CH, Rodriguez-Noriega E, et al. Oral ciproflaxacin vs parenteral cefotaxime in the treatment of difficult skin and skin structure infections. Arch Intern Med 1989; 149: 2579–2583.

....

5

Recent Advances in Lyme Disease

Russell C. Johnson
University of Minnesota Medical School, Minneapolis, Minnesota

INTRODUCTION

Lyme disease is a tickborne zoonosis caused by three closely related species (genospecies) of *Borrelia: B. burgdorferi* sensu stricto, which will be referred to as *B. burgdorferi* hereafter; *B. garinii,* and *B. afzelii* (1–3). The spirochetes are transmitted by the nymph and adult female *Ixodes* (hard) ticks. Infection of humans by these *Borrelia* may result in a broad spectrum of clinical syndromes collectively referred to as Lyme disease or Lyme borreliosis. The most common clinical manifestation is a skin lesion, erythema migrans, followed in some patients by rheumatological, cardiac, and neurological abnormalities.

PARASITE-HOST-VECTOR INTERACTION

Borrelia are extracellular, obligate parasites that have adapted to alternating life in arthropod vector ticks and mammalian and avian hosts. *B. burgdorferi* is a slow-growing pathogen with a generation time of 12 to 24 hours in laboratory media. The cells are slender (0.2 µm to 0.25 µm × 8 to 30 µm) and have the same basic structural features and unique motility shared by other spirochetes. The internal location of flagella, in combination with the spirochetes' ability to bind and activate host-derived proteases, may facilitate their rapid dissemination in the host. The genome of *Borrelia* differs from most other bacteria in that it is composed of a linear chromosome and linear plasmids, as well as the usual supercoiled bacterial plasmids (4–6). In addition to its linearity, the chromosome of

37

B. burgdorferi is characterized by its small size of 950 to 1000 kb. This is similar in size to the chromosomes of *Mycoplasma*, which are the smallest recorded genomes among extracellular bacterial pathogens (7). No mechanism of genetic exchange has been reported for *Borrelia*, and the lack of techniques for gene transfer has been a major impediment for investigating the molecular biology of these spirochetes. The absence of lateral genetic exchange among chromosomal genes suggests that *B. burgdorferi* is strictly clonal (8). In the absence of a mechanism for genetic exchange, any change in DNA sequences (mutation) is transmitted only by direct inheritance to the progeny cell.

A fresh isolate of *B. burgdorferi*, B31, contains eight linear plasmids and three circular plasmids (9). The largest plasmid (50 to 57 kb) is linear and encodes two major outer surface proteins, Osp A and B. *B. burgdorferi* binds human plasminogen on its surface, and Osp A has been identified as the major binding site (10). The bound plasminogen is converted to bioactive plasmin by a urokinase-type activator, facilitating the dissemination of the spirochetes in the host (11). The Lyme disease spirochete is the first tickborne bacterial pathogen shown to alter its expression of a specific surface protein during tick feeding (12). In unfed ticks, *B. burgdorferi* produces the outer surface protein, Osp A, but not Osp C, whereas during infection of humans, immunological data suggest the spirochete has changed its surface. It is now expressing Osp C and little or no Osp A. Although Osp A but not Osp C is expressed by spirochetes in the unfed tick, once the tick receives a blood meal, Osp C is expressed. This major change in outer surface proteins of *B. burgdorferi* appears to be regulated by temperature because Osp C is expressed at body temperature but not at 24°C. The presence of blood is also necessary to trigger this change in surface antigens. The rapid synthesis of Osp C in the feeding tick may be essential for these spirochetes to infect mammalian hosts. In support of this hypothesis is the observation that in unfed ticks, spirochetes expressing Osp A but not Osp C fail to cause infections in experimentally inoculated rodents, whereas spirochetes from fed ticks expressing Osp C are infectious (12). The apparent lack of Osp A in humans has important implications for the effectiveness of the recombinant outer surface protein A Lyme disease vaccine being evaluated for human use (13).

CLINICAL MANIFESTATIONS

Lyme disease is a multisystem infection; although for convenience of discussion the clinical manifestations are commonly described as early localized, early disseminated, and late persistent disease, individual presentations can vary considerably. A variety of prodromal features such as fever, chills, headache, stiff neck, arthralgias, myalgias, and lymphadenopathy precede or accompany the more definitive cases of Lyme disease. Most infections, however, affect one or some combination of four organ systems: skin, heart, nervous, and musculoskeletal. The first sign of early disease is usually erythema migrans, a minimally symptomatic but pathognomonic rash occurring 3 to 30 days (median 7 days) after exposure to an infected tick. The skin lesions usually appear as reddish macules that expand centrifugally and expand to diameters of 6 to 65 cm or greater. The lesions are flat or slightly elevated and vary in site, size, shape, color, number, duration, and recurrence. It is estimated that erythema migrans may be absent in 20% or more of clinical cases of Lyme disease, but clinical studies to validate this estimate are lacking (14). In the untreated patient, the erythema migrans resolves in an average of 28 days (range, 1 day to 14 months), while in the treated patient the lesion diminishes within several days of therapy. The erythema migrans may be difficult to identify, especially if it is atypical in appearance or if the physician's experience with this disease is limited. The erythema migrans must be distinguished from other dermatological conditions such as hypersensitivity reaction to arthropod bites, streptococcal and staphylococcal cellulitis, plant dermatitis, tinea, and granuloma annulare. Puritic or painful erythema migrans lesions may occur, but are generally mild.

Primary erythema migrans lesions begin at the site of the tick bite as red macules or papules that expand centrifugally to form a patch with varying intensities of redness or with bands of normal-appearing skin (15). Sunlight or warming of the skin sometimes makes the erythema migrans more obvious. One study reported the lesion area expands in area at approximately 20 cm^2/day and is probably due to the outward movement of the spirochetes from the tick bite site, because they can be isolated from the peripheral and periperipheral regions of the lesion (16). The shape of the lesion is most commonly round or oval, but a variety of forms may occur. Central clearing of the solidary erythema migrans lesion occurs less frequently in the United States (37%), as compared to Europe (80%), and may be due to early initiation of treatment (14). Also, the occurrence of secondary skin lesions differs in the United States and Europe. The multiple erythema migrans are seen more often in the United States (48% of patients), but has decreased to less than 25% as a result of early recognition and treatment of Lyme disease. It has been estimated that only 60% to 80% of patients with clinical Lyme disease have a history of a prior erythema migrans; however, the true incidence remains unknown.

Approximately 20% or more of patients with erythema migrans lack systemic symptoms that would cause them to see a physician. The remaining 80% of patients with erythema migrans experience a spectrum of systemic symptoms (14), which are more pronounced in patients with multiple lesions. The most common systemic symptoms experienced by a series of 79 patients with culture-confirmed infections were fatigue (54%), myalgia (44%), arthralgia (44%), headache (42%), fever and or chills (39%), and stiff neck (35%). Regional lymphadenopathy (23%) and fever (16%) were the most common objective physical findings (14). In untreated patients, arthritis usually occurs weeks to months (mean 6 months) after resolution of the skin lesion (14). Cranial nerve abnormalities (facial palsy) and meningitis generally are manifested earlier and may accompany the skin lesion.

The chronic skin lesion of Lyme disease, acrodermatitis chronica atrophicans, occurs in the United States but is rare at this time.

LABORATORY METHODS FOR THE DIAGNOSIS
OF LYME DISEASE

The diagnosis of Lyme disease should be based primarily on the clinical presentation and epidemiological information. Laboratory tests can be an important adjunct for the diagnosis, especially when the erythema migrans lesion is atypical or lacking. Direct detection of the spirochete in patients' specimens provides the most definitive diagnosis of infection. Unfortunately, one of the characteristics of Lyme disease is the paucity of spirochetes in the patient. This characteristic in combination with the requirement for special media has made isolation a procedure restricted to reference laboratories and a low yield test for most patient specimens. Culture of skin biopsy material from the periphery of the erythema migrans lesion provides the highest yield. Skin biopsy specimens obtained 4 mm inside the erythema migrans margin provide the best specimens for culture, with up to 86% of specimens culture positive (16). Although *B. burgdorferi* is migrating centrifugally from the lesion, isolation success declines to 60% if the skin biopsy is taken 4 mm outside the margin of the erythema migrans (16). Antimicrobial therapy for as short as 1 day before obtaining the skin specimen will probably result in negative culture results (16). Adequate antimicrobial therapy will eliminate spirochetes from the erythema migrans lesion. Skin biopsies obtained from the site of the previously culture positive region were culture-negative after therapy (17). In contrast to these results, Lyme disease spirochetes have been isolated from erythema migrans skin biopsies of two treated patients in Europe (18), suggesting either the patients were inadequately treated or some inherent differences exist in these spirochetes. Antibiotic resistance has not been reported for any of the Lyme disease spirochetes, even those isolated from patients who did not respond well to therapy (19). If patients with erythema migrans are not treated, the lesion will eventually resolve. Skin biopsies from the site of the erythema migrans remain culture-positive weeks to years after the lesion resolves (20). The propensity of Lyme disease spirochetes to survive in dermal tissue is exemplified by their isolation from an acrodermatitis chronica atrophicans lesion that had been present for 10 years (21). The infecting Lyme disease spirochete was probably *B. afzelii*, which is isolated more frequently from chronic skin lesions than *B. burgdorferi* or *B. garinii*.

Spirochetes have been isolated from other sites, but the yield is very low. Early in the disease, *B. burgdorferi* can be isolated from the blood, but only 2% to 7% of specimens are culture-positive. Spirochetes were cultured from the cerebral spinal fluid of 4 of 38 (11%) clinically selected patients with neuroborreliosis. These four patients had pleocytosis in their cerebrospinal fluid and a history of neurological symptoms of only 4 to 10 days (22). *B. burgdorferi* has rarely been isolated from synovial fluid specimens (23).

Another direct method for the detection of the Lyme disease spirochete is the polymerase chain reaction (PCR). The PCR detects specific target DNA sequences of the spirochete and may be a promising adjunct to existing diagnostic tests. It is an extremely sensitive assay and can detect the DNA of as few as 1 to 10 spirochetes. This high level of sensitivity, however, has presented problems with false-positive results caused by contamination of PCR laboratories or specimens with spirochetal DNA. When the PCR is conducted by an experienced laboratory, results can be very useful. Goodman et al. (24) compared culture and PCR for the detection of spirochetemia during early disease. Only 4 of 76 (5.3%) of the blood specimens of patients with erythema migrans were culture-positive, whereas 14 of 76 patients (18.4%) had *B. burgdorferi* DNA present in the blood. The plasma was the optimal blood fraction for detection by both culture and PCR. Polymerase chain reaction has also demonstrated the intraarticular persistence of *B. burgdorferi* DNA in culture-negative Lyme arthritis. These results suggest that persistent organisms and their components are important in maintaining ongoing immune and inflammatory processes even among some antibiotic-treated patients (25). Currently, PCR should be restricted for investigational use because it has not been evaluated rigorously for diagnostic use.

Serology is the most useful laboratory test that is readily available as an adjunct to the clinical diagnosis of Lyme disease. Maximum value of serological results are achieved when they are used in combination with clinical history, patient presentation, and an understanding of the antibody response in Lyme disease. Serological testing in Lyme disease can be performed with a high degree of sensitivity and specificity; however, results have varied among laboratories because testing was not standardized. This lack of standardization resulted in false-negative and false-positive results.

To minimize these testing discrepancies, the Centers for Disease Control and Prevention and the Association of State and Territorial Public Health Laboratory Directors recommend that all serum specimens submitted for Lyme disease serology be analyzed by a two-test procedure. The first test is a sensitive screening test (e.g., enzyme-linked immunosorbent assay [ELISA] or immunofluorescent antibody [IFA]), and all samples judged equivocal or positive should be confirmed by the second test, the Western blot. Specimens that test negative by a sensitive ELISA or IFA need not be tested further (26).

Patients with Lyme disease rarely have negative ELISA or IFA results. They can occur when specimens are obtained before the patient has developed a significant antibody response. Approximately one half of patients that present with erythema migrans are seronegative. The probability that a patient will be seropositive increases the longer the erythema migrans has been present and the more marked the clinical manifestations. Both IgM and IgG antibodies are present in early Lyme disease. Patients that are reinfected may have an IgG response only in early disease. Initiation of adequate antimicrobial therapy will abort the antibody response in about 20% of patients, and these patients will be susceptible to reinfection. The peak antibody response occurs 8 to 12 days into treatment. Antibody titer cannot be used to monitor the patients' response to therapy. Although most adequately treated patients will have a declining antibody titer, approximately 25% of successfully treated early Lyme disease patients will remain seropositive by ELISA or IFA at least for 1 year after treatment (27). If a patient suspected of having Lyme disease is seronegative, a second serum sample should be tested 2 weeks later.

Untreated late Lyme disease patients, particularly those with arthritis, have a strong antibody response, with a predominance of IgG antibody. Treated patients will have slowly decreasing antibody titers, but they may persist for years despite successful antibiotic treatment. For neuroborreliosis, testing of the cerebrospinal fluid can be useful because IgM or IgG antibody specific for the spirochete may be produced intrathecally (28).

False-negative ELISA or IFA results occur when the serological assay lacks adequate sensitivity. False-positive ELISA or IFA assays can result from overly sensitive tests and if the patient has cross-reaching antibodies. These antibodies can occur with certain viral infections, such as infectious mononucleosis, and bacterial infections, such as syphilis and relapsing fever.

The Western blot detects antibodies that are reactive with specific antigens of *B. burgdorferi*. This serological assay is used to confirm border-line (equivocal) and positive serologies obtained by ELISA or IFA. As presently used, the Western blot does not determine antibody concentration (titer); rather it determines only the presence of *B. burgdorferi*-specific antibodies. The Western blot must be used in conjunction with quantitative ELISA or IFA because antibodies can be detected with the Western blot years after treatment (29).

The Centers for Disease Control and Prevention and the American State and Territorial Public Health Laboratory Directors recommend (26) that for the interpretation of the Western blot, an IgM immunoblot be considered positive if two of the following three bands are present: 24 kDa (Osp C), 39 kDa (Bmp A), and 41 kDa (Fla) (27). An IgG immunoblot should be considered positive if five of the following 10 bands are present: 18 kDa, 21 kDa (Osp C), 28 kDa, 30 kDa, 39 kDa (Bmp A), 41 kDa (Fla), 45 kDa, 58 kDa (not GroEL), 66 kDa, and 93 kDa (30). Not all strains of *B. burgdorferi* express adequate amounts of immunoreactive proteins of diagnostic importance, especially those that have been passaged many times in culture media. Only strains of *B. burgdorferi* expressing adequate amounts of the proteins of diagnostic importance should be used for the immunoblot.

TREATMENT

Most patients presenting with erythema migrans respond exceptionally well to treatment. In vitro studies of the antimicrobial susceptibility of the Lyme disease spirochete (31–36) show that these spirochetes are susceptible to the macrolides, tetracyclines, semisynthetic penicillins, and the late second- and third-generation cephalosporins. *Borrelia burgdorferi* was moderately sensitive to penicillin G and chloramphenicol and relatively resistant to the aminoglycosides, trimethoprim, sulfamethoxazole, quinolines, and rifampicin. First-generation cephalosporins generally possessed a low level of activity. There is no documented report of the development of antimicrobial resistance in *Borrelia* (35). Antimicrobials that displayed good in vitro activity against *B. burgdorferi* also had good in vivo activity with the exception of erythromycin (33–36).

Effective oral drugs for treating patients with erythema migrans include amoxicillin, penicillin, tetracycline, doxycycline, and cefuroxime axetil (37,38). Studies comparing amoxicillin and doxycycline (39) and tetracycline and doxycycline (40) found no significant difference in outcome of patients treated with these drugs. A randomized, multicenter, investigator-blinded clinical trial of cefuroxime axetil and doxycycline found the drugs to be equally effective for treatment of patients with erythema migrans and in preventing subsequent development of late Lyme disease (41). A satisfactory clinical outcome was achieved in 88% to 93% of patients. A similar clinical trial was conducted comparing amoxicillin and azithromycin. Amoxicillin was significantly more effective than azithromycin in resolving the signs and symptoms of patients with erythema migrans and preventing subsequent relapse (42). Patients with early disease with cardiac or neurological manifestations are treated parenterally with ceftriaxone. Cefotaxime and penicillin are alternative and second choice drugs, respectively (37,38). Duration of oral and parenteral treatments is 14 to 30 days, depending on the severity of disease. At this time, there is no scientific evidence to support long-term oral or parenteral therapy.

Ixodes scapularis, in addition to being the vector for Lyme disease, also may carry the agents of babesiosis and human granulocytic ehrlichiosis. The possibility of concurrent infection should be considered if patients do not respond to therapy. In areas where both ehrlichiosis and Lyme disease are present, doxycycline is considered the drug of choice because it is effective against both agents.

REFERENCES

1. Baranton G, Postic D, Saint Girons I, et al. Delineation of *Borrelia burgdorferi* sensu stricto, *Borrelia garinii* sp. nov. and group VS461 associated with Lyme borreliosis. Int J Syst Bacteriol 1992; 42: 378–383.
2. Canica MM, Nato F, du Merle L, et al. Monoclonal antibodies for identification of *Borrelia afzelii* sp. nov. associated with late cutaneous manifestations of Lyme borreliosis. Scand J Infect Dis 1993; 25: 441–448.
3. Postic D, Assous MV, Grimont PAD, Baranton G. Diversity of *Borrelia burgdorferi* sensu lato evidenced by restriction fragment length polymorphism on rrf (5S)-rrl (23S) intergenic spacer amplicons. Int J Syst Bacteriol 1994; 44: 743–752.
4. Ferdows MS, Barbour AG. Megabase-sized linear DNA in the bacterium *Borrelia burgdorferi*, the Lyme disease agent. Proc Natl Acad Sci USA 1989; 86: 5969–5973.

5. Barbour AG, Garon CF. Linear plasmids of the bacterium *Borrelia burgdorferi* have covalently closed ends. Science 1987; 237: 409–411.

6. Hyde F, Johnson RC. Genetic relationship of Lyme disease spirochetes to *Borrelia, Treponema* and *Leptospira* spp. J Clin Microbiol 1984; 20: 151–154.

7. Pyle LE, Corcoran LN, Cocks BC, et al. Pulsed-field electrophoresis indicates larger-than-expected sizes for mycoplasma genomes. Nucleic Acids Res 1988; 16: 6015–6025.

8. Dykhuizen DE, Polin DS, Dunn JJ, et al. *Borrelia burgdorferi* is clonal: implications for taxonomy and vaccine development. Proc Natl Acad Sci USA 1993; 90: 10163–10167.

9. Xu Y, Johnson RC. Analysis and comparison of plasmid profiles of *Borrelia burgdorferi* sensu lato. J Clin Microbiol 1995; 33: 2679–2685.

10. Fuchs H, Wallich R, Simon MM, Kramer MD. The outer surface protein A of the spirochete *Borrelia burgdorferi* is a plasmin(ogen) receptor. Proc Natl Acad Sci 1994; 91: 12594-12598.

11. Klempner MS, Noring R, Epstein MP, et al. Binding of human plasminogen and urokinase-type plasminogen activator to the Lyme disease spirochete, *Borrelia burgdorferi*. J Infect Dis 1995; 171: 1258–1265.

12. Schwan TG, Piesman J, Golde WT, et al. Induction of an outer surface protein on *Borrelia burgdorferi* during tick feeding. Proc Natl Acad Sci 1994; 92: 2909–2913.

13. Keller D, Koster FT, Marks DH, et al. Safety and immunogenicity of a recombinant outer surface protein A Lyme vaccine. JAMA 1994; 271: 1764–1768.

14. Nadelman RB, Wormser GP. Erythema migrans and early Lyme disease. Am J Med 1995; 98(4A): 15S–22S.

15. Berger BW. Erythema chronicum migrans of Lyme disease. Arch Dermatol 1984; 120: 1017–1021.

16. Berger BW, Johnson RC, Kodner C, Coleman L. Cultivation of *Borrelia burgdorferi* from erythema migrans lesions and perilesional skin. J Clin Microbiol 1992; 30: 359–361.

17. Berger BW, Johnson RC, Kodner C, Coleman L. Failure of *Borrelia burgdorferi* to survive in the skin of patients with antibiotic-treated Lyme disease. J Am Acad Dermatol 1992; 27: 34–37.

18. Preac-Mursic V, Weber K, Pfister HW, et al. Survival of *Borrelia burgdorferi* in antibiotically treated patients with Lyme borreliosis. Infection 1989; 17: 355–359.

19. Berger BW, Johnson RC. Clinical and microbiologic findings in six patients with erythema migrans of Lyme disease. J Am Acad Dermatol 1989; 21:1188–1191.

20. Strle F, Chen Y, Cimperman J, et al. Persistence of *Borrelia burgdorferi* sensu lato in resolved erythema migrans. Clin Infect Dis 1995; 21: 380–389.

21. Asbrink E, Hovmark A. Early and late cutaneous manifestations in Ixodes-borne borreliosis. Ann NY Acad Sci 1988; 539: 4–16.

22. Karlsson M, Hovind-Hougen K, Svenungsson B, Stiernstedt G. Cultivation and characterization of spirochetes from cerebrospinal fluid of patients with Lyme borreliosis. J Clin Microbiol 1990; 28: 473–479.

23. Schmidli J, Hunziker T, Moesli P, Schaad UB. Cultivation of *Borrelia burgdorferi* from joint fluid three months after treatment of facial palsy due to Lyme borreliosis. J Infect Dis 1988; 158: 905–906.
24. Goodman JL, Bradley JF, Ross AE, et al. Bloodstream invasion in early Lyme disease: prospective, controlled study utilizing the polymerase chain reaction. Am J Med 1995; 99: 6–12.
25. Bradley JF, Johnson RC, and Goodman JL. The persistence of spirochetal nucleic acids in active Lyme arthritis. Ann Intern Med 1994; 120: 487–489.
26. Centers for Disease Control. Recommendations for test performance and interpretation from the second national conference on serologic diagnosis of Lyme disease. MMWR 1995; 44: 590–591.
27. Engstrom SM, Shoop E, Johnson RC. Immunoblot interpretation criteria for the serodiagnosis of early Lyme disease. J Clin Microbiol 1995; 33: 419–427.
28. Steere AC, Berardi VP, Weeks KE, et al. Evaluation of the intrathecal antibody response to *Borrelia burgdorferi* as a diagnostic test for Lyme neuroborreliosis. J Infect Dis 1990; 161: 1203–1209.
29. Feder HM, Gerber MA, Luger SW, Ryan RW. Persistence of antibodies to *Borrelia burgdorferi* in patients treated for Lyme disease. Clin Infect Dis 1992; 15: 788–793.
30. Dressler F, Whalen JA, Reinhardt BN, Steere AC. Western blotting in the serodiagnosis of Lyme disease. J Infect Dis 1993; 167:392–400.
31. Agger WA, Callister SM, Jobe DA. In vitro susceptibilities of *Borrelia burgdorferi* to five oral cephalosporins and ceftriaxone. Antimicrob Agents Chemother 1992; 36: 1788–1799.
32. Dever LL, Jorgensen JH, Barbour AG. Comparative in vitro activities of clarithromycin, azithromycin, and erythromycin against *Borrelia burgdorferi*. Antimicrob Agents Chemother 1993; 37: 1704–1706.
33. Johnson RC, Kodner C, Russell ME. In vitro and in vivo susceptibility of the Lyme disease spirochete, *Borrelia burgdorferi* to four antimicrobials. Antimicrob Agents Chemother 1987; 31: 164–167.
34. Johnson RC, Kodner C, Russell M, Girard D. In vitro and in vivo susceptibility of *Borrelia burgdorferi* to azithromycin. J Antimicrob Chemother 1990; 25(suppl A): 33–38.
35. Johnson RC, Kodner CB, Jurkovich PJ, Collins JJ. Comparative in vitro and in vivo susceptibilities of the Lyme disease spirochete *Borrelia burgdorferi* to cefuroxime and other antimicrobial agents. Antimicrob Agents Chemother 1990; 34: 2133–2136.
36. Preac-Mursic V, Wilske B, Shierz G, et al. Comparative antimicrobial activity of the new macrolides against *Borrelia burgdorferi*. Eur J Clin Microbiol Infect Dis 1989; 8: 651–681.
37. American Academy of Pediatrics. Section 5: Antimicrobials and related therapy. In: Peter G. ed. 1994 Red Book: Report of the Committee on Infectious Diseases. 23d ed. Elk Grove Village: American Academy of Pediatrics, 1994: 541–557.
38. Treatment of Lyme Disease. Medical Letter 1992; 34: 95–97.

39. Dattwyler RJ, Volkman DJ, Conaty SM, et al. Amoxycillin plus probenecid versus doxycycline for treatment of erythema migrans borreliosis. Lancet 1990; 336: 1404–1406.
40. Nowakowski J, Nadelman RB, Forseter G, et al. Doxycycline versus tetracycline therapy for Lyme disease associated with erythema migrans. J Am Acad Dermatol 1995; 32: 223–227.
41. Nadleman, RB, Luger SW, Frank E, et al. Comparison of cefuroxime axetil and doxycycline in the treatment of early Lyme disease. Ann Intern Med 1992; 117: 273–280.
42. Luft BJ, Luger SW, Rahn DW, et al. Azithromycin and amoxicillin for the treatment of erythema migrans. Preliminary analysis of a double-blind trial (abstr). In: Program and Abstracts of the Fifth International Conference on Lyme Borreliosis; May 30–June 2, 1992; Arlington, VA, Washington DC: Federation of American Societies for Experimental Biology, 1992; A56.

6
Antimicrobial Soaps: Their Role in Personal Hygiene

Bruce H. Keswick, Cynthia A. Berge, Robert G. Bartolo, and Deborah D. Watson

The Procter & Gamble Company, Cincinnati, Ohio

INTRODUCTION

This chapter provides an update on antimicrobial soaps and the role they play in personal hygiene. As background, a brief history is appropriate. Antimicrobial soaps have been used widely by consumers since their introduction in the 1960s. At first, the predominate product forms were bar soaps like Safeguard and Dial. In the ensuing years, however, increasing public concern over preventing disease has stimulated the growth of the antimicrobial-soap market. Many new product forms such as liquids and gels for hand and body washing have been developed to meet this growing consumer need.

The familiar products currently found in US households are regulated as over-the-counter (OTC) drugs. In the 1960s, antimicrobial soaps were regulated under the New Drug Application (NDA) process. At that time, several clinical studies were conducted to demonstrate the potential of antimicrobial soaps to mitigate skin infections. Beginning in 1971, these studies were reviewed by an Advisory Review Panel as part of the process to develop an OTC monograph to define permissible ingredients, efficacy testing, and claims for topical antimicrobial products. In 1974, the Advisory Review Panel reported its review of all of the data on topical antimicrobial products including that on antimicrobial soaps (1). The Panel had questions on some of the various methodologies used in these early antimicrobial soap clinical tests, and they concluded that although not all of these studies were definitive, some supported indications. The results from these clinical studies, combined with the results from laboratory in vivo testing, provided the Panel with enough data to recommend that antimicrobial soaps be included in the monograph on OTC Antimicrobial Drug Products for Repeated Daily Human Use. In 1978 a proposed Tentative Final Monograph was published (2).

Since 1978, there have been several reports on the development of suitable model efficacy tests to demonstrate the effectiveness of an antimicrobial soap product in reducing the numbers of bacteria on the skin (3). However, there have been no recent reports of clinical studies specifically focused on the reduction of skin infections.

In contrast, there have been numerous publications on the role of handwashing in the reduction of disease transmission (4–7). As a result of this vast amount of information on handwashing, we can conclude that handwashing is recognized as an important means of infection control (8).

In 1994, the Food and Drug Administration (FDA) proposed changes to the Tentative Final Monograph (9). The changes included elimination of the antimicrobial soap category by its reclassification as antiseptic handwash category. It also proposed elimination of the currently used active ingredients, leaving only consumer-unfriendly alcohol and povidone–iodine as approved active ingredients. The proposed changes are under review and comment before final rule making.

This chapter reviews and updates the current state of knowledge supporting the role of antimicrobial soaps in personal hygiene by reexamining the evidence for handwashing and whole body cleansing.

POTENTIAL BENEFITS OF ANTIMICROBIAL SOAPS

The potential benefits to consumers of antimicrobial soaps in addition to cleaning are (a) reduction in the incidence of pyogenic infections, (b) removal of potentially pathogenic transient organisms, and (c) reduction of body odor (10,11). Washing with antimicrobial soaps or with non-medicated soaps removes bacteria from the skin because of the surfactancy of the soap base and the mechanical action of the wash procedure. These soaps, however, also deposit an active ingredient on the skin that can control the number of surviving organisms and help prevent the colonization of potential pathogens such as *Staphylococcus aureus*. Washing with a nonmedicated soap does not provide this reservoir of antimicrobial activity.

THE USE OF ANTIMICROBIAL SOAPS FOR PERSONAL HYGIENE

Because one of every three purchases of a personal cleansing product by consumers involves an antimicrobial soap product (12), it is evident that consumers view these soaps as an important product class. Further, they view these soaps as appropriate for the entire family, and they believe it provides a cleaner feeling and more germ removal than nonmedicated soap. This high level of acceptance and consumer need is reflected in the marketplace, where approximately half (47%) the households in the United States use antimicrobial soap products. Consumer acceptance is also reinforced by recommendations from physicians. For example, 60% of pediatricians surveyed have recommended an antimicrobial soap to their patients for a variety of needs.

At the 1995 Annual Meeting of the American Academy of Dermatology, 93% of dermatologists surveyed said they have recommended antimicrobial soaps. Additionally, 82% responded that their ability to help manage their patient's medical conditions would be adversely affected if OTC antimicrobial cleansing products were not available (13). Antimicrobial soaps are available in many forms (e.g., bars, liquids, gels) and may contain one of several different active ingredients. They are basically used for two different purposes: handwashing and whole body washing. When antimicrobial soap is used for handwashing, the primary objective is to reduce the numbers of contaminating organisms on the hands to prevent the transmission of disease. When antimicrobial soap is used for whole body washing, the objective is to help prevent skin infections and to reduce body odor. Although these two purposes indicate different modes of action and could potentially use different antimicrobial ingredients with different spectrums of activity, these differences might not be easily distinguished by the consumer. It is clear, however, that consumers do recognize the following:

1. In everyday life, they are exposed to a wide variety of bacteria that have a potential to harm them.
2. Bathing, showering, and handwashing with an antimicrobial soap can help reduce the risk of infection and spread of disease that could result from exposure to these bacteria.

PUBLIC HEALTH IMPACT OF SKIN INFECTIONS

Frequency of Occurrence for the Public

Skin infections due to gram-positive organisms are recognized as a common and significant public health problem. These skin diseases are most commonly caused by staphylococci and streptococci. They include pustules, folliculitis, impetigo, furuncles, and infection of cuts and scrapes. In addition to the staphylococci and streptococci, other gram-positive bacteria such as *Corynebacterium minutissimum* can cause skin infections such as erythrasma (14). Up to 8% of visits to dermatology clinics are a result of some form of pyoderma (15,16). Skin related problems constitute about 6.8% of the visits to general pediatric clinics (17). Of these, about half are cutaneous infections, some of which can lead to frequent recurrence and intrafamilial spread. Data from one survey (16) estimated that 5.5 million office visits a year are due to skin infections. In a survey of a pediatric dermatology clinic, the second, third, and fifth most frequently diagnosed conditions were infectious diseases (18). Of all diagnoses, 33.6% were infections or infestations, of which 29.0% were bacterial, 42% were fungal, and 23.2% were viral. According to data obtained from the National Disease and Therapeutic Index (NDTI) (19), from 1992 to 1994, there were approximately 2 million diagnostic visits a year to dermatologists, pediatricians, general or family practitioners, and others for impetigo, pyoderma, and carbuncles/furuncles. Of the 2 million visits, pediatricians made 38% of these diagnoses, dermatologists made 10%, general or family practitioners made 31%, and others made 21%. These diagnostic visits are detailed by specialty in Table 1.

Table 1   Number of Physician Visits (Thousands) for Skin Infections by Specialty

Year	1992	1993	1994
Pediatrics	902	681	743
Impetigo	846	645	719
Carbuncle/Furuncle	33	25	18
Pyoderma	23	11	7
Family/General	635	638	579
Impetigo	406	445	385
Carbuncle/Furuncle	149	158	143
Pyoderma	80	36	51
Dermatology	205	212	199
Impetigo	91	119	96
Carbuncle/Furuncle	42	40	17
Pyoderma	72	54	87
Total Other Specialties	304	473	470

Source: Reference 19.

Effect of Climate and Geography

The occurrence of skin infections is highly correlated to geography and climate (20,21). There is a higher frequency of infections in areas with high temperatures and humidity. The conditions found year round in the tropics or during the summer months in more temperate climates are conducive to both fungal and bacterial infections. A report of a survey of troops in Vietnam suggested that streptococci were the most prevalent cause of skin infections in the tropics where climate, life-style, and insect bites play an important role in the initiation of infections (22).

Special occurrences, such as natural disasters, can lead to a decline in hygiene, affecting many households and resulting in an increase in the incidence of skin infections. In the United States, Quinn et al. (23) reported on the medical care of families affected by Hurricane Andrew in 1992. "During the two weeks following the storm, there were noted increases in pediatric dermatologic infections including impetigo, wound infections and cellulitis."

Effect of Age and Personal Hygiene

In addition to geography and climate, age and personal hygiene also have an important influence on skin infections. Children overwhelmingly con-stitute the population at greatest risk for bacterial skin infection, with those under 9 years of age having the greatest incidence (20). A higher frequency of impetigo among children was reported by Aly and Maibach (24). The number of children worldwide with skin infections is estimated to be in the millions, and they constitute a significant load on medical services (20); however, the elderly are also at risk. A survey of skin problems in elderly noninstitutionalized adults, ages 68 and older, iden-tified skin infections as a common occurrence (25). The authors further suggested that these skin problems may be exacerbated when the bathing and shampooing ability of older adults becomes substantially limited by physical incapacity.

Effect of Carriage of S. aureus

Atopic dermatitis affects approximately 10% to 15% of the population. Clinical studies have shown that the skin flora of atopics is quantitatively and qualitatively different from the skin of the normal population. It has been reported that these patients have increased numbers of skin flora and a higher frequency of colonization with S. aureus, not only on their skin, but also in their nares (26). The skin of 95% of atopic patients (versus about 5% of normal controls) was colonized with *S. aureus*. In the acute lesions and chronic plaques associated with this disease, the density of *S. aureus* was higher than on the unaffected skin (27). Because of the chronic presence of this organism, it is not surprising that patients with atopic dermatitis experience increased numbers of skin infections.

Chronic, asymptomatic carriage of *S. aureus* in the nares occurs in 20% to 40% of the normal population (28). Nasal carriage of *S. aureus* can be correlated to higher rates of infection in individuals, because this organism can be transferred from the nose to other skin sites (29). Many normal daily activities that result in minor cuts and scrapes have the potential to become contaminated with these transferred *S. aureus* and with other organisms from environmental sources.

Intrafamilial Transfer

Transmission of skin infections among family members is well recognized. Kay (30) reported that half the cases of staphylococcal infection originating in one family member can later spread to other family members. In almost every case, a single strain was responsible. The axilla and perineum, in addition to the nares, were identified as potential sources of the organisms. In half the cases, another member of the patient's family was found to carry the infecting strain even if the patient was not a nasal carrier.

Impetigo is frequently spread in families. Dillon (31) found 497 cases of impetigo that involved intrafamilial transmission in 347 families. In another study, the mean interval from index to secondary skin acquisition was 4.8 days, and recovery of a serotype from normal skin was associated with a high risk (76%) of infection (32).

Ben-Amitai and Ashkenazi (17) recommended that "prophylaxis of chronic recurrent furunculosis should be attempted. One of the most important factors in prevention is avoidance of autoinoculation and intra-familial spread. The patient should be instructed to follow a strict regimen of personal hygiene, including frequent handwashing, showers rather than baths, daily use of antimicrobial soap with special attention to the axillae and crotch, and daily laundering of bedding and clothing."

Zimakoff et al. (33) pointed out the importance of reinfection on the transmission of *Staphylococcus* within families and concluded that a residual antimicrobial effect is desirable to help prevent reacquisition of *Staphylococcus* that is shed into the household environment on sheets towels, and other linen.

Other skin sites on the body may also represent sources of bacteria. Elsner and Maibach (34) suggested that the dispersion of S. *aureus* from the vulvar skin may be important in the epidemiology of cross-infection between individuals as well as a focus of chronic infection.

Athletic Activities

Sevier (35) reviewed the causes of infectious diseases in athletes. He stated that bacterial infections in athletes often involve a history of lacerations, abrasions, or irritation from equipment, dirt, sweat, occlusion, or contact with other infected athletes. Impetigo, furuncles, folliculitis, erythrasma, and pitted keratolysis are the most common bacterial infections.

Summary: The Public Health Impact of Skin Infections

Skin infections constitute a significant public health issue, affecting millions of households. Improving personal hygiene has the potential to be an important control measure. From the preceding examples, we infer that there is an indication for an antimicrobial soap with an active ingredient that is substantive and provides residual activity primarily against staphylococci and streptococci.

THE POTENTIAL FOR ANTIMICROBIAL SOAPS TO MITIGATE SKIN INFECTIONS

The preceding discussion establishes that the consumer encounters a number of situations in everyday life at home, work, school, and play in which good personal hygiene is important to reduce the risk of infection. The next sections review the historic evidence (i.e., the results from a number of clinical studies) that demonstrates that antimicrobial soaps have the potential to provide this benefit. These clinical studies can be divided into two groups.

The first group consists of the studies that show a reduction in the numbers of bacteria on the skin. Results from these studies imply that control or reduction of bacteria on the skin is related to a reduction in disease. The second group consists of the studies that attempted to identify an actual reduction in skin infection.

Standard Evaluation Techniques: Measurement of Reduction or Control of Bacteria on the Skin

A wide variety of procedures and methods have been used to measure a reduction in the numbers of bacteria on the skin. Some of these studies were controlled experiments that involved regimented washes, inoculation of the skin with bacteria, and even occlusion with plastic wrap. Others were clinical field studies, with less controlled wash methods and test procedures. The results of these studies are summarized in Table 2.

Currently in the United States, three standard, experimental test procedures are used by manufacturers of antimicrobial soap to demonstrate that their products control or reduce the numbers of bacteria on the skin. Recently, the industry members of the Soap and Detergent Association and Cosmetics, Toiletries & Fragrance Association wrote these methods in a standardized format and submitted them to the American Society for Testing Materials for incorporation into their official manual of test procedures. These test procedures are (a) the modified Cade Handwash test, (b) the Cup Scrub test, and (c) the Agar Patch test. In addition, a number of other models have demonstrated the effectiveness of washing with antimicrobial products (Table 2).

Modified Cade Handwash Test

The objective of this test is to determine the effectiveness of an antimicrobial test product in reducing the level of aerobic resident flora on the hands after exclusive use of the test product for at least 5 days. This test consists of a wash-out period followed by a test period when subjects use the antimicrobial product.

This test is a modification of a procedure developed by Price (36) and Cade (37) and reported in OTC Topical Antimicrobial Products TFM (2). The bacterial sampling procedure used in the study involves collecting the lather, after a series of five handwashes, into a basin of sterile water. Studies showed that after four consecutive handwashes, the transient, contaminating bacteria are removed, but the resident bacteria remain (36). The microbial population collected from the fifth wash is representative of the resident flora. Efficacy is determined by comparing the numbers of resident bacteria on the hands before and after using an antimicrobial test product.

Using the above procedure of comparing the fifth basin wash from the baseline count to the fifth basin wash from the test count, Cade (37) reported a 98% reduction in a study done with a soap product containing 2% hexachlorophene. The 1978 OTC tentative final monograph stipulates that to demonstrate efficacy, an antimicrobial soap should show at least a 1 log or 90% reduction in bacterial flora (2).

Cup Scrub Test

The objective of this test is to compare the residual antimicrobial effectiveness of an antimicrobial soap product to a placebo or another antimicrobial soap product to reduce the numbers and control the regrowth of bacteria on the skin. The term *Cup Scrub Test* refers to the sampling method used to recover the bacteria from the subjects' skin. The cup scrub bacterial sampling method was developed by Williamson and Kligman (38) in 1965. In this procedure, an aliquot of buffer solution is pipetted into a sterile glass cylinder that is held firmly against skin. The area of skin inside of the cylinder is then scrubbed with the flat end of a rubber policeman for approximately 30 to 60 seconds. The buffer solution is decanted into a sterile test tube, and the scrubbing procedure is repeated with another aliquot of buffer. Microbiological analyses are performed on the combined sample solution.

There are several variations of the Cup Scrub Test. It can be used to measure reductions in the normal bacterial flora, or it can be used to measure the effect of a test product on pathogenic bacteria, which are inoculated onto skin (39,40). There have also been studies, using this basic procedure, that involved occlusion of the skin for a specified period of time (41). Most of the cup scrub tests use the skin on the volar surface of the forearm. However, this procedure can be done on the axilla in evaluations of axillary degerming efficacy (42).

Finkey et al. (39) used the occlusion variation of the procedure to demonstrate the antimicrobial efficacy of two bar soap formulations containing (TCC) against *S. aureus* and *C. minutissimum*. The results of this study indicated that both products produced significantly lower counts for both test organisms when compared to a placebo bar. Scala et al. (40) reported similar results.

Agar Patch Test

The objective of this test is to determine the residual bacteriostatic activity of antimicrobial soap products by measuring the reduction of bacteria streaked on an agar plate (patch) pressed against the volar surface of the forearm skin surface. The Agar Patch Test can be used to evaluate bar and liquid soap products.

Results from studies using this method have shown that the forearms washed with an antimicrobial soap containing 1.5% TCC had a

Table 2 Experimental Studies Reporting the Reduction of Bacteria on the Skin by Antimicrobial Soaps

Author	Year	Active ingredient	Study summary	Results
Finkey et al. (39)	1984	TCC	Cup scrub (Test organisms added to skin under occlusion)	Significant reduction in skin pathogens vs placebo
Scala et al. (40)	1994	TCC	Cup scrub (Test organisms added to skin under occlusion)	Significant reduction in skin pathogens vs placebo
Leyden et al. (41)	1979	HXP, CHX, others	Cup scrub test (occlusion test, expanded flora test, persistence test, ecological shift test)	Significant differences vs placebo
Yackovich et al. (43–45)	1985	TCC	Agar Patch Method	Significantly greater residual bacteriostatic activity than placebo
Bannan (102)	1969	TBS/TCC/TFC	Modified Cade Test — Children's hands were washed 2x/d	Personal hygiene use resulted in 5% reduction in *S. aureus* carriage
Paulson et al. (103)	1994	PCMX, others	Healthcare Personnel Hand Wash Test (*Serratia marcescens* seeded onto hands)	Antimicrobial lotion soap was statistically more effective than plain soap in both immediate and persistent antimicrobial properties
Ansari et al. (104)	1989	CHX, ALC, PCMX Liquid Soap, others	Finger pad technique	Demonstrated antiseptic effects of hand washing
Rotter et al. (105, 106)	1986	PI, ALC, Phenolic Soap	Vienna test model	Test demonstrates hygienic hand disinfection
Leyden et al. (107)	1993	CHX, PI, TCS, CBC	Full-hand touch plates method	Demonstrated the effectiveness of some but not all of the products tested

Reference	Year	Agent	Description	Results
Bannan (108)	1967	TBS/TCC/TFC	Surgeons and nurses used for scrub and personal hygiene	Personal hygiene use resulted in 5% reduction in S. aureus carriage
Wilson (109)	1970	TCC, HXP	18 months trial in a hospital ward	Both antibacterial soaps showed significant reductions in skin flora. Transmission of staphylococci in the ward was reduced by the TCC soap.
Voss (110)	1975	TCC/TFC	225 subjects used bars for personal hygiene over 2 to 7 months	Reductions in total aerobic flora of 47% to 77% vs plain soap were reported
Aly and Maibach (111)	1976	CHX	Daily use for 6 months by 40 subjects	Lower total microbial counts were detected from each of four areas vs nonantibacterial soap group
Aihara et al. (112)	1993	1:100 PI	Used antimicrobial solutions to prevent the colonization of skin in a premature infants unit	No additional MRSA infections occurred
Hedin and Hambraeus (113)	1993	CHX	Daily use of CHX wash	Prevented colonization by antibiotic resistant S. epidermidis

CBC = chlorbenzarconium, CHX = chlorhexidine, HXP = hexachlorophene, TCC = triclocarban, TBS = tribromsalan, TCS = triclosan, TFC = clofucarban, ALC = alcohols, PCMX = chloroxylenol, PI = povidone iodine, MRSA = methacillin-resistant S. aureus

79% to 88% reduction in the colony-forming unit (CFU) count compared to forearms washed with a placebo product (43). Studies to compare a liquid soap containing triclosan (TCS) to a liquid placebo soap showed complete inhibition (100%) with the TCS product compared to the placebo product (44). In addition to showing differences between antimicrobial and placebo products, this method can be sensitive enough to detect differences in the efficacy of two antimicrobial products containing different levels of active ingredients (45). This method evaluates only the presence of the antimicrobial on the skin. Interaction of the organism and antimicrobial ingredient occurs on the agar plate, not on the skin. This method is sensitive to different diffusion rates of antimicrobial ingredients.

Clinical Studies Reporting the Effect of Antimicrobial Soap on Skin Infection

Superficial Cutaneous Pyogenic Infections
(S. aureus and Streptococcus pyogenes)

In the late 1960s, work began to determine whether the regular use of antimicrobial soaps would prevent bacterial infections on the skin. For the most part, these studies examined sizable populations of individuals who were living in controlled environments, such as boarding schools, institutions, and prisons, where it was possible to enforce some type of restrictions and thereby control some of the confounding variables. Although a variety of study designs were used, the studies that required daily examinations were the most successful because potential episodes of infection were tracked more thoroughly. Obviously, these studies were complicated, expensive, and difficult to conduct; and some of the results were not as conclusive and as easy to interpret as expected (1). Some of the preliminary studies, however, demonstrated that antimicrobial soaps were effective in reducing primary *S. aureus* skin infections, including furunculosis, impetigo, paronychia, and infections of blisters, insect bites, and lacerations. These studies are summarized in Table 3. Several of these studies were reviewed (11) in the proceedings from the last session of this symposium.

Erythrasma Corynebacterium minutissimum

In the late 1960s, a few studies were conducted that clearly demonstrated the efficacy of antimicrobial bars in treating erythrasma (3). Erythrasma is a superficial bacterial infection of the skin caused by *C. minutissimum*, which can be detected by its coral red fluorescence under long wave ultraviolet light. Classically, erythrasma is a localized infection that can be found on the toe webs, groin, trunk, and limbs. It is usually successfully treated with systemically administered antibiotics; however, infections in the toe web area can be resistant to this type of treatment regimen.

The 1974 OTC panel (1) also reviewed the erythrasma studies that are presented in Table 3. They concluded that the studies provided definitive evidence of the therapeutic effectiveness of antimicrobial soaps against erythrasma, but that the results could not be extrapolated to other skin disease-causing organisms.

Summary

Several experimental studies have demonstrated that antimicrobial soaps can decrease and control populations of both resident and transient bacteria on the skin to a greater degree than plain soap. This view was summarized as "antimicrobial soaps as presently formulated effectively reduce the normal flora of the skin and have significant protective powers against colonization with *S. aureus*" (46).

Several clinical studies have reported the ability of antimicrobial soaps to reduce the incidence of skin infection (Table 3). Although some of these studies were viewed as equivocal by the OTC panel (1) because of methodological questions, they did provide a strong suggestion of potential benefit. We conclude that there is reason to expect that antimicrobial soaps can play a role in skin hygiene.

HANDWASHING: INTERRUPTING DISEASE TRANSMISSION FROM TRANSIENT FLORA

Hands and Transient Flora

The hands can be viewed as unique in three respects:

1. More than any other part of the body, the hands are in constant contact with the environment and are exposed to transient contaminants from many sources.
2. Their various parts, such as the nail folds and interdigital spaces, provide microenvironments that can support organisms with specific growth requirements.

Table 3 Studies Reporting the Effect of Antimicrobial Soaps on Skin Infections

Name	Place	Active ingredient	Study duration	Wash freq.	Population	Results
Kooistra 1965 (114)	Volunteers, OH	TBS/TCC/ TFC	8–11 months	daily	71 males with erythrasma 38 test, 33 control	At 11 months, 71% of control vs 21% of test subjects exhibited toe web infection; "split foot" 0/7 test vs 6/7 control subjects were still infected after a 5-day treatment.
Dubow and Winter 1967 (115)	Juvenile detention home, NY	HXC/TCC	not reported	bathed daily	160 treated, 160 control (8 to 16 yr olds)	Decreased the infection frequency of moderate to severe wounds.
Leonard 1967 (116)	US Military Academy, NY	TBS/TCC/ TFC	2 months	not mentioned	474 treated, 609 control (new cadets)	Decreased the incidence of superficial cutaneous infections by 44%.
Dodge et al. 1968 (117)	Patients, TX	TBS/TCC/ TFC	21 days	2×/day	28 patients with erythrasma	Positive effect on resolution of infection in 9/9 test vs 2/4 control subjects.
Dodge et al. 1968 (117)	Prison, TX	TBS/TCC/ TFC	8 months	daily	2600 males, 70 with erythrasma	51/51 cleared with antibacterial bar.
Duncan et al. 1969 (118)	Prison farm(s), TX	TBS/TCC/ TFC	9 months	shower 1×/day or ad libitum	2550 w/crossover, 1275 treated/ control (adults)	Positive effect reported for use under regulated conditions.

Study	Location	Agents	Duration	Frequency	Number	Results
Taber et al. 1969 (119)	Volunteers	HXP/TCC	13 days	daily	50 males	In 27/38 subjects the infection resolved in the treated foot before the control foot.
Wheatley et al. 1969 (120)	State School, MS	TBS/TCC/TFC	14–16 week cross over	bathed daily and as needed	169 (ages 6–20)	Decreased infections by 50% vs plain soap.
MacKenzie 1970 (121)	US Naval Academy, MD	HXP/TCC	6 months	shower 3×/day	602 treated, 599 control (1st year midshipmen)	Fewer infections were reported in the treatment group.
Sharrett et al. 1974 (122)	Homes, Trinidad	HCX, TCC	2 months	wash lesions and legs 2×/day	135 patients (13 years)	Not significantly different from placebo, but "prevalence of streptococcal skin lesions was relatively decreased in the treated group."
Taplin 1981 (11)	Navajo Boarding School, AZ	TCC/TFC	2 months	shower 1×/day	322 treated, 311 control (7 to 12 yr olds)	Neither plain soap nor anti-microbial soap reduced group A streptococci infections.

CHX = chlorhexidine, HXP = hexachlorophene, TCC = triclocarban, TBS = tribromsalan, TCS = triclosan, TFC = clofucarban, ALC = alcohols, PCMX = chloroxylenol, PI = povidone iodine

3. The flora on the hands are highly subject to modification because of exposure to a number of varied daily activities.

Aly and Maibach (15) showed that as many as 10^6 CFUs can be recovered from the hands. Basically, these are the transient bacteria that lie free on the skin or are loosely attached with dirt (47). Separate from these are the stable population of resident flora that live in the surface layers of the stratum corneum.

The factors that influence both kinds of flora on the hands have been studied extensively. Peterson (48) presented data to show that the normal resident microbial population on the hands is relatively stable over time and not significantly influenced by season, diet, or climate. The numbers and types of resident flora can be influenced by exposure to solvents, systemic and topical antibiotics, hormones, and disinfecting agents. In contrast, the transient flora found on hands are directly related to the source of contamination that is touched during activities such as gardening, food preparation, and animal handling. There is consensus in medical and scientific communities that the transfer of transient bacteria via hands is a major factor in the spread of disease. The potentially infectious sources of transient contamination that the consumer can be exposed to are examined below.

Sources of Transient Contamination

Home Environment

In the home, consumers can expect to encounter a wide variety of organisms. Surveys of the bacteria found in the home environment suggested four major sites of household contamination: dry areas (floors, linens, furniture, clothing), wet areas (baths, sinks, toilets, drains), food, and people (49–53). In many homes, animals (pets, farm animals) and outside work (gardening, yard work) also should be included. The survey found that high bacterial colony counts were mainly in wet areas associated with sinks, bath tiles, and diaper pails. High bacterial colony counts were also frequently recovered from washcloths, dishcloths, and cleaning towels. *Escherichia coli*, pseudomonads, *S. aureus*, and streptococci were the organisms most commonly isolated.

Marples and Towers (54) established a model to study the transfer of staphylococci from contact with objects. Mackintosh and Hoffman (55) extended the model to include gram-negative bacteria, *Staphylococcus saprophyticus* and *S. pyogenes*. Although it is accepted that the risk of infection in the general community is lower than that associated with hospitalized patients, Scott et al. (49) noted there have been a significant number of outbreaks of household food poisonings in which hand contamination may have played a role. A study of 10 family households to detect infectious enteritis causing organisms found that 267 of 4683 samples of food contained staphylococci (56). They also found that hard surfaces and utensils were contaminated.

Impact of Day Care Centers

The shift in recent years from home-based child care to group day care has effectively extended the boundaries of the household, resulting in an increased risk of the transmission of disease. Infectious bacteria from one household environment can be transmitted to another household by the interaction of the children (56–61). Furthermore, studies (59,62) have also demonstrated that diseases in day care centers can be brought home and transferred among other family members.

Surveys of the day care center environment have found contamination on the surfaces of toys, food areas, diaper changing areas, and on the hands of children and adults (62–66). An increased risk of diarrhea associated with elevated fecal contamination levels was demonstrated by Laborde et al. (66). They found that the incidence of diarrhea was strongly effected by contamination of hands and toys with high levels of coliform bacteria. Because dry surfaces are generally less likely to be sources of enteropathogens, they suggested that "hands can be primary vehicles of enteric disease transmission."

With 5.3 to 11 million children in the United States currently in out-of-home day care, many families are potentially affected by their children's exposure to conditions where sanitation may be less than satisfactory. Compounding the problem are inadequate personal hygiene practices among children and facility personnel. One study estimated that the staff in only 75% of the centers studied complied with handwashing recommendations (67). The recent work of Laborde et al. (66) that demonstrated the correlation between contamination level and increased risk of disease reemphasized that handwashing and disinfection should continue to be enforced as primary intervention measures to interrupt infectious cycles in day care centers.

Home Care of the Ill and Elderly

In addition to the consumer risk that changes in day care have brought, Simmons et al. (68) stated, "Recent trends in medical care have resulted in increasing numbers of patients being cared for in the home health setting."

When the elderly or ill family members are cared for at home, the patient, other family members, and the home health care professional may be at risk of transmitting and developing infections. For example, *Clostridium difficile* is the most important cause of antibiotic-associated colitis. Using selective media, it is possible to detect contamination with C. *difficile* in the environment of patients with the disease. Because this organism is a hardy spore former, it was most frequently found in areas that were in contact with patients known to carry this organism, such as floors, hoppers, toilets, bedding, mops, scales, and furniture. The organism was also isolated from the hands and stools of asymptomatic hospital personnel. Although the importance of the spread of the organisms from these various sources was not known, it has been suggested that "enteric isolation precautions, and careful handwashing and cleansing of potentially contaminated surfaces and objects may be worthwhile when cases of antibiotic-associated colitis are identified" (69).

Gram-negative bacteria can be found on the hands of nurses after performing activities similar to the activities done at home, such as bed making, handling a patient's wash cloths and towels, and after handling dirty linen (70). Gram-positive organisms are also found on the hands. Nishijima et al. (71) reported an increased frequency of carriage of S. *aureus* on hands of patients with atopic dermatitis and the possibility of transmission of staphylococci by the hands. Roth and Land (72) instructed family members to wash hands immediately after touching contaminated objects and surfaces such as soiled laundry to help keep home care from becoming a health hazard to other family members. Handwashing is an important part of home infection control practices. Antimicrobial soaps may be useful in these situations (73,74).

Handwashing and Food Preparation

Household outbreaks of foodborne illness are a common occurrence (49). When Bryan (75) reviewed the causes of foodborne illness, he found that colonized persons were implicated in 18% of outbreaks. He also found that most outbreaks of staphylococcal food poisoning followed the handling of cooked foods by persons carrying enterotoxigenic staphylococcal strains on their skin or in their nares. Reviews by Reed (76) identify the household conditions that can lead to the transfer of disease-causing organisms. For example, food handlers who cough or sneeze, or have "careless hand habits" (touching body parts) and do not wash their hands frequently, can transmit "staph" bacteria in the kitchen.

In another report, 'salmonella were recovered from fingertips after handling artificially contaminated eggs (77). Once acquired, bacteria can remain viable on the skin for significant periods. Pether and Gilbert (78) reported that "salmonellas can survive on the fingertips for several hours, and during this time, they can be transmitted to cause infection." Reed (79) pointed out that preventing salmonellosis is based on four principles, one of which is "cleanliness, especially of the hands." It has also been noted that infection from contaminated food poses an increased risk to the elderly (80).

It is well accepted that the failure to wash hands after toilet use can lead to foodborne illness (81). In one recent report, E. coli was detected from 4% of the samples from hands before stools and 25% of the samples taken after stools (81). Handwashing reduced the E. coli counts. Gilman et al. (82) demonstrated that most unwashed fingers remain contaminated during the first several hours of observation. Because more than 20% of individuals with contaminated fingers handled food within an hour, there was a potential for pathogens to be transferred to new individuals. In 25% of the observed occurrences of contamination, the hands were not washed before the opportunity to transfer the bacteria occurred.

The general public also has been affected, outside of the home, by large outbreaks of foodborne illness that result from inadequate handwashing. The investigation of an outbreak of shigellosis by Lee (83) demonstrated the "need for surveillance and prompt public health intervention when Shigella infections are recognized in persons attending mass outdoor gatherings, the singular importance of handwashing in reducing secondary transmission of shigellosis, and the potential for explosive outbreaks when communal meals are prepared by large numbers of food handlers."

In a summary of food handling practices, Foulke (84) in the FDA Consumer recommends, "Thorough hand washing with soap and water after using the toilet or changing a baby's diaper can prevent person-to-person transmission. Proper food handling . . . will help avoid cross contamination."

Summary

Although the outbreak of disease resulting from poor personal hygiene is most often associated with the preparation and handling of food and with activities such as diaper changing in day care centers, other activities in every day life can lead to exposure to potentially harmful microorganisms. Handshaking; exposure to ill colleagues in close quarters such as meetings; shared objects such as public toilets, telephones, or exercise equipment; and general contact with the public are all examples. The importance of handwashing has been reinforced by a report from the Mayo Clinic (85) that pointed out that it is especially critical to wash hands after using the bathroom, handling food, handling money, coughing, and sneezing.

Effect of Handwashing with Antimicrobial Soap

Because transient flora are found on the skin on a temporary basis and do not normally establish colonization, washing will readily remove most transients. The resident bacteria are removed more slowly. McGinley et al. (86) pointed out that many types of bacteria found in the subungual region of the hands can still be detected after handwashing. Antimicrobial soaps can help reduce the numbers of these bacteria.

Because the surfactancy action of the soap will remove much of the organism load, it may not be as important for the active ingredient to have an immediate killing effect as it is for the active to provide residual activity that works over time. In effect, the surfactancy mechanism is broad spectrum and, if the washing is sufficiently vigorous, is fairly effective (87,88) at removing organisms.

Residual action is desirable because consumer handwashing is rarely as thorough as in the hospital settings. We know from hospitals that bland soaps are not always effective in preventing the transmission of disease (89). Ehrenkranz (88) points out that "a pervasive misconception in infection control circles is that a simple handwash reliably prevents hand transmission of transiently acquired bacteria." Studies by Huttly et al. (90) and Aulia et al. (91) point to a need for better handwashing in areas where hygiene is poor. Additionally, Bartzokas et al. (92) reported that the efficacy of an antimicrobial handwash preparation "was significantly augmented" with repeated handwashing. They concluded that "such cumulative action must be attributed to the deposition of the active antimicrobial on the skin during handwashing and retention following rinsing."

STUDIES OF HANDWASHING EFFICACY

The importance of handwashing and the role of antimicrobial soap for infection control have been reviewed thoroughly for settings outside the home (4,7,93). Although no definitive studies on the use of currently marketed products in the home setting have been reported in the literature, it can be logically inferred from the totality of data that antimicrobial soaps have a role in personal hygiene. Because of the ability to better control experimental conditions, most studies have been conducted in hospitals. Larson (94) reported, "What we know now from natural experiments, epidemiologic studies and experimental models is that clean hands are associated with reduced risk of contact-spread infection in a variety of settings." Based on this hospital evidence, we conclude that antimicrobial soaps also have a potential role in the control of diseases that can be transmitted from routine everyday activities.

The next sections review the standard test for handwashing effectiveness and recent literature supporting the importance of handwashing in reducing the spread of infection.

Experimental Studies: Health Care Personnel Handwash Test (General Use Handwash Test)

A laboratory test method used to evaluate antimicrobial handwash products for health care workers is included in the 1994 version of the TFM (9). This method is known as the Healthcare Personnel Handwash Test. Recently, a modification of this method has been proposed as the General Use Handwash Test. In the modified version for consumer products, the number of washes and log reduction requirements are lower.

The objective of this test is to evaluate the efficacy of an antimicrobial soap product to reduce the level of transient microbial flora (contaminants) on the hands after a single or multiple handwashes. Subjects' hands are contaminated with a predetermined number of marker bacteria, *Serratia marcescens* or *E. coli*.

Antimicrobial activity is determined by comparing the number of bacteria removed from the hands after washing with the antimicrobial product to the number of bacteria removed from unwashed hands.

Washing with antimicrobial soaps or with nonmedicated soaps will remove a significant number of bacteria from the skin because of the surfactancy of the soap base and the mechanical action of the wash procedure. Results from studies conducted with a one-wash procedure have sometimes shown little difference between the antimicrobial containing product and the placebo product. The advantage of the active ingredient deposited on the skin, however, can be demonstrated when a multiple contamination and wash procedure is used. In a study conducted by Bartzokas (92), antimicrobial products containing TCS and chlorhexidine gluconate were compared to a nonmedicated soap product. The effect of the TCS and chlorhexidine product progressively increased with repeated washings despite multiple hand recontaminations.

Studies in Developing Countries and Noninstitutional Settings

Several handwashing studies have been conducted in developing countries with environments that are conducive to the spread of disease. The data generated from these studies are relevant to conditions found in areas of the United States where hygiene is poor, such as border city shanty towns and migrant worker camps (95). They are also relevant to situations in which sanitation is not optimal, as in day care facilities (58) and outdoor festivals (83). For example, the shigellosis outbreak at an outdoor festival in the United States that was caused by inadequate sanitation and poor hygiene practices (83) indicates that unsanitary conditions are not limited to developing countries.

Bryan et al. (7) recently updated a previous literature review (4) on the importance of handwashing in reducing the spread of infection. Thirteen nonexperimental studies and five experimental studies in a variety of environmental settings were identified and reviewed. Four of these, which were conducted in developing countries, are summarized in Table 4. In addition, a number of other studies, summarized in Table 5, have provided an indication of the positive impact of handwashing.

Studies from Day Care, Institutions, and Schools

Black et al. (96) first demonstrated the effectiveness of handwashing to prevent diarrhea in day care centers. After the initiation of a handwashing program in several day care centers, the incidence of diarrhea among children in the study was significantly and consistently lower (approximately half) than the incidence in two control centers over the 35-week study period (Table 6).

Bartlett et al. (97) studied the incidence of diarrheal illness among day care children. They followed 10 randomly selected centers that received staff training and follow-up surveillance in procedures to reduce diarrhea transmission and 11 other centers as controls. Although the children in the 21 centers had higher rates of diarrheal disease than children in home care, the centers in the surveillance group had significantly lower rates than the control centers. In addition, the authors suggested that further attention must be directed to effective promotion of hygienic practices among day care center workers without external monitoring.

It is often difficult to attribute independent specific effectiveness to an intervention and control program because they are inherently multifaceted. For example, Butz et al. (98) evaluated the effectiveness of an intervention program in day care homes that included handwashing

Table 4 Literature from 1986–1993 Reporting Strong Evidence (7) Linking Handwashing and Infection

Investigator	Year	Summary
Stanton and Clemens (123)	1987	In a report of a randomized trial in urban Bangladesh to study the effects of an educational intervention program on hygiene and diarrhea rates, the incidence of diarrhea in the intervention group was 26% lower than in the control group. After intervention, 49% of test families vs 33% of control families washed their hands before food preparation. The improvement in personal hygiene was related to improvement in diarrhea incidence.
Clemens and Stanton (124)	1987	Significantly more diarrhea occurred in those children in urban Bangladesh whose mothers did not wash hands before food preparation.
Leroy and Garenne (125)	1991	Results of a study on risk factors of neonatal tetanus in Senegal concluded that teaching mothers and birth attendants simple hygienic principles and basic techniques may have a significant impact on neonatal tetanus mortality. Risk factors associated with the skill and behavior of the birth attendant and mother were highly significant and were associated with high odds ratio and included whether the hands of the person cutting the cord were washed with soap.
Hlady et al. (126)	1992	Found a significantly lower risk of neonatal tetanus in rural Bangladesh when the person cutting the umbilical cord had washed his or her hands.

education, the use of vinyl gloves, disposable diaper changing pads, and an alcohol-based hand rinse. Symptoms of enteric illness were lower in the intervention homes, but it was not possible to separate out the effects of each component of the intervention. Additional study is needed to identify specific practices, in addition to handwashing, that reduce introduction and transmission of infectious agents in child care groups.

Nahata (99), in reviewing disease transmission in day care centers, wrote: "it has been clearly shown that handwashing can prevent diarrhea and respiratory disease."

Harris et al. (100) studied the person-to-person transmission in an outbreak of enteroinvasive *E. coli* at a school for mentally retarded adults

Table 5 Additional Studies Suggesting the Importance of Handwashing for Personal Hygiene and Infection Control

Investigator	Year	Summary
Kaltenhaler et al. (127)	1991	A study in Zimbabwe demonstrated that washing with soap is more effective for reducing fecal bacterial contamination of the hands than not using soap.
Khan (128)	1982	Handwashing had a positive effect on interrupting shigellosis transmission even in unsanitary environments in rural Bangladesh.
Wilson and Chandler (129)	1993	Determined from their education program, which encouraged handwashing with soap among 57 mothers in Indonesia, that 2 years after the intervention (a) 79% of mothers were still using hand soap, despite the fact that they now had to buy it themselves and (b) the community seemed to be benefiting from a sustained reduction in diarrhea episodes due to improved hygiene practices.
Wilson et al. (130)	1991	Indonesian children experienced an 89% reduction in diarrhea episodes vs the control period, when their mothers were given soap for handwashing and an explanation of the fecal-oral route of diarrhea transmission.
Verweij et al. (131)	1991	Suggested that improving the water supply alone did not correlate with an improvement in infectious disease, but the prevalence of infectious skin disease was negatively correlated with the frequency of washing. It was concluded that personal hygiene appears to play an essential role in keeping the prevalence of infectious disease low.
Pinfold (132)	1990	Found that the rates of diarrhea were seasonal and correlated with levels of cross contamination in the domestic environment.
Lee et al. (83)	1991	An estimated 3175 women attending a 5-day outdoor music festival contracted shigella gastroenteritis. Limited access to soap and running water by the more than 2000 volunteer food preparers was suggested as a contributing factor.

Table 6 Literature Reporting the Effectiveness of Handwashing in Day Care Centers

Investigator	Year	Illness/ Condition	Summary
Black et al. (96)	1984	Diarrhea	Concluded a handwashing program will probably prevent at least some diarrhea in day care centers.
Bartlett et al. (97)	1988	Diarrhea	Further attention must be directed to effective promotion of hygienic practices among day care center workers.
Holaday et al. (65)	1990	Fecal contam- ination	Centers with formal hand-washing procedures had lower recovery rates (fecal coliforms) than those without such practices.
Van et al. (64)	1991	Diarrhea	Fecal contamination might be reduced by emphasizing the importance of hand washing.
Butz et al. (98)	1990	Diarrhea	Handwashing by providers is con- sidered to be the single most impor- tant preventive measure in day care facilities.
Laborde et al. (66)	1993	Diarrhea	Increased attention to handwashing by day care providers and the use of disposable diaper changing pads may reduce the incidence of diarrheal disease. Handwashing and disinfection should continue to be emphasized as primary intervention measures to interrupt infectious cycles in day care centers.
Thompson (133)	1994	Diarrhea	Prevention and control measures include training and education in good personal hygiene, emphasis on the need for frequent hand- washing.
Mohle-Boetani et al. (134)	1995	Shigellosis	Increased handwashing, caring for convalescing children in day care centers as a separate group, and rapid diagnosis and treatment probably all contributed to curtailment of the shigellosis epidemic.

and children in Missouri. Although they emphasized handwashing as an infection control measure, they also stated that control measures to interrupt the transmission of *E. coli* should include the separation of symptomatic or culture-positive students from those who were well.

Summary of the Impact of Handwashing on Disease Transmission from Transient Flora

The recent literature has examined the role of handwashing under a wide variety of conditions. The collective conclusion is that handwashing is a primary infection control measure. Several studies have further demonstrated the effectiveness of antimicrobials in handwashing (7,93,101).

SUMMARY

This review clearly indicates that improved hygiene can help prevent skin infections and interrupt the transmission of infectious disease transferred by the hands. Thus, the regular use of soap for personal cleansing has a recognized role in the prevention of disease. Further, residual antimicrobial activity may help extend this efficacy by mitigating against specific bacterial sources of infection.

Handwashing is repeatedly cited as the most important infection control measure in hospitals. It is no less important in the home. It can be demonstrated that with regular use, antimicrobial soaps reduce the numbers of organisms on the skin to a greater extent than nonmedicated soap. In addition, model systems have demonstrated the control of potentially pathogenic organisms on the skin. Antimicrobial ingredients deposited on the skin, also can be of benefit when washing is inadequate and leaves behind organisms that can cause infection or can be transferred to other skin sites. Thus, soap has a role in personal hygiene for cleaning the skin, and antimicrobial soaps can potentially expand this role and provide consumers with important health benefits.

REFERENCES

1. Department of Health, Education, and Welfare. OTC Topical Antimicrobial Products and Drug and Cosmetic Products, Fed Reg 1974; 39: 33102–33141.
2. Department of Health, Education and Welfare. OTC Topical Antimicrobial Products, 21 CFR Part 333. Fed Reg 1978; 43: 1243–1244.

3. Hall LC, Daniels JI, Aly R, et al. Recommendation of showering frequencies for preventing performance degrading nonsytemic microbial skin infections in military personnel in the field. US Army Med Res Devlp Command 1991; No. 90PP0826.

4. Larson E. A casual link between handwashing and risk of infection? Examination of the evidence. Infect Control Hosp Epidemiol 1988; 9: 28–36.

5. Larson E. Draft guideline for handwashing and hand antisepsis in health care settings. Am J Infect Control 1994; 22: 25A–47A.

6. Larson E. Handwashing and skin: physiologic and bacteriologic aspects. Infect Control 1985; 6: 14–23.

7. Bryan J, Cohran J, Larson E. Handwashing: a ritual revisited. In: Rutala WA, ed. Chemical Germicides in Healthcare International Symposium 1994. Assoc. for Professionals in Infection Control and Epidemiology, Washington, DC: Morin Heights, PQ, Canada: Polyscience Publishers, 1995, pp. 163–178.

8. Nokes KM. Prevention of nosocomial infections through handwashing. Med Ultrasound 1983; 7: 113–115.

9. Department of Health and Human Services. Tentative Final Monograph for Healthcare Antiseptic Drug Products; Proposed Rule 21 CFR Pts. 333 and 339. Vol. 59, No. 116, June 17, 1994, pp. 31402–31452.

10. Marzulli FN, Bruch M. Soaps: Benefits versus risks. In: Maibach HI, Aly R, eds. Skin Microbiology, Relevance to Clinical Infection. New York: Springer-Verlag, 1981; 125–134.

11. Taplin D. Chlorhexidine and clinical infections. In: Maibach H, Aly R eds. Skin Microbiology: Relevance to Clinical Infection. New York: Springer-Verlag, 1981: 113–124.

12. Procter & Gamble. Internal Data, 1995.

13. Dial Corporation. Internal Data, 1995.

14. Roth RR, James WD. Microbiology of the skin: resident flora, ecology, infection 1989; 20: 367–390.

15. Aly R, Maibach HI. Comparative antibacterial efficacy of a 2 minute surgical scrub with chlorhexidine gluconate, povidone iodine, and chloroxylenol sponge-brushes. Am J Infect Control 1988; 16: 173–177.

16. Stern RS, Nelson C. The diminishing role of the dermatologist in the office-based care of cutaneous diseases. J Am Acad Dermatol 1993; 29: 774–777.

17. Ben-Amitai D, Ashkenazi S. Common bacterial skin infections in childhood. Pediatr Ann 1993; 22: 225–233.

18. Schachner L, Simons Ling N, Press S. A statistical analysis of a pediatric dermatology clinic. Pediatr Dermatol 1983; 1: 157–164.

19. National Disease and Therapeutic Index. Plymouth Meeting, PA: IMS America, Ltd. 1995.

20. Taplin DL, Lansdell AM, Allen R, et al. Prevalence of streptococcal pyoderma in relation to climate and hygiene. Lancet 1973; I: 501–503.

21. Allen AM, Taplin D. Skin infections in eastern Panama. Survey of two representative communities. Am J Public Health 1974; 23: 950–956.

22. Talpin D. Fungous and bacterial skin infections in the tropics. US Army Research and Development Command 1978; DADA-17-17-C-1084.
23. Quinn B, Baker R, Pratt J. Hurricane Andrew and a pediatric emergency department. Ann Emerg Med 1994; 23: 737–741.
24. Aly R, Maibach HI. Skin Infections—fungal and bacterial. Diseases, Diagnoses, Therapy, Sommerville, NJ: Hoechst Roussel Pharmaceutical, 1987.
25. Beauregard S, Gilchrest GA. A survey of skin problems and skin care regimens in the elderly. Arch Dermatol 1987; 12: 1638–1643.
26. Sampson HA. Atopic dermatitis. Ann Allergy 1992; 69: 469–483.
27. Lacour M, Hauser C. The role of microorganisms in atopic dermatitis. Crit Rev Allergy 1993; 11: 491–522.
28. Williams REA, Mackie RM. The staphylococci: importance of their control in the management of skin disease. Dermatolo Ther 1993; 11: 201–206.
29. Noble WC, Staphylococci on the skin. In: Noble WC ed. The Skin Microflora and Microbial Skin Disease. Cambridge, UK: Cambridge University Press, 1993: 135–152.
30. Kay CR. Sepsis in the home. Br Med J 1962; 1: 1048–1052.
31. Dillion HC. Impetigo contagiosa: supparative and non-supparative complications. I. Clinical, bacteriologic and epidemiologic characteristics of impetigo. Am J Dis Child 1968; 115: 530–541.
32. Ferrieri PA, Jajani S, Wannamaker LW, Chapman SS. Natural history of impetigo. 1. Site sequence of acquisition and familial patterns of spread of cutaneous streptococci. J Clin Invest 1972; 51: 2851–2862.
33. Zimakoff J, Thamdrup V, Petersen W, Scheibel J. Recurrent staphylococcal furunculosis in families. Scand J Infect Dis 1988; 20: 403–405.
34. Elsner P, Maibach HI. Microbiology of specialized skin: the vulva. Seminars Dermatol 1990; 9: 300–304.
35. Sevier TL. Infectious disease in athletes. Sports Med 1994; 78: 389–412.
36. Price PB. The bacteriology of normal skin: a new quantitative test applied to a study of the bacterial flora and the disinfection action of mechanical cleansing. J Infect Dis 1938; 63: 301–318.
37. Cade AR. A method for testing degerming efficacy of hexachlorophene soaps. J Soc Cosmet Chem 1951; 2: 281–291.
38. Williamson P, Kligman AM. A new method for the quantitative investigation of cutaneous bacteria. J Invest Dermatol 1965; 45: 498–503.
39. Finkey MB, Corbin NC, Aust LB, et al. In vivo effect of antimicrobial soap bars containing 1.5% and 0.8% trichlorocarbanilide against two strains of pathogenic bacteria. J Soc Cos Chem 1984; 35: 351–355.
40. Scala DD, Fishler GE, Morrison BM et al. Evaluation of antibacterial bar soaps containing triclocarban. Abstract of the Annual Meeting of the American Academy of Dermatology, New Orleans, LA, 1994.
41. Leyden JJ, Stewart R, Kligman AM. Updated in-vivo methods for evaluating topical antimicrobial agents on human skin. J Invest Dermatol 1979; 72: 165–170.
42. Leyden JJ, McGinley KJ, Holzle E, et al. The microbiology of the human axilla and its relationship to axillary odor. J Invest Dermatol 1981; 77: 413–416.

43. Yackovich F, Heinze JE. Evaluation of substantivity and antibacterial activity of soap bars on human skin by an in-vivo agar patch method. J Soc Cosmet Chem 1985; 36: 231–236.
44. Yackovich F, Wagner CA, Heinze JE. Validation of the agar patch test with an antibacterial liquid soap and comparison with the finger imprint method. J Soc Cosmet Chem 1989; 40: 265–271.
45. Yackovich F, Poulsen NK, Heinze JE. Validation of the agar patch test using soap bars which deposit different amounts of triclocarban. J Soc Cosmet Chem 1986; 37: 99–104.
46. Marples RR. Antibacterial cosmetics and the microflora of human skin. Devel Industrial Microbiology 1971; 12: 178–187.
47. Rayan GM, Flournoy DJ. Microbiologic flora of human fingernails. J Hand Surg 1987; 12A: 605–607.
48. Peterson AF. Microbiology of the hands: factors affecting the population. In Developments in Industrial Microbiology Volume 26, Proceedings of the 41st General; Meeting of the Soc. for Industrial Microbiology August, 1984. Society for Industrial Microbiology, Washington, D.C. 1985; 503–507.
49. Scott E, Bloomfield SF, Barlow CG. An investigation of microbial contamination in the home. J Hyg (Camb.) 1982; 89: 279–293.
50. Finch JE, Prince J, Hawksworth M. A bacteriological survey of the domestic environment. J Appl Bacteriol 1978; 45: 357–364.
51. Mendes MF, Lynch DJ. A bacteriological survey of washrooms and toilets. J Hyg (Camb.) 1976; 76: 183–190.
52. Bloomfield SF. A review: the use of disinfectants in the home. J Appl Bacteriol 1978; 45: 1–38.
53. Roach M. How to win at germ warfare. Health 1994; 26: 77–80.
54. Marples RR, Towers AG. A laboratory model for the investigation of contact transfer of microorganisms. J Hyg (Lond) 1979; 82: 237–248.
55. Mackintosh CA, Hoffman PN. An extended model for transfer of micro-organisms via the hands: differences between organisms and the effect of alcohol disinfection. J Hyg (Lond) 1984; 92: 345–355.
56. Borneff J, Wittig JR, Borneff M, Hartmetz G. Untersuchungen uber das vorkommen von Enteritis—Erreggen in Haushalt—eine Pilotstudie. Zbl Bakteriol Microbiol Hyg-B 1985; 180: 319–334.
57. Goodman RA, Osterholm MT, Granoff DM, Pickering LK. Infectious diseases and child care. Pediatrics 1984; 74: 134–139.
58. Pickering LK, Bartlett AV, Woodward WE. Acute infectious diarrhea among children in day care. Epidemiol Control Rev Infect Dis 1986; 8: 539–547.
59. Morrow AL, Townsend IT, Pickering LK. Risk of enteric infection associated with child day care. Pediatr Ann 1991; 20: 427–433.
60. Chorba TL, Meriwether RA, Jenkins BR et al. Control of a non-foodborne outbreak of salmonellosis: day care isolation. Am J Public Health 1987; 77: 979–981.

61. Fornasini M, Reeves RR, Murray BE, Pickering LK. Trimethoprim-resistant *Escherichia coli* in households of children attending day care centers. J Infect Dis 1992; 166: 326–330.
62. Osterholm MT, Reeves RR, Murph JR, Pickering LK. Infectious diseases and child day care. Pediatr Infect Dis J 1992; 11: 531–541.
63. Ekanem E, Dupont HL, Pickering LK, et al. Transmission dynamics of enteric bacteria in day care centers. Am J Epidemiol 1983; 118: 562–572.
64. Van R, Morrow AL, Reves RR, Pickering LK. Environmental contamination in child day-care centers. Am J Epidemiol 1991; 133: 460–470.
65. Holaday B, Pantell R, Lewis C, Gillis CL. Patterns of fecal coliform contamination in day-care centers. Publ Health Nurs 1990; 7: 224–228.
66. Laborde DJ, Weigle KA, Weber DJ, Kotch JB. Effect of fecal contamination on diarrheal illness rates in day-care centers. Am J Epidemiol 1993; 138: 243–255.
67. Adis DG, Sacks JJ, Kresnow M, et al. The compliance of licensed US child care centers with National Health and Safety Standards. Am J Public Health 1994; 84: 1161–1163.
68. Simmons B, Trusler M, Roccaforte J, et al. Infection control for home health. Infect Control Hosp Epidemiol 1990; 11: 362–370.
69. Fekety R, Kim KH, Brown D, et al. Epidemiology of antibiotic-associated colitis. Isolation of *Clostridium difficile* from the hospital environment. Am J Med 1981; 70: 906–908.
70. Sanderson PJ, Weissler S. Recovery of coliforms from the hands of nurses and patients: activities leading to contamination. J Hosp Infect 1992; 21: 85–93.
71. Nishijima S, Namura S, Kawa S, et al. *Staphylococcus aureus* on hand surface and nasal carriage in patients with atopic dermatitis. J Am Acad Dermatol 1995; 32: 677–679.
72. Roth K, Land GK. How to prevent infection in a home care patient. RN 1987: 50: 61–70.
73. Ahmed NI, Abbas S, Shaaban E. Family care of elderly problems. J Egypt Public Health Service 1993; 68: 161–177.
74. Smith PW. Infection Control in Long Term Care Facilities. New York: John Wiley & Sons, 1984.
75. Bryan FL. Risks practices, procedures and processes that lead to outbreaks of foodborne diseases. J Food Protection 1988; 51: 663–673.
76. Reed GH. Foodborne illness (Part 1) Staphylococcal ("Staph") food poisoning. Dairy Food and Environmental Sanitation 1993; 13: 642.
77. Humphrey TJ, Martin KW, Whitehead A. Contamination of hands and work surfaces with *Salmonella enteriditis* PT4 during the preparation of egg dishes. Epidemiol Infect 1994; 113: 403–409.
78. Pether JVS, Gilbert RJ. The survival of salmonella on fingertips and transfer of the organisms to foods. J Hyg (Lond) 1971; 69: 673–681.
79. Reed GH. Foodborne illness (Part 2). Salmonellosis. Dairy Food and Environmental Sanitation 1993; 13: 706.
80. Yen PK. Playing it safe with food. Geriatr Nurs 1993; 14: 221–222.

81. DeWit JCD, Roumbouts FM. Faecal microorganisms on the hands of carriers: *Escherichia coli* as a model for salmonella. Zbl Hyg 1992; 193: 230–236.

82. Gilman RH, Marquis GS, Ventura G, et al. Water cost and availability: key determinants of family hygiene in a Peruvian shantytown. Am J Public Health 1993; 83: 1554–1558.

83. Lee LA, Ostroff SM, McGee HB, et al. An outbreak of shigellosis at an outdoor music festival. Am J Epidemiol 1991; 133: 608–615.

84. Foulke J. How to outsmart dangerous *E. coli* strain. FDA Consumer 1994; 28: 7–11.

85. Mayo Clinic Health Letter. Handwashing 1993; 11(6): 4.

86. McGinley KJ, Larson ET, Leyden JJ. Composition and density of microflora in the subungual space of the hand. J Clin Microbiol 1988; 26: 950–953.

87. Ayliffe GAJ. The effect of antibacterial agents on the flora of skin. J Hosp Infect 1980; 1: 111–124.

88. Ehrenkranz NJ. Bland soap handwash or hand antisepsis? The pressing need for clarity. Infect Control Hosp Epidemiol 1992; 13: 299–301.

89. Ehrenkranz NJ, Alfonso BC. Failure of bland soap handwash to prevent hand transfer of patient bacteria to urethral catheters. Infect Control Hosp Epidemiol 1991; 12: 654–662.

90. Huttly SRA, Lanata CF, Gonzales H, et al. Observations on handwashing and defecation practices in a shanty town of Lima, Peru. J Diarrhoeal Dis Res 1994; 12: 14–18.

91. Aulia H, Surapaty S, Bahar E, et al. Personal and domestic hygiene and its relationships to the incidence of diarrhoea in South Sumetera. J Diarrhoeal Res 1994; 12: 42–48.

92. Bartzokas CA, Corkill JE, Makin T. Evaluation of the skin disinfecting activity and cumulative effect of chlorhexidine and triclosan handwash preparations on hands artificially contaminated with serratia marcescens. Infect Control 1987; 8: 163–168.

93. Doebbeling BD, Stanley GL, Sheetz CT, et al. Comparative efficacy of alternative hand-washing agents in reducing nosocomial infections in intensive care units. N Engl J Med 1992; 327: 88–93.

94. Larson E. Guideline for use of topical antimicrobial agents. Am J Infect Control 1988; 16: 253–263.

95. Mintz ED, Reiff FM, Tauxe RV. Safe water treatment and storage in the home. J Am Med Ass 1995; 273: 948–953.

96. Black RE, Dykes AC, Andersen KE. Handwashing to prevent diarrhea in day care centers. Am J Epidemiol 1981; 113: 445–451.

97. Bartlett AV, Jarvis BA, Ross VK, et al. Diarrheal illness among infants and toddlers in day care centers: effects of active surveillance and staff training without subsequent monitoring. Am J Epidemiol 1988; 127: 808–817.

98. Butz AME, Larson E, Fosarelli P, Yolken P. Occurrence of infectious symptoms in children in day care homes. Am J Infect Control 1990; 6: 347–353.

99. Nahata MC. Handwashing prevents infection. Drug Intell Clin Pharm 1985; 19: 738.

100. Harris JR, Mariano J, Wells JG, et al. Person-to-person transmission in an outbreak of enteroinvasive *Escherichia coli*. Am J Epidemiol 1985; 122: 245–252.
101. Zafar AB, Butler RC, Reese DJ, et al. Use of 0.3% triclosan (Bacti-Stat) to eradicate an outbreak of methicillin-resistant *Staphylococcus aureus* in a neonatal nursery. Am J Infect Control 1995; 23: 200–208.
102. Bannan EA, Jones DV, Kooistra JA. Degerming the hands of children. Cutis 1969; 5: 704–706.
103. Paulson DS. A comparative evaluation of different hand cleansers. Dairy, Food and Environmental Sanitization 1994; 14: 524–528.
104. Ansari S, Sattar S, Springthorpe V, et al. In vivo protocol for testing efficacy of hand-washing agents against viruses and bacteria: experiments with rotavirus and *Escherichia coli*. Applied and Environmental Microbiology 1989; 55: 3113–3118.
105. Rotter ML, Killer W, Wewalka G, et al. Evaluation of procedures for hygienic hand-disinfection: controlled parallel experiments on the Vienna test model J Hyg (Camb.) 1986; 96: 27–37.
106. Rotter ML, Koller W. Test models for hygienic handrub and hygienic hand-wash: the effects of two different contamination and sampling techniques. J Hosp Infect 1992; 20: 163–171.
107. Leyden JJ, McGinley KJ, Kaminer MS, et al. Computerized image analysis of full-hand touch plates: a method for quantification of surface bacteria on hands and the effect of antimicrobial agents. J Hosp Infect 1991; 18: 13–22.
108. Bannan EA. Surgical scrub degerming: the effect of personal bar soaps. Ohio State Med J 1967; 63: 1322–1324.
109. Wilson PE. A comparison of methods for assessing the value of antibacterial soaps. J Appl Bacteriol 1970; 33: 574–581.
110. Voss JG. Effects of an antibacterial soap on the ecology of aerobic bacterial flora of human skin. Appl Microbiol 1975; 3: 551–556.
111. Aly R, Maibach H. Effect of antimicrobial soap containing chlorhexidine on the microbial flora of skin. Appl Environ Microbiol 1976; 31: 931–935.
112. Aihara M, Sakai M, Iwasaki M, et al. Prevention and control of nosocomial infection caused by methicillin-resistant *Staphylococcus aureus* in a premature infant ward—preventive effect of a povidone iodine wipe of neonatal skin. Postgrad Med 1993; 69: S117–S121.
113. Hedin G, Hambraeus A. Daily scrub with chlorhexidine reduces skin colonization by antibiotic-resistant *Staphylococcus epidermidis*. J Hosp Infect 1993; 24: 47–61.
114. Kooistra JA. Prophylaxis and control of erythrasma of the toe webs. J Invest Dermatol 1965; 48: 399–400.
115. Dubow E, Winter L. Effect of an antibacterial soap in the management of scratches, cuts and abrasions. Curr Ther Res 1967; 9: 631–633.

116. Leonard RR. Prevention of superficial cutaneous infections. Arch Dermatol 1967; 95: 520–523.
117. Dodge BG, Knowles WR, McBride MW, et al. Treatment of erythrasma with an antibacterial soap. Arch Dermatol 1968; 97: 548–552.
118. Duncan WC, Dodge G, Knox JM. Prevention of superficial pyogenic skin infections. Arch Dermatol 1969; 99: 465–468.
119. Taber D, Ward AB, Yackovich F. Use of an antimicrobial soap in the treatment of erythrasma of the toe webs. Cutis 1969; 5: 991–993.
120. Wheatley ML, Oden GB, de la Bretonne GA, Kooistra JA. Antibacterial soap bar usage for the prevention of superficial pyogenic infections. P&G Internal Report, 1969.
121. Mackenzie AR. Effectiveness of antibacterial soaps in a healthy population. JAMA 1970; 211: 973–976.
122. Sharrett AR, Finklea JF, Potter EV, et al. The control of streptococcal skin infections in South Trinidad. Am J Epidemiol 1973; 99: 408–413.
123. Stanton BF, Clemens JD. An educational intervention for altering water-sanitation behaviors to reduce childhood diarrhea in urban Bangladesh II. A randomized trial to assess the impact of intervention on hygienic behaviors and rates of diarrhea. Am J Epidemiol 1987; 125: 292–301.
124. Clemens JD, Stanton BF. An educational intervention for altering water-sanitation behaviors to reduce childhood diarrhea in urban Bangladesh I. Application of the case control method for development of an intervention. Am J Epidemiol 1987; 125: 284–291.
125. Leroy O, Garenne M. Risk factors of neonatal tetanus in Senegal. Int J Epidemiol 1991; 20: 521–526.
126. Hlady W, Bennett JV, Samadi A, et al. Neonatal tetanus in rural Bangladesh: risk factors and toxoid efficacy. Am J Public Health 1992; 82: 1365–1369.
127. Kaltenhaler E, Waterman R, Cross P. Faecal indicator bacteria on the hands and the effectiveness of handwashing in Zimbabwe. J Trop Med Hyg 1991; 94: 358–363.
128. Khan MU. Interruption of shigellosis by handwashing. Trans R Soc Trop Med Hyg 1982; 76: 164–168.
129. Wilson JM, Chandler GN. Sustained improvements in hygiene behavior amongst village women in Lombok, Indonesia. Trans R Soc Trop Med Hyg 1993; 87: 615–616.
130. Wilson JM, Chandler GN, Mushlihatun, Samiluddin. Handwashing reduces diarrhea episodes study in Lombok, Indonesia. Trans R Soc Trop Med Hyg 1991; 85: 819–821.
131. Verweij PE, van Egmond M, Bac DJ, et al. Hygiene, skin infections and types of water supply in Venda South Africa. Trans R Soc Trop Med Hyg 1991; 85: 681–685.
132. Pinfold JV. Faecal contamination of water and fingertip rinses as a method for evaluating the effect of low-cost water supply and sanitation activities on faeco-oral disease transmission. II. Hygiene intervention study in rural northeast Thailand. Epidemiol Infect 1990; 105: 377–389.

133. Thompson SC. Infectious diarrhoea in children: controlling transmission in the child care setting. J Paediatr Child Health 1994; 30: 210–219.

134. Mohle-Boetani JC, Stapelton M, Finger R, et al. Community-wide shigellosis: control of an outbreak and risk factors of child day-care centers. Am J Public Health 1995; 85: 812–816.

7

Do Antiseptic Agents Reduce Surgical Wound Infections? Preoperative Bathing, Operative Site Preparation, Surgical Hand Scrub

Edna K. Kretzer
Johns Hopkins Bayview Medical Center, Baltimore, Maryland

Elaine L. Larson
Georgetown University School of Nursing, Washington, D.C.

INTRODUCTION

Skin antisepsis practices are based on sound theoretical principles of infection prevention, but are also fraught with ritual. A review of the biomedical literature through February 1994 was conducted to examine evidence of a causal association between risk of infection and three aspects of preoperative skin preparation: preoperative whole body patient bathing, preoperative patient skin preparation of the operative site, and the hand scrub of the surgical team. This chapter summarizes and evaluates the research relating preoperative skin preparation practices with infection rates.

By permission, adapted from The Association for Professionals in Infection Control and Epidemiology, Inc.: Edna K. Kretzer and Elaine L. Larson, *Chemical Germicides in Health Care*, 1995, pp. 149–161.

METHODS

The full computerized Medline System database was searched using the following terms: nosocomial, cross infections, skin, antiinfective agents, bacterial infections (prevention and control of), and infection control. Articles were limited to those in English only, with human subjects, and covered the years 1960 to February, 1994. Those articles available through the National Library of Medicine, Bethesda, Maryland, were incorporated into this literature review.

RESULTS

Preoperative Whole Body Patient Bathing

Thirteen articles were found in which the effect of preoperative patient bathing regimens on surgical wound infection rates or levels of bacterial colonization was evaluated (Table 1).

Several blinded, randomized trials were reported. In one (10), two groups of patients received three preoperative showers with either a 4% chlorhexidine detergent solution ($n = 57$) or a placebo soap ($n = 58$). The chlorhexidine group had a 20-fold reduction in skin flora as compared to no change in skin flora in the placebo group ($p < 0.01$). There was a 5-day median time to recolonization in the chlorhexidine group and a 2-day median time in the placebo group. The sample size was too small to allow a meaningful comparison of infection rates.

In a second trial (19) of 575 surgical patients, chlorhexidine, povidone-iodine and medicated soap were compared. Two preoperative showers using four applications of chlorhexidine were significantly more effective in reducing levels of bacterial colonization than showering with either of the other treatments in like manner. Postshower cultures from patients using chlorhexidine yielded no growth on 43% of the surgical sites preoperatively as compared to 16% with the povidone-iodine group and 6% in the soap group ($p < 0.001$).

In a prospective, randomized observer-blinded study of 39 patients, chlorhexidine, povidone-iodine and lotion soap were evaluated in one-stage (evening only) versus two-stage (both evening and morning) showers (26). Chlorhexidine was associated with a significant reduction in staphylococcal colonization, while the results obtained from povidone-iodine were inconsistent. Showering with soap actually increased staphylococcal colony counts. Repeated applications of chlorhexidine were superior to a single application.

Table 1 Studies of Effects of Preoperative Patient Bathing and Skin Preparation on Colonization and Infection Rates

Author/Year	Prep type Bath/Scrub	Agents[a] A/I/C/O	Outcome:[b] Col/Inf	Results
Brandberg (1981)	Bath	C	Inf	Significant decrease in inf in C Group
Ayliffe (1983)	Bath	C	Inf	No significant differences
Rotter (1988)	Bath	C	Inf	No significant differences
Hayek (1988)	Bath	C	Inf	Significant decrease in inf
Leclair (1988)	Bath	C, I	Col	Decrease with C
Kaiser (1988)	Bath	C, I	Col	Greater decrease with C— Repeated applications superior
Garibaldi (1988)	Bath	C, I, O	Col	Greater decrease with C
Mannion (1989)	Bath	C, I	Col	Decrease with C
Earnshaw (1989)	Bath	C	Inf	No significant differences between C and plain soap
Byrne (1990)	Bath	C	Col	Significant decrease with 2 showers
Byrne (1991)	Bath	C	Col	20-fold decrease in skin colonization
Lynch (1992)	Bath	C	Col/Inf	Col significantly reduced; no difference in inf
Ichida (1993)	Bath	C	Col/Inf	Lower, but no significant differences in col or inf in C Group

[a] A = alcohol, I = povidone-iodine or iodophor, C = chlorhexidine, O = other
[b] Col = bacterial colonization, Inf = infection rates

Mannion et al. (37) studied the bacterial flora of 12 cardiac patients preparing for aortic grafts and 3 patients undergoing abdominal herniorrhaphies. The patients undergoing vascular grafts were divided into group A, who received 2% aqueous povidone-iodine soaks to the groin at least one hour before surgery, and group B, who received two baths with a 4% chlorhexidine gluconate product, one the day before and one the morning of surgery. The three patients undergoing repair of abdominal hernias served as controls. All groups received the same preoperative skin site preparation. Groups A and B also received antibiotic prophylaxis. A total of 1106 isolates (892 staphylococci) were obtained from the 15 patients studied. Bacterial counts from all patients were 20-fold higher from perianal swabs than from groin swabs and increased with hospital stay, except in group B. Perianal bacterial counts from patients in group B 1 week and 2 weeks postsurgically were lower than on admission. No statistical analyses were reported, probably because of the small number of patients studied.

Byrne et al. (9) evaluated chlorhexidine showering or bathing in 10 volunteers. A significant reduction (p <0.005) in skin flora was evident after two preoperative showers with 4% chlorhexidine. The authors recommended three showers using 4% chlorhexidine for optimum antiseptic activity.

Leclair et al. (29) randomized 151 patients undergoing neurosurgery into four groups to compare the efficacy of shampoo and/or site preparations using chlorhexidine in groups A and B and iodophor in groups C and D. All groups received surgical site preparation with their respective antiseptics while groups A and C also received shampoos with chlorhexidine or iodophor, respectively. Patients receiving both the chlorhexidine shampoo and site preparation had significantly fewer positive scalp cultures at the end of surgery. There were no reported postoperative infections from any group.

Hayek and Emerson (23) studied 2015 patients assigned to one of three preoperative bathing regimens, each taking two showers: (a) chlorhexidine (n = 689), (b) placebo (n = 700), and (c) plain soap (n = 626). Infection rates were chlorhexidine, 9%; placebo, 11.7%; and plain soap, 12.9% (p <0.05). The initial placebo product was found to have some antibacterial effect, which might have explained the lower infection rate with placebo rather than soap.

Two randomized groups of patients undergoing prosthetic vascular grafts (16) received two baths: one group used chlorhexidine (n = 31) and the other group used a nonmedicated soap (n = 35). All patients received chlorhexidine for skin site preparation just before surgery. Wound infection rate in the chlorhexidine group was 26%, as compared to 11% in the soap group (p = 0.12). The small sample size in the study increased the risk of a type II error.

A randomized, double-blind, placebo-controlled study of 3482 general surgery patients (34) was conducted to measure the efficacy of whole body disinfection with chlorhexidine as compared with plain soap. After three showers, the patients using chlorhexidine had significantly reduced skin colony counts when compared with those showering with the detergent. Wound infection rates were similar in both groups (5.79% and 5.75%, respectively), and no economic benefit was obtained from using the chlorhexidine suppression of skin flora.

Ichida et al. (24) compared routine bathing of 71 burn patients (historical control group) to a total body chlorhexidine bath for 84 patients. The chlorhexidine group had overall lower colonization counts, rate of infection was 55% higher, and median length of hospital stay was longer for the historical control group. However, no differences were statistically significant. A larger sample size would have been needed to increase the statistical power to 80%.

A nonrandomized, prospective study was conducted in Sweden (8) to examine the effects of whole body bathing with chlorhexidine on wound infection rates. Half of the patients (n = 171) received the standard preoperative site preparation and the others (n = 170), in addition to the standard preparation, took three to eight showers with chlorhexidine. In the standard group, 17.5% of patients developed wound infections as compared to 8% of patients in the shower-bath group (p <0.05).

Rotter et al. (46) compared two groups of patients in a prospective, randomized, double-blind, placebo-controlled whole body bathing study. In one group, 1413 patients bathed twice using a chlorhexidine detergent, and the other group of 1400 patients used a nonchlorhexidine detergent. There was no significant difference in infection rates between the groups (2.6% and 2.4%, respectively).

In a similar study, chlorhexidine preoperative bathing was compared with nonmedicated soap bathing (4) in 5536 patients. The majority of patients (92.6%) had one bath, while 7.4% had either two or three baths. There was no significant difference (p = 44) in infection rates among those patients using chlorhexidine (48.8%) as compared with those patients using the nonmedicated soap (51.2%).

Preoperative Patient Skin Preparation

Most of the studies assessing preoperative patient skin preparation have compared the effects of various products on bacterial colonization rates (Table 2). Agents used in the past have included mercury-containing and quaternary ammonium compounds, iodine, and hexachlorophene. For various reasons, including low bactericidal activity, narrow spectrum of activity, or toxic side effects, these agents are rarely used today. Primary alternatives currently include alcohols, chlorhexidine gluconate, and

Table 2 Studies of Preoperative Patient Skin Preparation and Infection Rates

Author/Year	Prep type Bath/Scrub	Agents[a] A/I/C/O	Outcome[b] Col/Inf	Results
Levy (1988)	Scrub	I	Col	Higher levels of contamination of IV catheters and glove tips without iodophor-impregnated film
Geelhoed (1983)	Scrub	A, I	Col	1-min A significantly better than 5 min I
Alexander (1985)	Scrub	A, I	Col, Inf	No significant difference in bacterial counts.
Johnston (1987)	Scrub	A, I, C	Col	A with iodophor drape had lowest bacterial count up to 3 hr after application
Dzubow (1988)	Scrub	A, I, C	Col	No significant differences in 10-sec A wipe and 60 sec application of A, I or C tincture immediately after application. Lower counts maintained after 1 hr with I and C
Payne (1989)	Scrub	I	Inf	Iodophor paint applied 12 hours before surgery associated with significant reduction in amputation site infections
Gilliam (1990)	Scrub	I	Col	Iodophor scrub plus tincture comparable to iodophor tincture alone
Longombe (1991)	Scrub	A	Inf	No infectious complication in 1027 injections and spinal taps or 127 surgical procedures
Robson (1992)	Scrub	I	Inf	No significant difference in infection rates with two or one step regimen of iodophor scrub and paint.

[a]A = alcohol, I = povidone-iodine or iodophor, C = chlorhexidine, O = other
[b]Col = bacterial colonization, Inf = infection rates

iodophors. These agents have been studied using a variety of protocols (35). This section contains a review of recent studies of these products for preparation of patient skin before surgery.

Geelhoed et al. (20) randomly assigned 178 thoracic and general surgery patients to receive one of three skin preparations: a traditional 5-minute scrub with iodophor soap followed by painting and cloth draping; the same 5-minute scrub followed by alcohol cleansing and application of an antimicrobial drape; a 1-minute alcohol cleansing followed by application of the antimicrobial drape. While all three protocols resulted in a significant reduction of skin flora, the 1-minute alcohol cleansing was associated with a significantly better reduction than the 5-minute iodophor scrub.

Thirty subjects undergoing total joint surgery had a traditional 5-minute iodophor scrub followed by application of iodophor paint. The skin of 30 comparison subjects was painted with an iodophor tincture solution. Both protocols were comparably effective in reducing bacterial counts at the operative site (21).

Similarly, three skin preparation methods were compared on the faces of 14 volunteers: a 10-second alcohol wipe, and 60-second applications of either alcohol, povidone-iodine, or tincture of chlorhexidine. There were no significant differences in reductions in bacterial counts between these four groups 5 minutes after application. One hour after application, the povidone-iodine and chlorhexidine-treated sites maintained lower bacterial counts than the alcohol sites. None of the products had much impact on anaerobic flora (15).

One British group simultaneously tested five different preoperative protocols in 15 volunteers: 3-minute paint with chlorhexidine in alcohol; 3-minute paint with povidone-iodine in alcohol; 1-minute paint with 70% isopropyl alcohol followed by application of a plastic adhesive drape; 1-minute paint with alcohol followed by application of a plastic adhesive drape containing slow-release iodophor; and a control. At all time periods tested (5, 30, 60, 180 minutes), the site prepared with the alcohol and iodophor drape had the lowest bacterial counts (25).

Levy et al. (30) also studied the effect of an iodophor-impregnated adhesive drape on the contamination of intravascular catheters and the glove tips of anesthesiologists. Among the 30 patients for whom iodophor alone was used, 83% of glove tips and 13% of catheters were contaminated; none were contaminated in the group prepared with the impregnated film. Kutarski and Grundy (27) concluded that there were no significant differences in bacterial reductions up to 2 hours after application of povidone-iodine whether the antiseptic was wiped off after 30 seconds or allowed to dry.

Evidence is clear that preoperative shaving of the surgical site, particularly the day before surgery, increases the risk of wound infection by creating nicks that are more readily colonized. Depilatories or, if necessary, clipping or shaving of the site in the operating room immediately before surgery are safer alternatives (2,11,12,22,43,47).

With the exception of shaving, little work has been done to assess the impact of other aspects of preoperative patient skin preparation on surgical wound infection rates. Such studies present difficult logistical and practical problems and would require large sample sizes at prohibitive costs. A few relevant studies are reviewed below.

One group (1) conducted three randomized clinical trials including 1324 patients to compare two skin preparation protocols: a 1-minute scrub with 70% alcohol and application of an iodophor-impregnated drape or a 1-minute scrub with 2% iodine in 90% alcohol followed by application of the drape. The investigators found that when drapes were lifted from the operative site during surgery, there was a significant increase in infection rates. Consistent with other studies, the infection rate was higher when hair was shaved and in clean-contaminated or contaminated cases. There were no infections in the 133 patients whose operations were shorter than 2 hours. However, there were no significant differences in bacterial counts at the site or in infection rates among patients receiving the alcohol or the iodophor preparation. In this study, the use of the drape rather than the antiseptic was a more important factor with regard to risk of wound infection.

Several investigators in Kenya tested the use of alcohol as an application to surgeons' hands before donning gloves and in a 2% iodine tincture for cleaning injection and operative sites. They reported no infectious complications associated with 1027 injections and spinal taps and 127 surgical procedures, primarily herniorrhaphies and laparotomies. They suggested that alcohol, which is extremely inexpensive and readily available in developing countries, can be safely used for preoperative skin preparation (31).

In a group of 19 patients, Payne et al. (39) applied povidone-iodine paint 12 hours before amputation and covered the extremity with a sterile towel. These patients had significantly lower infection rates and shorter hospital stays than a comparison group of patients who received the same paint preparation just before surgery. However, nursing time to do the preparation was greatly increased, and the investigators had difficulty with accrual to the study protocol because of a nursing shortage.

Two Canadian investigators compared a two-step regimen with povidone-iodine scrub followed by povidone-iodine paint to a one-step paint alone. In 752 clean and clean-contaminated cases, there were no significant differences in surgical wound infection rates among those randomly assigned to either treatment group (45).

Two studies comparing products used for cleansing of intravascular catheter sites also have examined infection rates. In one study, 150 patients receiving brachial vein cutdowns were randomly assigned to daily site care with one of three products: 70% ethyl alcohol, 1% chlorhexidine cream, or 5% iodophor cream. The chlorhexidine group had more infectious complications and significantly higher incidence of positive catheter tip cultures (13). However this was associated with daily application rather than initial site preparation and therefore has limited relevance to preoperative patient skin preparation.

In a prospective randomized trial, Maki et al. (36) compared local site infection and bacteremia rates associated with central line site preparation using either povidone-iodine, alcohol, or chlorhexidine gluconate. They reported a significantly lower rate of local infection and bacteremia in the aqueous chlorhexidine group. However, confounding variables may have had an impact on the results (50). Additionally, aqueous chlorhexidine is not available in the United States.

Surgical Hand Scrub

The rationale for surgical hand scrub is to afford maximum reduction in total microbial populations on the hands of the surgical team member to minimize the possibility of patient wound contamination. To that end, a variety of techniques and products have been tested for their relative efficacy in reducing skin colonization. Elaborate efforts to reduce the quantity of skin flora on surgeons' hands were of paramount importance before the onset of universal use of gloves by surgical personnel. The wearing of sterile gloves has reduced by many fold the exchange of microorganisms between patient and surgical staff. However, the presence of undetected pinholes and leaks that occur during glove wearing has served as the rationale for a continued requirement for the preparation of the surgical team's hands with a lengthy application of an antimicrobial agent. The Association of Operating Room Nurses, for example, publishes prescriptive standards for the surgical hand scrub (3).

Studies of surgical hand antisepsis are limited primarily to evaluations of bacterial colonization. Examples of such studies, in chronological order, that compare products or variations in technique are found in the

reference list (5,6,17,28,32,38,42,48) and (14,33,40,41,44,49), respectively
(Table 3). Murie and Macpherson (38) reported no significant differences in infection rates when chlorhexidine was used in a detergent or a
methanol base, although their sample size was insufficient for adequate
statistical power.

DISCUSSION

Preoperative Patient Bathing

Preparation of patients' skin before surgery has been a common practice
since the late nineteenth century. It has two purposes: physical cleansing
and removal of dirt, microorganisms, and residue; and antisepsis to minimize the total microbial load. Protocols for preoperative patient skin preparation are based on our understanding of the physiology of the skin and
on the fact that the majority of surgical wound infections are associated
with skin flora, often that of the patient. Hence, it is reasonable to expect
that minimizing numbers of microorganisms on the skin immediately

Table 3 Studies of Skin Preparation of Hands of Surgical Team

Author/Year	Agents[a] A/I/C/O	Outcome[b] Col/Inf	Results
Peterson (1978)	I, C, O	Col	Initial reductions: C > I > O (Hexachlorophene). Significant regrowth under gloves with I, but not with C or hexachlorophene
Eitzen (1979)	I, O	Col	Significant post-scrub reductions with I, triclosan, and hexachlorophene
Murie (1980)	C	Col, Inf	C in 95% methanol > aqueous deter- gent of C. No significant difference in wound infection rates
Ayliffe (1984)	I, C, O	Col	Alcoholic C > C in detergent > I
Soulsby (1986)	C, O	Col	C comparable to PCMX
Larson (1990)	A, I, C, O	Col	A > C > I > triclosan
Babb (1991)	A, I, C, O	Col	A > I > triclosan C products varied considerably by brand

[a]A = alcohol, I = povidone-iodine, C = chlorhexidine, O = other
[b]Col = bacterial colonization, Inf = infection rates

before surgery would reduce the risk of wound contamination and subsequent infection.

A series of clinical trials evaluating the effects of preoperative chlorhexidine showers on subsequent postoperative wound infection rates has been published over the past two decades; yet results remain equivocal. Initial evidence of a reduction in risk of wound infection emanated from Sweden with the work reported by Brandberg et al. (8). Subsequent European controlled trials with large sample sizes by Rotter et al. (46) (2813 patients) and Ayliffe et al. (4) (5536 patients) failed to demonstrate any protective effect. Hayek and Emerson (23) (2015 patients), on the other hand, reported a significantly lower infection rate among the chlorhexidine-bathed group. None of these three studies used similar definitions or surveillance systems. Additionally, intervention varied from one to three applications, and there was little attempt to monitor patient compliance with the prescribed regimens.

Because chlorhexidine requires several applications before its substantive effect is evident, it is not surprising that there would be little or no effect with one or perhaps even two applications. Even if two or three applications were effective, practical issues such as compliance and the fact that many of the highest risk surgical procedures are not elective (and therefore no preoperative showers could be planned) would limit the value of the practice of antimicrobial preoperative patient bathing. One component that needs to be added to the evaluation of this practice is a cost/benefit analysis.

Preoperative Patient Skin Preparation

Recent work assessing preoperative patient skin preparation has focused on incremental changes that could potentially result in time or cost savings (15,20,21,25,27,30). In general, shorter scrubs with agents containing alcohols or using antimicrobial-impregnated films are reported to have equivalent, and sometimes better, effectiveness as compared to longer procedures. Protocols that increase the need for either staff time or patient adherence, such as the one described by Payne et al. (39) are unlikely to gain wide acceptance.

Variations in preoperative skin preparation, including type of product used, drape, and duration and method of product application, have an impact on levels of bacterial colonization and wound infection rates. However, too few studies with comparable protocols are available to assess the ideal components of the preparation. This area of patient care practice is fraught with ritual and deserves thoughtful reconsideration to combine maximum efficacy with cost effectiveness and patient comfort.

Surgical Hand Scrub

Boyce et al. (7) recently reported a common-source outbreak of *Staphylococcus epidermis* infections among patients undergoing cardiac surgery. The epidemic strain was traced to the hands of a surgeon, and the outbreak ceased when the surgeon changed his hand scrub practices. Such case studies, anecdotally common but rarely published in the 1950s and 1960s, are clear evidence of a causal link between the hand preparation of the surgical team and preoperative wound infection rates. Nevertheless, less than 2% of wound infections are associated with exogenous sources (18). Ayliffe (5) suggested that although preoperative surgical hand scrub protocols may be rational, it is also reasonable to reconsider their impact on preventing infections. There may be ways to streamline and improve the regimens prescribed.

SUMMARY

Despite more than a century of clinical experience, research relating antiseptic skin practices in surgery to postoperative wound infection rates continues. Evidence of the value of preoperative whole body patient bathing with an agent such as chlorhexidine is weak, and this practice is likely to be cost effective only in situations of high patient compliance and high risk. Preoperative preparation of patient skin and surgeon's hands seems important, but procedures should be streamlined for cost and time efficiency and for patient comfort as products and protocols that are fast acting and/or slow release are tested and improved.

REFERENCES

1. Alexander JW, Aerni S, Plettner JP. Development of a safe and effective one-minute preoperative skin preparation. Arch Surg 1985; 120: 1357–1361.
2. Alexander JW, Fischer JE, Boyajian M, et al. The influence of hair-removal methods on wound infections. Arch Surg 1983; 118:347–351.
3. Association for Operating Room Nurses. AORN Standards and Recommended Practices for Perioperative Nursing-1992. Denver: AORN, 1992, pp. II:8-1–8.5.

4. Ayliffe GAJ, Noy MF, Babb JR, et al. A comparison of pre-operative bathing with chlorhexidine-detergent and non-medicated soap in the prevention of wound infection. J Hosp Infect 1983; 4: 237–244.
5. Ayliffe GAJ. Surgical scrub and skin disinfection. Infect Control 1984; 5:23–27.
6. Babb JR, Davies JG, Ayliffe GAJ. A test procedure for evaluating surgical hand disinfection. J Hosp Infect 1991; 18(suppl B): 41–49.
7. Boyce JM, Potter-Bynoe G, Opal SM, et al. A common-source outbreak of *Staphylococcus epidermis* infections among patients undergoing cardiac surgery. J Infect Dis 1991; 161: 494–499.
8. Brandberg A, Holm J, Hammarsten, Schersten T. Postoperative wound infections in vascular surgery: effect of preoperative whole body disinfection by shower-bath with chlorhexidine soap. In: Maibach H, Aly R, eds. Skin Microbiology Relevance To Clinical Infection. New York: Springer Verlag 1981: 98–102.
9. Byrne DJ, Napier A, Cuschieri A. Rationalizing whole body disinfection. J Hosp Infect 1990; 15: 183–187.
10. Byrne DJ, Napier A, Phillips G, Cuschieri A. Effects of whole body disinfection on skin flora in patients undergoing elective surgery. J Hosp Infect 1991; 17: 217–222.
11. Court-Brown CM. Pre-operative skin depilation and its effect on post-operative wound infections. J R Coll Surg Edinb 1981; 26: 238–241.
12. Cruse PJE, Foord R. A five-year prospective study of 23,649 surgical wounds. Arch Surg 1973; 107: 206–210.
13. Danchaivijitr S, Theeratharathorn R. Comparison of effects of alcohol, chlorhexidine cream, and iodophore cream on venous catheter-associated infections. J Med Assoc Thai 1989; 72(suppl 2): 39–43.
14. Dineen P. An evaluation of the duration of the surgical scrub. Surg Gynecol Obstet 1969; 129: 1181–1184.
15. Dzubow LM, Halpern AC, Leyden JJ, et al. Comparison of preoperative skin preparations for the face. J Am Acad Dermatol 1988; 19: 737–741.
16. Earnshaw JJ, Berridge DC, Slack RCB, et al. Do preoperative chlorhexidine baths reduce the risk of infection after vascular reconstruction? Eur J Vasc Surg 1989; 3: 323–326.
17. Eitzen HE, Ritter MA, French MLV, Gioe TJ. A microbiological in-use comparison of surgical hand-washing agents. J Bone Joint Surg 1979; 61A: 403–406.
18. Emmerson AM. The role of skin in nosocomial infections: a review. J Chemother 1989; 1(suppl n.1): 12–18.
19. Garibaldi RA, Skolnick D, Lerer T, et al. The impact of preoperative skin disinfection on preventing intraoperative wound contamination. Infect Control Hosp Epidemiol 1988; 9: 109–113.
20. Greelhoed GW, Sharpe K, Simon GL. A comparative study of surgical skin preparation methods. Surg Gynecol Obstet 1983; 157: 265–268.
21. Gilliam DL, Nelson CL. Comparison of a one-step iodophor skin preparation versus traditional preparation in total joint surgery. Clin Orthopa Relat Res 1990; 250: 258–260.

22. Hamilton HW, Hamilton KR, Lone FJ. Pre-operative hair removal. Can J Surg 1971; 20: 269–275.
23. Hayek LJ, Emerson JM. Preoperative whole body disinfection—a controlled clinical study. J Hosp Infect 1988; 11(supplement B): 1–19.
24. Ichida JM, Wassell JT, Keller MD, Ayers LW. Evaluation of protocol change in burn-care management using the cox proportional hazards model with time-dependent covariates. Stat Med 1993; 12: 301–310.
25. Johnston DH, Fairclough JA, Brown EM, Morris R. Rate of bacterial recolonization of the skin after preparation: four methods compared. Br J Surg 1987; 74: 64.
26. Kaiser AB, Kernodle DS, Barg NL, Petracek MR. Influence of preoperative showers on staphylococcal skin colonization: a comparative trial of antiseptic skin cleansers. Ann Thorac Surg 1988; 45: 35–38.
27. Kutarski PW, Grundy HC. To dry or not to dry? An assessment of the possible degradation in efficiency of preoperative skin preparation caused by wiping skin dry. Ann R Coll Surg Engl 1983; 75: 181–185.
28. Larson EL, Butz AM, Gullette DL, Laughon BA. Alcohol for surgical scrubbing? Infect Control Hosp Epidemiol 1990; II; 139–143.
29. Leclair JM, Winston KR, Sullivan BF, et al. Effect of preoperative shampoos with chlorhexidine or iodophor on emergence of resident scalp flora in neurosurgery. Infect Control Hosp Epidemiol 1988; 9: 8–12.
30. Levy JH, Nagle DM, Curling PE, et al. Contamination reduction during central venous catheterization. Crit Care Med 1988; 16: 165–167.
31. Longombe AO, Knight P, Kunangbangate N. 'Traditional' alcohol in surgical antisepsis in a rural African setting: a kind of intermediate technology? Trop Doc 1991; 21: 133–134.
32. Lowbury EJL, Lilly HA. Disinfection of the hands of surgeons and nurses. Br J Med 1960; I: 1445–1450.
33. Lowbury EJL, Lilly HA. The effect of blood on disinfection of surgeons' hands. Br J Surg 1974; 61: 19–21.
34. Lynch W, Davey PG, Malek M, et al. Cost-effectiveness analysis of the use of chlorhexidine detergent in preoperative whole-body disinfection in wound infection prophylaxis. J Hosp Infect 1992; 21: 179–191.
35. Mackenzie I. Preoperative skin preparation and surgical outcome. J Hosp Infect 1988; II(suppl B): 27–32.
36. Maki DG, Ringer M, Alvarado CJ. Prospective randomised trial of povidone-iodine, alcohol, and chlorhexidine for prevention of infection associated with central venous and arterial catheters. Lancet 1991; 338: 339–343.
37. Mannion PT, Thom BT, Reynolds CS, Strachan CJL. The acquisition of antibiotic resistant coagulase-negative staphylococci by aortic graft recipients. J Hosp Infect 1989; 14: 313–323.
38. Murie JA, Macpherson SG. Chlorhexidine in methanol for the preoperative cleansing of surgeons' hands: a clinical trial. Scot Med J 1980; 25: 309–311.
39. Payne JE, Breust M, Bradbury R. Reduction in amputation stump infection by antiseptic pre-operative preparation. Aust N Z J Surg 1989; 59: 637–640.

40. Pereira LJ, Lee GM, Wade KJ. The effect of surgical handwashing routines on the microbial counts of operating room nurses. Am J Infect Control 1990; 18: 354–364.
41. Peterson AF. The microbiology of the hands: effects of varying scrub procedures and times. In: Development in Industrial Microbiology, Vol. 19. Society for Industrial Microbiology, Arlington, 1978: 325–334.
42. Peterson AF, Rosenberg A, Alatary SD. Comparative evaluation of surgical scrub preparations. Surg Gynecol Obstet 1978; 146: 63–65.
43. Powis SJA, Waterworth TA, Arkell DG. Preoperative skin preparation: clinical evaluation of depilatory cream. Br Med J 1976; 2: 1166–1168.
44. Rehork B, Ruden H. Investigations into the efficacy of different procedures for surgical hand disinfection between consecutive operations. J Hosp Infect 1991; 19: I15–I27.
45. Robson D, Harding GKM. Antiseptic preparation of patients' skin at the operative site. Proceedings of 19th Annual Educational Conference, Association of Practitioners in Infection Control, San Francisco, 1992: 98.
46. Rotter ML, Larsen SO, Cooke EM, et al. A comparison of the effects of preoperative whole-body bathing with detergent alone and with detergent containing chlorhexidine gluconate on the frequency of wound infections after clean surgery. J Hosp Infect 1988; 11: 310–320.
47. Seropian B, Reynolds BM. Wound infections after pre-operative depilatory versus razor preparation. Am J Surg 1971; 12I: 251–254.
48. Soulsby ME, Barnett JB, Maddox S. Brief report: the antiseptic efficacy of chlorxylenol-containing vs. chlorhexidine gluconate-containing surgical scrub preparations. Infect Control 1986; 7: 223–226.
49. Tucci VJ, Stone AM, Thompson C, et al. Studies of the surgical scrub. Surg Gynecol Obstet 1977; 145: 415–416.
50. Wilcox MH, Spencer RC. Antiseptic catheter care (letter). Lancet 1991; 338: 635.

8

Prevalence of Wound Infection Under Occlusive Dressings

Jerry J. Hutchinson
ConvaTec, Ltd., Deeside, Clwyd, Wales

INTRODUCTION

Since 1962, when Winter (1) reported that occluding a skin wound with a moisture-retentive dressing accelerated healing by up to 50%, there has been concern that the conditions that led to enhanced healing also would lead to an increased risk of infection (2,3). Moisture and warmth, the conditions that accelerate healing, are precisely those required by microorganisms for optimal proliferation. It was perceived that this would inevitably lead to infection through enhanced invasion of wound tissue. Winter stated that ". . . in human clinical practice a moist wound surface may not be desirable because of the risk of infection" (4).

After some 30 years of clinical experience, it is clear that Winter's prediction is not valid. On the contrary, a moist wound environment is associated with a reduced risk of infection (5–7). In practice, in venous ulcers the type of dressing appears to exert little influence on the contaminating microbial flora, in terms of either the species found or the viable counts (6). This is in direct contradiction to the expectation from occluded human normal skin (8) and experiments conducted in acute pig wounds (9), both of which showed higher microbial counts under occlusive dressings. Furthermore, clinical evidence clearly shows that although ulcers are usually colonized by often very high viable counts of a wide range of microorganisms, there is no correlation between the types of organisms found, their numbers, and healing rates of ulcers (10,11).

99

The published literature provides some clues as to the reason for a reduced risk of infection under occlusive wound dressings. This chapter examines the microbial flora of wounds, the reported rate of clinical infection as deduced from a retrospective literature review and a prospective trial, and the properties of occlusive dressings and the activities of host defenses under occlusion that lead to a reduced risk of clinical infection under occlusive dressings compared with conventional wound care materials.

WOUND COLONIZATION AND INFECTION

Definitions

To understand the microbiology of wounds, it is critical to differentiate contamination and colonization, from infection. Throughout this review, the term *colonization* is used to describe the state wherein microorganisms exist harmlessly in a wound, often in great numbers, but without attendant signs of clinical infection, and over prolonged periods. The term *contamination* refers to small numbers of organisms present only transiently, but causing no morbidity. The term *infection* is used to describe the state wherein microorganisms have invaded the wound tissue and elicited an inflammatory response greater than that normally observed in wound healing.

In contrast to colonization, infection is characterized by heat, redness, swelling, and pain evident in the affected tissue site. Severe infection in which systemic spread occurs is associated with lymph involvement as evidenced by inflamed lymph ducts seen as redness tracking toward the site of a lymph gland. Histologically, infection is characterized by massive polymorphonuclear leukocyte (PMN) infiltration and microorganisms visible in tissue sections. Infection exerts a deleterious effect on healing (12) and can lead to a reduced repair rate or in severe cases dehiscence of suture lines or even death. Infection results in most cases from well-recognized predisposing factors in wounds (7,13) such as anoxic tissue, dead space, necrotic or foreign material, or an underlying pathology such as uncontrolled diabetes that impairs host defense function (14).

Colonization

All wounds are likely to be at least contaminated with microorganisms (15), and many remain heavily colonized throughout the entire healing process. Wound organisms may originate from the host skin, host fecal flora, or the air. Wounds such as partial-thickness skin donor sites are widely believed to be sterile, but in fact become contaminated through the surgical process that severs hair follicles and other skin adnexae in which organisms survive even after presurgical skin disinfection. This releases organisms from the deeper parts of the adnexae.

Most wounds contain gram-positive cocci such as *Staphylococcus* spp, *Streptococcus* spp, and diphtheroids. Acute wounds may yield gram-negative organisms such as *Escherichia coli* or *Pseudomonas* spp, but anaerobic organisms are less frequently isolated from acute wounds unless necrotic tissue is present or the wound is deep. Chronic ulcers contain a wide range of organisms (6,16,17). Up to 60% contain anaerobic organisms (18,19) including *Peptococcus, Peptostreptococcus, Fusobacterium, Bacteriodes*, and pathogens such as *Clostridium perfringens*. Gram-negative organisms isolated from chronic wounds include species of *Achromabacter, Acinetobacter, Citrobacter, Enterobacter, Klebsiella, Proteus*, and *Pseudomonas* (6,19). Yeasts may be isolated from up to 85% of burns (20) and are reported in up to 11% of venous ulcers (19,21). Filamentous fungi are not usually associated with the wound itself, but have been reported on the surrounding skin (21).

Characteristically, wound organisms present at the start of healing persist throughout treatment, although in acute wounds the viable count reduces quickly as the wound exudes less as healing progresses. This process can result in moisture-dependent gram-negative bacteria decreasing faster than gram-positive organisms. In chronic wounds such as venous and pressure ulcers, the flora persists virtually unchanged in type and viable count throughout treatment (6,18,19) unless significant healing is seen. It is not uncommon for ulcers to be colonized by three or more species (6,19) and to harbor total viable counts of between 10^6 and 10^8/ml of wound fluid.

Although ulcers are usually colonized by many species of organism at high viable counts, an unequivocal association between presence of specific organisms or high microbial counts and impaired healing has not been established. On the contrary, it is becoming increasingly evident that there is no association in the absence of clinical infection. Some reports purporting to show links with specific bacteria and impaired healing have emerged (22) but are unsubstantiated. The weight of evidence now indicates that even heavy wound colonization is relatively benign (6,10,18,23).

THE RATE OF INFECTION UNDER OCCLUSION

In contradistinction to the prediction of Hinman et al. (4), the rate of wound infection under occlusive dressings has not been elevated compared with conventional treatments. In an extensive retrospective review of the published literature on clinical experience, with occlusive dressings of all types used to treat both acute and chronic wounds, the risk of infection under occlusion was shown to be reduced compared with nonocclusive modalities (7). The reported rate of infection under conventional, nonocclusive dressings was 5.36%, whereas that under occlusive dressings was 2.08% (P = <0.05). All categories of occlusive product reported (hydrocolloids, films, foams, and hydrogels) were associated with lower infection rates compared with conventional dressings (P = <0.05). The same outcome was documented when the data were analyzed for infection rates by wound type (ulcers, burns, donor sites, and others).

Retrospective reviews are subject to limitations. It is not possible to state with certainty that the methods used in all studies reviewed were equivalent (7). Further, some studies reviewed were small, some were controlled whereas others were not, and different nonocclusive controls were used. For these reasons, a prospective, randomized, controlled multicenter trial was conducted to evaluate the rate of clinical infection under one occlusive dressing, a hydrocolloid wafer, in comparison with impregnated gauze in venous ulcers, partial-thickness burns, and donor site wounds (6). Results of this study confirmed the data from the retrospective review. The occlusive dressing was associated with an overall infection rate of 1.9%, whereas the impregnated gauze group was associated with an infection rate of 5.38%

Occlusion not only does not lead to increased risk of infection, it offers the potential to reduce the risk of infection. The conditions required for optimal wound healing are also those required for optimal proliferation of microorganisms. Wound healing is optimized under occlusion through the provision of conditions that permit optimal function of the cells involved in healing, including host defense cells such as PMNs. This characteristic and the physical properties of occlusive dressings lead to a reduced risk of infection. These factors are examined in the next section.

THE MECHANISM OF REDUCED RISK OF INFECTION

Dressing-Related Factors

For a wound to become infected, microorganisms must gain access to it. As discussed earlier, all wounds are likely to be contaminated or colonized by a natural flora derived chiefly from the host. In some circumstances, however, it is desirable to limit potential contamination by new organisms. This is the case in extended care facilities with critically ill patients, especially burn care centers in which patients are likely to have impaired defenses as a result of their injuries. Occlusive dressings present a barrier to the passage of bacteria and viruses such as human immuno-deficiency virus (HIV) and hepatitis B virus (HBV) as shown in in vitro tests (24–26). In vivo it has been shown that occlusive dressings such as hydrocolloid wafers (HCD) and polyurethane films (PUF) may present a barrier to bacteria (27), and clinical evidence shows hydrocolloid wafers to be bacterial barriers (24).

Both HCDs and PUFs have been associated with the disappearance of strict aerobes such as *Pseudomonas* and *Klebsiella* spp (18,28,29). This obser-vation has been attributed to the hypoxic environment known to develop under occlusive dressings used for prolonged periods (18,30).

It has been demonstrated in a simulated in vitro wound model and in a clinical study of patients with small burns that an HCD is associated with reduced airborne dispersal of bacteria at dressing change (31). This finding has implications for the practice of infection control, particularly in high-risk clinical settings.

Host Factors

Winter's original work (1) unwittingly provided evidence of biological activity in moist wounds, which is now recognized as perhaps the key factor in reducing the risk of infection in occluded wounds. It was reported that moist wounds were infiltrated by PMNs to a greater degree than were dry wounds. This phenomenon also was reported by Saymen et al. (32). Polymorphonuclear leukocytes are the key nonspecific host defense cells which enter wounds by chemotaxis early in the inflam-matory phase of healing to protect against tissue invasion by wound microorganisms (33,34), and large numbers are seen in infected tissue.

The activity of PMNs is evident in occluded wounds. Wound fluid collected from occluded wounds contains PMNs in which stainable bac-terial inclusions may be observed, indicating previous phagocytic activity (35), and the numbers of PMNs seen under occlusion are normal relative to circulating blood (30).

CONCLUSIONS

Clinical evidence shows that many of the fears and concerns surrounding the use of occlusive dressings on skin wounds are unfounded. The type of dressing applied to wounds such as chronic ulcers appears not to influence the bacterial load or range of species. Chronic wounds heal in the presence of often very high microbial viable counts, and there is no unequivocal evidence linking specific bacteria with an increased risk of infection or healing impairment.

In direct contrast to early expectations, the risk of wound infection as distinct from colonization under occlusive dressings is not greater than with conventional products. It is in fact reduced. This finding is attributed to the barrier properties of occlusive dressings, the reduced risk of airborne dispersal at dressing change, and the efficient function of the host defenses in the moist environment created under occlusion.

REFERENCES

1. Winter GD. Formation of the scab and the rate of epithelialization of superficial wounds in the skin of the young domestic pig. Nature 1962; 193: 293–294.
2. Laforet EG. Wound dressing or window dressing? Arch Surg 1974; 109: 457.
3. Bennett RG. The debatable benefit of occlusive dressings for wounds. Dermatol Surg Oncol 1982; 8: 166–167.
4. Hinman CC, Maibach HI, Winter GD. Effect of air exposure and occlusion in experimental human skin wounds. Nature 1963; 200: 377–379.
5. Hutchinson JJ. Prevalence of wound infection under occlusive dressings: a collective survey of reported research. Wounds 1989; 2: 123–134.
6. Hutchinson JJ. A prospective clinical trial of wound dressings to investigate the rate of infection under occlusion. In: EDS. Proceedings of the Fourth European Symposium on Advances in Wound Management. London: MacMillan, 1994: 93–96.
7. Hutchinson JJ, Lawrence JC. Wound infection under occlusive dressings. J Hosp Infect 1991; 17: 83–94.
8. Aly R, Shirley C, Cunico B, Maibach HI. Effect of prolonged occlusion on the microbial flora, pH, carbon dioxide and transepidermal water loss on human skin. J Invest Dermatol 1978; 71: 378–381.
9. Mertz PM, Eaglstein WH. The effect of a semiocclusive dressing on the microbial population in superficial wounds. Arch Surg 1984; 119: 287–289.
10. Annoni F, Rosina M, Chiurazzi D, Ceva M. The effects of a hydrocolloid dressing on bacterial growth and the healing process of leg ulcers. Int Angiol 1989; 8: 224–228.
11. Friedmann PS, Pryce DW, Hutchinson JJ. Manuscript submitted for publication.
12. Robson MC, Stenberg BD, Heggers JP. Wound healing alterations caused by infection. Clin Plast Surg 1990; 17: 485–492.
13. Cruse PJE, Foord R. The epidemiology of wound infection. A ten year prospective study of 62939 wounds. Surg Clin North Amer 1980; 60: 27–40.

14. Rayfield EJ, Ault MJ, Keusch GT, et al. Infection and diabetes: the case for glucose control. Am J Med 1982; 72: 439–450.
15. Longe RL. Current concepts in clinical therapeutics: pressure sores. Clin Pharm 1986; 5: 679–681.
16. Lookingbill DP, Miller SH, Knowles RC. Bacteriology of chronic leg ulcers. Arch Dermatol 1978; 114: 1765–1768.
17. Daltrey DC, Rhodes B, Chattwood JG. Investigation into the microbial flora of healing and non-healing decubitis ulcers. J Clin Pathol 1981; 34: 701–705.
18. Gilchrist B, Reed C. The bacteriology of leg ulcers under hydrocolloid dressings. Br J Dermatol 1989; 121: 337–344.
19. Hansson C, Hoborn J, Möller Å, Swanbeck G. The microbial flora in venous leg ulcers without clinical signs of infection. Acta Derm Venereol 1995; 75: 24–30.
20. Neely AN, Odds FC, Basatia BK, Holder IA. Characterization of *Candida* isolates from pediatric burn patients. J Clin Microbiol 1988; 26: 1645–1649.
21. English MR, Smith RJ, Harman RRM. The fungal flora of ulcerated legs. Br J Dermatol 1971; 84: 576–581.
22. Schraibman IG. The significance of β-hemolytic streptococci in chronic leg ulcers. Ann R Coll Surg Engl 1990; 72: 123–124.
23. Handfield-Jones SE, Gratton CEH, Simpson RA, Kennedy CTC. Comparison of hydrocolloid dressing and paraffin gauze in the treatment of venous ulcers. Br J Dermatol 1988; 118: 425–427.
24. Wilson P, Burroughs D, Dunn L. Methicillin-resistant *Staphylococcus aureus* and hydrocolloid dressings. Pharm J 1988; 241: 787–788.
25. Lawrence JC, Lilly HA. Are hydrocolloid dressings bacteria-proof? Pharm J 1987; 239: 184.
26. Bowler PG, Delargy H, Prince D, Fondberg L. The viral barrier properties of some occlusive dressings and their role in infection control. Wounds 1993; 5: 1–8.
27. Mertz PM, Marshall DA, Eaglstein WH. Occlusive wound dressings to prevent bacterial invasion and wound infection. J Am Acad Dermatol 1985; 12: 662–668.
28. Katz S, McGinley K, Leydon JJ. Semipermeable occlusive dressings. Effects on growth of pathogenic bacteria and reepithelialization of superficial wounds. Arch Dermatol 1986; 122: 58–62.
29. Mulder GD, Kissil MT, Mahr JJ. Bacterial growth under occlusive and non-occlusive wound dressings. Wounds 1989; 1: 63–69.
30. Varghese MC, Balin AK, Carter DM, Caldwell D. Local environment of chronic wounds under synthetic dressings. Arch Dermatol 1986; 122: 52–57.
31. Lawrence JC. Reducing the spread of bacteria. J Wound Care 1993; 2: 48–52.
32. Saymen DG, Nathan P, Holder IA, et al. Control of surface wound infection: skin versus synthetic grafts. Appl Microbiol 1973; 25: 921–934.
33. Clarke RAF. Cutaneous tissue repair: basic biologic considerations I. J Am Acad Dermatol 1985; 13: 701–725.

34. Mimms CA, ed. The Pathogenesis of Infectious Disease. 3d ed. London: Academic Press, 1987: 63–91.
35. May SR. Physiology, immunology and clinical efficacy of an adherent polyurethane wound dressing; OpSite[R]. In Wise DL, ed. Burn Wound Coverings. Boca Raton, Florida: CRC Press, 1984: 53–78.

9

Handwashing: A Ritual Revisited

Jacalyn L. Bryan
Association of State and Territorial Health Officials, Washington, D.C.

Jackie Cohran
Prince George's Hospital Center, Cheverly, Maryland

Elaine L. Larson
Georgetown University School of Nursing, Washington, D.C.

INTRODUCTION

In 1988, a review of evidence for a causal link between handwashing and infection included literature published over 107 years, 1879 through 1986 (1). Interestingly, very little experimental data were evidenced for the century between Semmelweis and the late 1970s; the four clinical trials reported were all published in the 1980s. Since then there appeared to be a resurgence of interest and study in the area of handwashing and infections; the review of literature in that area was extended for six years to include January 1987 through June 1993. This chapter presents a comprehensive review of the literature published from January 1987 to June 1993 linking handwashing and infections.

By permission, adapted from The Association for Professionals in Infection Control and Epidemiology, Inc.: Jacalyn L. Bryan, Jackie Cohran, and Elaine L. Larson, *Chemical Germicides in Health Care*, 1995, pp. 163–178.

Methods

Two databases were searched under the subject heading of "Hand-washing": The Cumulative Index to Nursing and Allied Health Literature (CINAHL) and the miniMEDLINE SYSTEM file at the Dahlgren Memorial Library, Georgetown University, which contained 1,224,907 citations from 1146 journals from January 1987 through June 1993, published in English language biomedical literature during this 78-month period.

Articles reviewed were divided into seven categories according to their primary focus: (a) methods, articles reporting development and testing of methods to study hand flora or handwashing; (b) products, articles reporting evaluations or comparisons of specific products; (c) behavior, articles in which the primary focus was the behavioral aspects of handwashing; (d) reviews, general discussions of handwashing, reviews of previous work, or other types of commentary; (e) infection, retrospective or prospective studies relating handwashing to infection; (f) microbiology, studies describing the microbial flora on the hands; and (g) other, articles that did not fit the other categories.

Categories of studies were compared between the first review spanning 107 years and this review, which spanned 6.5 years. Research articles were also categorized, into six study designs: (a) experimental, (b) observational, (c) survey (self-report), (d) case-control, (e) case study or report, and (f) other.

RESULTS

From January 1987 through June 1993, 91 publications specifically related to handwashing were found. The average number of publications per year was 13.7 (range: 8 to 17) for the past 6 years as compared with an average of 3.8 publications per year (range 0 to 12) in the prior century, a 72.3% increase. The percentage of behavioral studies nearly doubled, and the studies examining the evidence of a link between handwashing and infections showed a fivefold increase. In contrast, studies of product evaluation and handwashing decreased by 30.6%. No substantial differences were observed in the other categories. (Figure 1.)

The most frequent categories of handwashing publications were review articles (30, 33.0%) (2–30), infections (18, 19.8%) (31–48), studies evaluating products (19, 20.9%) (49–67), behavior (18, 19.8%) (68–85), and microbiological flora on hands (5, 5.5%) (86–90), and one other (91). These are sorted by category and referenced at the end of the article. Some review articles cited anecdotal evidence that handwashing reduced infections or the lack of handwashing increased risk, but these were not

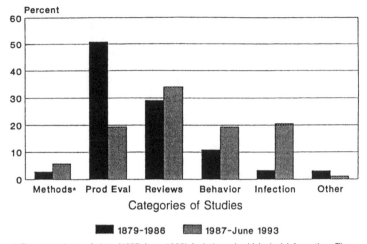

Figure 1   Categories of studies specifically related to handwashing.

included in our analysis. Publications linking handwashing and infections included 13 retrospective studies in which interruption in the spread of outbreak strains of microorganisms was attributed to handwashing and five prospective studies in which handwashing was the independent variable and infection was the dependent variable. The following is a review and critique of the 18 studies linking handwashing to the risk of infection.

REVIEW OF THE EVIDENCE

Nonexperimental Evidence

There have been 13 published nonexperimental studies since 1986 in which a link between handwashing and infection was studied. Seven of these were of the case study type and six were case control studies (Table 1). In two studies conducted in the rural areas of Bangladesh and Senegal, the incidence of neonatal tetanus was linked to the contaminated hands of the birth attendant (40,43). In a survey conducted between March 1989 and March 1990, subjects were systematically selected from the census (40). A total of 43,791 households were surveyed and the mothers of 6148 eligible infants interviewed. One hundred twelve of the 330 neonates met the case definition for tetanus, 21 (18.8%) of whom were seen at a

Table 1 Nonexperimental Studies Linking Handwashing and Infections

Year published	Investigator	Setting	Study type		Results
			Case study	Case-control	
1987	Rubio	Operating room	X		0.3% postoperative infection rate (no comparison group)
1987	Clemens	Urban Bangladesh		X	Significantly more diarrhea in children whose mothers did not wash hands before food preparation
1987	Chorba	Day care center	X		Outbreak control measure including handwashing limited spread of infection
1989	Issacs	Neonatal nursery	X		Outbreak resolved without any other intrervention other than rein-forcing handwashing
1990	Boyce	Operating room	X		Outbreak of surgical infections attributed to hands of surgeon carrier
1990	Guiguet	Intensive care unit		X	Simple control measures including reinforcement of handwashing decreased rate of MRSA colonization and infection
1990	Raad	Pediatric unit	X		Use of ineffective handwashing agent may have contributed to continued nosocomial spread
1991	Lee	Outdoor festival	X		Outbreak of shigellosis attributed to lack of handwashing facilities (circumstantial)
1991	Leroy	Rural Senegal		X	Significantly lower risk of neonatal tetanus when hands of person cutting umbilical cord were washed
1991	Ehrenkranz	Surgical intensive care units		X	Significant decrease in deep sternal wound infections attributed solely to improved infection control practices including handwashing
1992	Coovadia	Neonatal nursery	X		Outbreak of amikacin-resistant *Klebsiella pneumoniae* following relaxation of control measures for prior MRSA outbreak: 3 hand carriers
1992	Hlady	Rural Bangladesh		X	Significantly lower risk of neonatal tetanus when hands of person cutting umbilical cord were washed
1993	Watson	Neonatal intensive care unit		X	Significantly greater risk of hepatitis A among staff not routinely washing hands after contact with infected infant

MRSA = methicillin-resistant *S. aureus*

health care facility. Three living infants—matched for sex, residence, and date of birth to control for effects of circumcision, regional variations in birth practices, and recall—were selected as controls for each case. Results of a multivariate analysis of risk factors demonstrated that attendant handwashing and the use of a cleaned tool to cut the umbilical cord were both associated with decreased risk of tetanus (odds ratio [OR] 0.49; $P = .005$).

The study conducted in rural Senegal (43) was a component of a more comprehensive study on mortality rates. All neonatal deaths were investigated to identify those caused by neonatal tetanus. Once they were properly identified, they were matched with two types of controls—all other births occurring in the same and in neighboring compounds in which the infant survived the neonatal period. In a multivariate analysis, failure to wash hands with soap before cord cutting was significantly and independently associated with higher risk of neonatal tetanus (OR 5.22; $P = 0.0001$).

Outbreaks attributed to poor hygiene, inadequate sanitary facilities, and lack of potable water are not unique to developing countries. In one case study, an estimated 3175 women attending a 5-day outdoor music festival became ill with gastroenteritis caused by *Shigella sonnei*. More than 2000 volunteer food handlers prepared the communal meals. Limited access to soap and running water for handwashing was one of the few sanitary deficits noted at the festival. Results of questionnaires completed by a sample of attendees systematically selected by choosing every third person by Zip Code from a mailing list were used to estimate attack rates. A tofu salad (uncooked and mixed with vegetables by hand) was implicated as the outbreak vehicle (OR = 3.4; $P < 0.0001$). In the analysis of the case-control data, however, reported frequency of food handlers' handwashing was not associated with illness (42).

A case-control study was performed to develop an empirically based intervention for improving water-sanitation practices and rates of childhood diarrhea among families residing in urban Bangladesh (35). The lack of handwashing by mothers preparing food significantly correlated with increased rates of childhood diarrhea over the 3-month observation interval. "Sentinel" families were randomly selected. A group of cases was created from families having rates of childhood diarrhea in the highest 25% of all families, and a group of controls was selected from among families with rates of childhood diarrhea in the lowest 25%. Both groups were comparable with respect to family size and level of education. Significantly more control than case mothers (82% versus 53%, respectively) were observed to wash hands before preparing food ($P < .01$).

Two case studies described interventions to curtail outbreaks of salmonellosis (34) and rotavirus (45). One study (34) of a nonfoodborne outbreak of salmonellosis in a day care center reported similar attach rates across age groups, but the nature of exposure for each child could not be determined. The few environmental cultures obtained were negative for *Salmonella*. Transmission among infants confined to cribs was attributed to the hands of attendants or inanimate objects, whereas transmission among toddlers probably occurred by direct spread from one infected child to another. A distinction would not be made between which prevention measures, if any, were successful in curtailing the spread of infection. Another study illustrated the failure of all infection control efforts to contain nosocomial rotavirus transmission in hospitalized pediatric patients during a community outbreak (45). Despite repair of malfunctioning handwashing dispensers and other control measures, the nosocomial outbreak continued. Thus, results of neither study provided evidence of a link between handwashing and reduction in spread of the infecting agent.

In a study by Rubio (46) of 3480 surgical cases performed over 8 years, the surgical team members used an agent containing 0.23% hexachlorophene in a 46% ethyl alcohol base (Septisol Antiseptic Foam) to prepare their hands and forearms before surgery. The author attributed a very low postoperative infection rate to this surgical hand preparation agent. The author's conclusion was weakened by the fact that no microbiological studies were performed and a comparison group was not used.

Two commons-source outbreaks were studied in which the authors described breaks in handwashing technique (32,48). A case-control study was undertaken to investigate an outbreak of *Staphylococcus epidermidis* infections among patients undergoing cardiac surgery. Noninfected patients served as controls. The prevalence of the epidemic strain of *Staphylococcus* was associated with one particular surgeon who was using a nonantimicrobial preparation for preoperative scrubbing. Use of an appropriate preoperative scrub solution eradicated the epidemic strain from the surgeon's hands and terminated the outbreak (32).

In an outbreak of hepatitis A virus (HAV) among neonatal intensive care unit (NICU) staff, infant-to-staff transmission was ascertained by reviewing NICU staffing records and each infected infant's medical record (48). A self-administered questionnaire on infection control practices was distributed to NICU nurses, respiratory therapists, and family members. Among the staff exposed to the index infant, HAV occurred in 8 (57.1%) of 14 NICU staff who reported rarely or never washing their hands immediately after care of the index infant compared with 2 (10.5%) of 19 who reported washing sometimes or often (relative risk = 5.4; P <.01). No statistically significant association was observed among NICU staff for HAV and other factors (e.g., age, experience, gloves, eating).

An intervention to reinforce the importance of handwashing practices was associated with the resolution of three outbreaks in intensive care units (36,39,41). In the first case study of an amikacin-resistant *Klebsiella pneumoniae* (ARKP) outbreak in a neonatal unit it appeared there was a breakdown in certain infection control practices implemented after a previous outbreak of methicillin-resistant *Staphylococcus aureus* (MRSA). Isolates of ARKP obtained from infected and colonized babies, a colonized physician, nurse, mother, and the environment were related to the outbreak strain. Several control measures were implemented including strict enforcement of handwashing with 0.5% chlorhexidine in 70% alcohol. Reintroduction and reenforcement of infection control procedures resulted in an abrupt end of the outbreak as evidenced by negative repeat cultures and the absence of cases. However, it was not possible to determine how much of the outbreak was eliminated by handwashing alone or in combination with other measures (36).

In a second study examining the effectiveness of simple infection control measures in controlling an outbreak of MRSA infections, an index case served as a source for subsequent hand-to-hand spread to other patients. Although the author attributed the sharp decrease of MRSA infection to reinforcement of handwashing precautions, a distinction could not be made between this and other control measures (i.e., isolation), and the evidence to support the conclusion was weak (39).

A third study (41) described a nosocomial echovirus 11 outbreak in a neonatal unit with concomitant echovirus 11 circulating in the community. Twelve (29%) of 41 babies exposed in the unit were infected, all of whom were 14 days old. This suggested horizontal transmission, presumably from one or more infected staff member. Except for emphasizing the importance of handwashing, other infection control interventions were not deemed practical (i.e., cohorting). The authors attributed the rapid resolution of the outbreak to the reinforcement of handwashing (41).

Ehrenkranz and Pfaff (38) conducted a case-control study to determine the causes of an excess frequency of deep sternal wound infections. The rate in hospital A was 4% as compared with 0.48% in hospital B ($P = .002$, Fisher exact test, two-tailed). The two hospitals were served by the same surgeons over the same time period. No breaches in operative technique were noted. Inspection of the two hospitals revealed important differences in handwashing sink location, use of antimicrobial soap, and isolation policies. Next, intervention were implemented over a 9-month period including enforcement of handwashing and use of alcohol antiseptics by surgical intensive care unit (SICU) personnel before manipulation of catheters, increased staffing, segregation of cardiac surgery patients, an increased presence by infection control practitioners, and feedback on handwashing practices. Frequency and type of infection control surveillance, as well as the general efficacies of infection control practices, were verified as comparable between the two hospitals. Results showed different rates of deep sternal wound infection at the two hospitals during the initial period and similar rates in the postintervention period. Because no bacteriological studies of the hands of SICU staff were performed, it was not clear whether changes in the inanimate environment or in antisepsis of hands led to outbreak control. However, the authors felt that they had sufficient evidence to conclude that the significant decrease in deep sternal wound infections (no cases; $P = .02$) in the postinterventional period among patients who underwent cardiac surgery in hospital A could be attributed to improved infection control practices, particularly handwashing, in the SICU.

Experimental Evidence

Five experimental studies have been (Table 2) published since 1986 in which handwashing was the independent variable and infection was the dependent/outcome variable.

Stanton and Clemens (47) conducted a randomized trial in urban Bangladesh to assess the impact of a multifaceted educational intervention program on hygienic behaviors and rates of diarrhea. The educational intervention was designed to improve three water sanitation behaviors empirically shown to be associated with high rates of childhood diarrhea in Dahka, Bangladesh. The educational intervention consisted of group discussions, pictorial demonstrations, posters, and games. These were targeted to improve handwashing before preparing food, decrease the incidence of open defecation, and draw attention to proper disposal of garbage and feces.

A total of 937 intervention families received the educational intervention, while 986 served as controls. Before intervention, the rates of diarrhea and frequency of behavioral practices were nearly identical. After intervention, 49% of the study families and 33% of the control group washed their hands before preparing food ($P <0.05$). The incidence of diarrhea in the intervention areas was 26% lower than that for the nonintervention areas (incidence ratio = 0.74; $P <0.0001$). Garbage and feces remained uncovered and the number of children who put the garbage in their mouths did not differ, but the amount of garbage and feces in the intervention households decreased.

Table 2 Prospective Studies of the Influence of Handwashing on Infection

Year published	Investigator	Setting	Elements of experimental design				Significant results
			Intervention?	Comparison group?	Randomization?	Blinding?	
1987	Stanton	51 communities in Bangladesh	Yes	Concurrent	Yes	No	Significant reduction in diarrhea
1988	Bartlett	21 day care centers	Yes	Concurrent	Yes	No	Surveillance without training associated with a significant decrease in diarrheal disease. One-time staff training led to no significant difference.
1989	Butz	24 family day care homes	Yes	Concurrent	Yes	No	Significant reduction in symptoms of enteric disease.
1991	Peters	Hospital maternity ward	Yes	Sequential	No	No	Significant reduction in puerperal mastitis.
1992	Doebbeling	Critical care unit	Yes	Crossover	No	No	Significant difference in nosocomial infection rate with one hand-washing product.

The fact that significantly more mothers washed their hands before preparing food in the study families as compared to controls seems to have contributed to the decreased incidence of diarrhea in the intervention group. The investigators concluded that a simple educational message could modify behavioral practices and lower the incidence of diarrheal disease.

In 1988, Bartlett et al. (31) conducted a 3-year longitudinal study of diarrhea among infants and toddlers attending day care centers. The authors evaluated the effects of staff training without external monitoring or active surveillance on the rates of diarrhea. Twenty-one day care centers were randomly assigned to intervention or control conditions.

Staff of the intervention day care centers ($n = 10$) received training in procedures to reduce transmission of infectious diarrhea. In the first phase, day care directors were trained. The directors then participated in training sessions for their classroom staffs. Sessions included information on schedules and procedures for caregiver tasks, including staff and child handwashing, diapering, food handling, environmental cleaning, and other child hygiene practices. No differences were found in diarrhea rates between pretraining and posttraining years or in diarrhea rates between intervention and control centers either before or after the training intervention. All of the 21 day care centers had significantly higher diarrhea rates than did day care homes or households not using day care, but significantly lower rates than day care centers not included in the active surveillance. It was not possible, however, to assess the independent effects of each component of the educational intervention, specifically handwashing.

In 1990, Butz et al. (33) evaluated the effectiveness of an intervention program in decreasing the incidence of symptoms associated with enteric and respiratory infectious diseases among children attending family day care homes. Twenty-four family day care homes were randomly assigned, 12 each to the intervention and control groups.

The intervention consisted of a handwashing educational program, instructions delineating indications for use of vinyl gloves, use of disposable diaper changing pads, and use of an alcohol-based hand rinse by the day care provider. The intervention group received a monthly supply of disposable diaper changing pads, vinyl gloves, and the alcohol-based hand rinse solution.

Diarrhea rates were reported in one of every 100 child care days, representing one diarrhea episode per month in a typical family day care home. Symptoms of enteric disease (diarrhea, vomiting, and fever) were significantly reduced in the intervention family day care homes. Again, however, it was not possible to assess the independent effects of each component of the intervention.

Peters and Flick-Filli'es (44) prospectively evaluated the incidence of puerperal mastitis during time periods with and without the availability of an additional hand hygiene product at the bedside for use by new mothers. During the two 12-month study periods, the authors found that without the additional hand rinse at the bedside, 32 mothers (2.9%) following 1095 births developed mastitis. In contrast, 8 of 1230 new mothers (0.65%) developed mastitis when the hand rinse was available at the bedside (P <0.001). These findings suggest that the mother herself contributed significantly to the risk of puerperal mastitis and that women should be advised to use hand disinfection as an essential step in the prevention of puerperal mastitis.

Doebbeling et al. (37) conducted an 8-month prospective multiple crossover trial to compare the efficacy of two agents—a 4% solution of chlorhexidine gluconate and a 60% isopropyl alcohol hand-rinsing agent with the optional use of a non-medicated soap—in reducing the risk of nosocomial infections in three intensive care units.

A total of 1352 patients were included in the chlorhexidine group and 1382 patients in the alcohol-soap group. The handwashing behavior of the staff was monitored over 152 hours, during which there were 1233 opportunities for handwashing. Handwashing compliance was 42% during chlorhexidine use and 38% during alcohol-soap use (P = 0.002). Overall, 152 nosocomial infections occurred in the chlorhexidine group, as compared to 202 nosocomial infections in the alcohol-soap group (incidence density ratio, 0.73; 95% confidence intervals, 0.59 to 0.90).

The authors concluded that chlorhexidine was superior to alcohol for reducing nosocomial infection rates. However, the differences could be explained by a lower rate of compliance among health care workers during alcohol use (less frequent and lower volumes used) rather than the lower efficacy of the product. The reason for better handwashing compliance with chlorhexidine may have been because it required only one step. The most important aspect of this study is the clear demonstration that handwashing practice can have a significant impact on nosocomial infection rates.

DISCUSSION

Handwashing has become an integral component of the tradition and ritual of infection prevention practice, but several factors make it difficult to evaluate its effectiveness. First, handwashing is only one of a myriad of practices that form the armamentarium of strategies to prevent the transmission of infection. These practices rarely occur singularly, and hence it is impossible to pinpoint the independent effects of one practice such as handwashing. This phenomenon was evident in a number of studies reviewed (31,33,34,36,38,39). Second, because handwashing is assumed to be efficacious, an association between handwashing and changes in infection rates or the termination of an outbreak is sometimes assumed to be causal, when, in fact, it may be circumstantial. This confusion of association with causality could have been at play in several of the outbreak investigations discussed here (41,46,48). Two studies reviewed demonstrated no effect of handwashing on outbreaks of salmonellosis (42) and rotavirus (45). Both of these studies, however, were fraught with methodological problems such as self-reporting, misclassification, lack of reliability, and so forth. Table 3 summarizes studies reviewed in light of the strength of their evidence of causality.

Other studies using careful case-control designs confirmed further that handwashing can result in significant reductions in infection transmitted

Table 3 Literature Linking Handwashing and Infection 1/86 through 6/93

Design	Strength of evidence	
	Strong	Weak
Experimental:		
1987 Stanton	x	
1988 Bartlett		x
1989 Issacs		x
1990 Butz		x
1991 Peters		x
1992 Doebbeling	x	
Case Control:		
1987 Clemens	x	
1987 Chorba		x
1990 Raad		x
1991 Leroy	x	
1992 Hlady	x	
1993 Watson		x
Case Studies:		
6		x

by the fecal–oral route and in situations of poor hygiene (35,40,43,47). More important in the setting of health care in developed and industrialized nations is the question of whether handwashing, in the presence of a variety of other advanced and sophisticated prevention techniques and ready availability of disposable products such as gloves and other protective clothing, provides any added benefit. That is, is handwashing a ritual that deserves now to be set aside or reevaluated in light of technological and hygienic advances?

Three studies reviewed since 1987 have relevance to the modern, high technological hospital environment. The prospective study reported by Boyce et al. (32) demonstrated that the eradication of an epidemic strain of *Staphylococcus* from a surgeon's hands by use of an antiseptic surgical scrub was followed by termination of an outbreak with that strain. The temporal sequence and the specificity and clear relationship between surgical wound infection and a single member of the surgical team lends strong evidence that the surgical hand scrub was causally related to a reduction in risk of wound infection. This evidence is consistent with the epidemiology of the nosocomial spread of staphylococcal disease as clearly elucidated during the outbreaks in neonatal units and operating rooms in the 1950s and 1960s associated with nasal and hand carriage of staphylococci by health care professionals.

The study by Peters and Flick-Filli'es (44) offers clear evidence that hand hygiene by new mothers can reduce the incidence of early postpartum mastitis and suggests that even in hospital settings, patient hygiene can influence nosocomial infection rates. The most important study to shed light on the question of whether handwashing adds any value to current infection control regimes was that of Doebbeling et al. (37). Even with methodological problems that make it difficult to conclude which product (if either) was more efficacious, the study clearly demonstrated that hand hygiene practices in a high risk critical care setting can have a significant impact on nosocomial infection rates.

The study also again confirmed that handwashing practices are suboptimal. It seems clear, based on the marginal success of many interventions in influencing handwashing behavior, that the handwashing practices of health care professionals will continue to be suboptimal without stronger mandates and monitoring. Such monitoring is probably not economically feasible, even if it were successful in significantly improving the frequency and/or quality of handwashing. It is unfortunate but not surprising that handwashing behavior is not optimal because the nature of the task if repetitive, tedious, and mundane.

It would be extremely helpful to be able to quantitate the full impact of handwashing on nosocomial infection rates and to develop predictive models against which infection outcomes in given units or institutions could be evaluated. Theoretically, an experiment could be designed with two test conditions in a high risk environment: one in which all health professionals washed their hands every time handwashing was indicated and a comparison group in which patients and other conditions were comparable but there was no handwashing practice change. Aside from the practical problems with such a study, it is likely that the single hand-washing intervention would be accompanied by other changes in person-nel behavior, again making it difficult to have a high level of assurance that the independent effects of handwashing were delineated.

Based on this review, we conclude that:

1. Hand hygiene of selected groups of patients may influence nosocomial infection rates and deserves increased attention.
2. Handwashing, even in this area of universal precautions and ready access to a variety of protective barriers, adds incremental value to infection prevention and control strategies in acute care as well as community settings.
3. It is highly desirable but unlikely that the impact of "ideal" hand-washing on nosocomial infection rates will be quantified.

REFERENCES

1. Larson E. A causal link between handwashing and risk of infection? Examination of the evidence. Infect Control Hosp Epidemiol 1988; 9: 28–36.
2. Ansari SA, Springthorpe SV, Sattar SA. Survival and vehicular spread of human rotaviruses: possible relation to seasonality of outbreaks. Rev Infect Dis 1991; 13: 448–461.
3. Beck WC. Handwashing, Semmelweis, and chlorine. Infect Control Hosp Epidemiol 1988; 9: 366–367.
4. Borgatta L, Fisher M, Robbins N. Hand protection and protection from hands: handwashing, germicides, and globes. Women Health 1989; 15: 77–92.
5. Cudworth K. A step-by-step guide to clean hands. RN 1987; 50: 22–23.
6. Edmond MB, Wenzel RP. Ethical considerations in the use of subliminal stimulation to improve handwashing compliance: scientific utility versus autonomy of the individual. Infect Control Hosp Epidemiol 1993; 14: 107–109.
7. Ehrenkranz NJ. Bland soap handwash or hand antisepsis? The pressing need for clarity. Infect Control Hosp Epidemiol 1992; 13: 299–301.
8. Geiss HK, Heeg P. Hand-washing agents and nosocomial infections [letter]. N Engl J Med 1992; 327: 1390.
9. Gidley C. Now, wash your hands. Nurs Times 1987; 83:40–42.

10. Goldmann D, Larson E. Hand-washing and nosocomial infections [editorial]. N Engl J Med 1992; 327: 120–122.
11. Gould D. Nurses' hands as vectors of hospital-acquired infection: a review. J Adv Nurs 1991; 16: 1216–1225.
12. Heenan A. Handwashing practices. Nurs Times 1992; 88: 70.
13. Johnson G. Scrubbing: a sacred cow? Nurs (Lond) 1991; 4: 19–21.
14. Lapides M. Emphasize handwashing benefits. Occup Health Safety 1993; 62: 72.
15. Larson E. Rituals in infection control: what works in the newborn nursery? J Obstet, Gynecol, Neonatal Nurs 1987; 16: 411–416.
16. Larson E, Rotter ML. Handwashing: are experimental models a substitute for clinical trials? Two viewpoints. Infect Control Hosp Epidemiol 1990; 11: 63–66.
17. Laufman H. Current use of skin and wound cleansers and antiseptics. Am J Surg 1989; 157: 359–365.
18. Maley MP. Extend handwashing to the forearms? [letter]. Am J Nurs 1989; 89: 1437.
19. McFarlane A. Why do we forget to remember handwashing? Prof Nurs 1990; 5: 250, 252.
20. Monsma M, Day R, St. Arnaud S. Handwashing makes a difference. J School Health 1992; 62: 109–111.
21. Mooney BR, Armington LC. Infection Control: how to prevent nosocomial infections. RN 1987; 50: 20–23.
22. Othersen MJ, Othersen HB. A history of handwashing: seven hundred years at a snail's pace. Pharos 1987; Spring: 23–28.
23. Perceval A. Wash hands, disinfect hand, or don't touch? Which, when, and why? Infect Control Hosp Epidemiol 1993; 14: 273–275.
24. Phillips C. Hand hygiene. Nurs Times 1989; 86: 76–79.
25. Silver MR. On washing up [letter]. N Engl J Med 1992; 326: 958.
26. Turner J. Hand-washing behavior versus hand-washing guidelines in the ICU. Heart Lung 1993; 22: 275–277.
27. Ward K. Infection Control. Why not wash? Nurs Times 1992; 88: 68.
28. Watts GT. Handwashing and horizontal spread of viruses [letter]. Lancet 1989; 2: 218.
29. Weymont G. Hands. Nurs Times 1989; 84: 76–77.
30. Zeitlyn S, Islam F. The use of soap and water in two Bangladeshi communities: implications for the transmission of diarrhea. Rev Infect Dis 1991; 13(suppl 4): S259–264.
31. Bartlett AV, Jarvis BA, Ros V, et al. Diarrheal illness among infants and toddlers in day care centers: effects of active surveillance and staff training without subsequent monitoring. Am J Epidemiol 1988; 127: 804–817.
32. Boyce JM, Potter-Byrne G, Opal SM, et al. A common-source outbreak of *Staphylococcus epidermidis* infections among patients undergoing cardiac surgery. J Infect Dis 1990; 161: 494–499.
33. Butz AM, Larson E, Fosarelli P, Yolken R. Occurrence of infectious symptoms in children in day care homes. Am J Infect Control 1990; 6: 347–353.

34. Chorba TL, Meriwether RA, Jenkins BR, et al. Control of a non-foodborne outbreak of salmonellosis: day care in isolation. Am J Public Health 1987; 77: 979–981.
35. Clemens JD, Stanton BF. An educational intervention for altering water-sanitation behaviors to reduce childhood diarrhea in urban Bangladesh. I. Application of the case-control method for development of an intervention. Am J Epidemiol 1987; 125: 284–291.
36. Coovadia YM, Johnson AP, Bhana RH, et al. Multiresistant *Klebsiella aerogenes* in a neonatal nursery. The importance of infection control policies and procedures in the prevention of outbreaks. J Hosp Infect 1992; 22: 197–205.
37. Doebbeling BN, Stanley GL, Sheetz CT, et al. Comparative efficacy of alternative hand-washing agents in reducing nosocomial infections in intensive care units. N Engl J Med 1992; 327: 88–93.
38. Ehrenkranz NJ, Pfaff SJ. Mediastinitis complicating cardiac operations: evidence of postoperative causation. Rev Infect Dis 1991; 13: 803–814.
39. Guiguet M, Rekacewicz C, Leclercq B, et al. Effectiveness of simple measures to control an outbreak of nosocomial methicillin-resistant *Staphylococcus aureus* infections in an intensive care unit. Infect Control Hosp Epidemiol 1990; 11: 23–26.
40. Hlady WG, Bennett JV, Samadi AR, et al. Neonatal tetanus in rural Bangladesh: risk factors and toxoid efficacy. Am J Public Health 1992; 82: 1365–1369.
41. Issacs D, Dobson SR, Wilkinson AR, et al. Conservative management of an echovirus 11 outbreak in a neonatal unit. Lancet 1989; 1: 543–545.
42. Lee LA, Ostroff SM, McGee HB, et al. An outbreak of shigellosis at an outdoor music festival. Am J Epidemiol 1991; 133: 608–615.
43. Leroy O, Garenne M. Risk factors of neonatal tetanus in Senegal. Int J Epidemiol 1991; 20: 521–526.
44. Peters F, Flick-Filli'es D. Hand disinfection to prevent puerperal mastitis [letter]. Lancet 1991; 338: 831
45. Raad II, Sheretz RJ, Russell BA, Reuman PD. Uncontrolled nosocomial rotavirus transmission during a community outbreak. Am J Infect Control 1990; 18: 24–28.
46. Rubio PA. Septisol antiseptic foam: a sensible alternative to the conventional surgical scrub. Int Surg 1987; 72: 243–246.
47. Stanton BF, Clemens JD. An educational intervention for altering water-sanitation behaviors to reduce childhood diarrhea in urban Bangladesh. II. A randomized trial to assess the impact of the intervention of hygienic behaviors and rates of diarrhea. Am J Epidemiol 1987; 125: 292–301.
48. Watson JC, Fleming DW, Borella AJ, et al. Vertical transmission of hepatitis A resulting in an outbreak in a neonatal intensive care unit. J Infect Dis 1993; 167: 567–571.
49. Ayliffe GAJ, Babb JR, Davies JG, et al. Hygienic hand disinfection test in three laboratories. J Hosp Infect 1990; 16: 141–149.
50. Bellamy K, Alcock R, Babb R, et al. A test for the assessment of hygiene hand disinfection using rotavirus. J Hosp Infect 1993; 24: 201–210.

51. Bendig JWA. Surgical hand disinfection: a comparison of 4% chlorhexidine detergent solution and 2% triclosan detergent solution. J Hosp Infect 1990; 15: 143–148.
52. Butz AM, Laughon BE, Gullette DL, Larson EL. Alcohol-impregnated wipes as an alternatives in hand hygiene. Am J Infect Control 1990; 18: 70–76.
53. Cronin WA, Groschel DHM. A no-rinse alcohol antiseptic and a no-touch dispenser for hand decontamination. Infect Control Hosp Epidemiol 1989; 10: 80–83.
54. Doebbeling BN, Pfaller MA, Houston AK, Wenzel RP. Removal of nosocomial pathogens from the contaminated glove. Implications for glove reuse and handwashing. Ann Intern Med 1989; 109: 394–398.
55. Ehrenkranz NJ, Alfonso BC. Failure of bland soap handwash to prevent hand transfer of patient bacteria to urethral catheters. Infect Control Hosp Epidemiol 1991; 12: 654–662.
56. Faix RG. Comparative efficacy of handwashing agents against cytomegalovirus. Infect Control 1987; 8: 158–162.
57. Holloway PM, Platt JH, Reybrouck G, et al. A multi-centre evaluation of two chlorhexidine-containing formulations for surgical hand disinfection. J Hosp Infect 1990; 16: 151–159.
58. Hoque BA, Briend A. A comparison of local handwashing agents in Bangladesh. J Trop Med Hyg 1991; 94: 61–64.
59. Kolari PJ, Ojajarvi J, Laluharanta J, Makela P. Cleansing of hands with emulsion—a solution to skin problems of hospital staff? J Hosp Infect 1989; 13: 377–386.
60. Larson EL, Butz AM, Gullette DL, Laughon BA. Alcohol for surgical scrubbing? Infect Control Hosp Epidemiol 1990; 11: 139–143.
61. Larson E, Bobo L. Effective hand degerming in the presence of blood. J Emerg Med 1992; 10: 7–11.
62. Meers PD, Leong KY. Hot air hand dryers. J Hosp Infect 1989; 14: 169–171.
63. Nicoletti G, Boghossian V, Borland R. Hygienic hand disinfection: a comparative study with chlorhexidine detergents and soap. J Hosp Infect 1990; 15: 323–337.
64. Rotter ML, Koller W. Surgical hand disinfection: effect of sequential use of two chlorhexidine and preparations. J Hosp Infect 1990; 16: 161–166.
65. Takahashi S, Terao Y, Nagano Y. The effectiveness of ethanol gauze for hand disinfection in surgical wards. J Hosp Infect 10: 40–46.
66. Webster J, Faoagali JL. An in-use comparison of chlorhexidine gluconate 4% w/v, glycol-poly-siloxane plus methylcellulose and a liquid soap in a special care baby unit. J Hosp Infect 1989; 14: 141–151.
67. Webster J. Handwashing in a neonatal intensive care nursery: product acceptability and effectiveness of chlorhexidine gluconate 4% and triclosan 1%. J Hosp Infect 1993, 21: 137–141.
68. Campbell C. Could do better. Nurs Times 1988; 84: 66–71.
69. Conly JM, Hill S, Ross J, et al. Handwashing practices in an intensive care unit: the effects of an educational program and its relationship to infection rates. Am J Infect Control 1989; 17: 330–339.

70. Davenport SE. Frequency of hand washing by registered nurses caring for infants on radiant warmers and in incubators. Neonatal Netw 1992; 11: 21–25.
71. De Carvalho M, Lopes JM, Pellitteri M. Frequency and duration of handwashing in a neonatal intensive care unit. Pediatr Infect Dis J 1989; 8: 179–180.
72. Donowitz LG. Handwashing technique in a pediatric intensive care unit. Am J Dis Child 1987; 141: 683–685.
73. Dubbert PM, Dolce J, Richter W, et al. Increasing ICU staff handwashing: effects of education and group feedback. Infect Control Hosp Epidemiol 1990; 11: 191–193.
74. Gould D, Ream E. Assessing nurses' hand decontamination performance. Nurs Times 1993; 89: 47–50.
75. Graham M. Frequency and duration of handwashing in an intensive care unit. Am J Infect Control 1990; 18: 77–81.
76. Larson E, Mayur K, Laughon BA. Influence of two handwashing frequencies on reduction in colonizing flora with three handwashing products used by health care personnel. Am J Infect Control 1992; 17: 83–88.
77. Larson E, McGeer A, Quraishi ZA, et al. Effect of an automated sink on handwashing practices and attitudes in high-risk units. Infect Control Hosp Epidemiol 1991; 12: 422–428.
78. Lohr JA, Ingram DL, Dudley SM, et al. Handwashing in pediatric ambulatory settings. An inconsistent practice. Am J Dis Child 1991; 145: 1198–1199.
79. Marcil WM. Handwashing practices among occupational therapy personnel. Am J Occup Ther 1993; 47: 523–528.
80. Pritchard V, Hathaway C. Patient handwashing practice. Nurs Times 1988; 84: 68–72.
81. Raju TN, Kobler C. Improving handwashing habits in the newborn nurseries. Am J Med Sci 1991; 302: 355–358.
82. Roe BH. Study of the effects of education on the management of urine drainage systems by patients and carers. J Adv Nurs 1990; 15: 517–524.
83. Simmons B, Bryant J, Neiman K, et al. The role of handwashing in prevention of endemic intensive care unit infections. Infect Control Hosp Epidemiol 1990; 11: 589–594.
84. Williams E, Buckles A. A lack of motivation. Nurs Times 1990; 84: 60–64.
85. Zimakoff J, Stormark M, Larsen SO. Use of gloves and handwashing behaviour among health care workers in intensive care units. A multicentre investigation in four hospitals in Denmark and Norway. J Hosp Infect 1993; 24: 63–67.
86. deWit JC, Rombouts FM. Faecal micro-organisms on the hands of carriers: *Escherichia coli* as model for *Salmonella*. Zentralbl Hyg Umweltmed 1992; 193: 230–236.
87. Larson EL, McGinley KJ, Foglia A, et al. Handwashing practices and resistance and density of bacterial hand flora on two pediatric units in Lima, Peru. Am J Infect Control 1992; 20: 65–72.
88. Mbithi JN, Springthorpe VS, Boulet JR, Sattar SA. Survival of hepatitis A virus on human hands and its transfer on contact with animate and inanimate surfaces. J Clin Microbiol 1992; 30: 757–763.

89. Newsom SW, Rowland C. Application of the hygienic hand-disinfection test to the gloved hand. J Hosp Infect 1989; 142: 245–247.
90. Rayan GM, Flournoy DJ. Microbiologic flora of human fingernails. J Hand Surg [Am] 1987; 12: 605–607.
91. Doring G, Ulrich M, Muller W, et al. Generation of *Pseudomonas aeruginosa* aerosols during handwashing from contaminated sink drains, transmission to hands of hospital personnel, and its prevention by use of a new heating device. Zentralbl Hyg Umweltmed 1990; 191: 494–505.

ADDITIONAL ANNOTATED BIBLIOGRAPHY*

Ehrenkranz NJ. Bland soap handwashing or hand antisepsis? The pressing need for clarity. Infect Control Hosp Epidemiol 1992; 13: 299–301. Review article discussing the fact that it was chlorinated lime, a strong antiseptic, and not plain soap that resulted in reductions in puerperal sepsis rates during Semmelweis' time. It is vital to distinguish between hand cleaning and disinfection.

Grinbaum RS, de Mendonca JS, Cardo DM. An outbreak of handscrubbing-related surgical site infections in vascular surgical procedures. Infect Control Hosp Epidemiol 1995; 16: 198–202. In an outbreak (rate: cases, 66.7%; controls, 16.7%) of surgical site infections after vascular surgery (limb amputations and arterial reconstruction), use of antiseptic hand scrub was the only significant difference between groups ($P < .00001$).

Lee YL, Cesario T, Lee R, et al. Colonization with *Staphylococcus* species resistant to methicillin or quinolone on hands of medical personnel in a skilled-nursing facility. Am J Infect Control 1994; 22: 346–351. Hands of patient care personnel ($n=129$) in a skilled nursing facility were significantly more likely to be colonized with methicillin- and quinolone-resistant strains of coagulase-negative staphylococci than hands of nonpatient care personnel ($n=40$).

Nystrom B. Impact of handwashing on mortality in intensive care: examination of the evidence. Infect Control Hosp Epidemiol 1994; 15: 435–436. Discusses difficulties of demonstrating a causal link between handwashing and infections. For example, it would take about 110,000 patients to show a statistically significant difference in nosocomial infection rates for pneumonia if proper handwashing halved the rate. Hands are readily contaminated during patient care; organisms are readily transferred (about 85%); washing reduces contamination; without washing, transfer of organisms occurs; with washing, transfer decreases. Therefore, all supporting and logical data lead one to conclude that handwashing plays an important role in reducing infections.

---

*References in alphabetical order according to category.

Perceval A. Wash hands, disinfect hands, or don't touch? Which, when, and why? Infect Control Hosp Epidemiol 1993; 14: 273–275. Handwashing is not benign. It can cause skin damage and increase costs. Hence, it is important to establish its most effective and appropriate use. The author suggests that it is preferable to emphasize no-touch technique and protection of patient entry sites when possible and that studies of handwashing should assess cost effectiveness and instances in which handwashing is actually required to prevent infections.

Zafar AB, Butler RC, Reese DJ, et al. Use of a 0.3% triclosan (Bacti-Stat) to eradicate an outbreak of methicillin-resistant *Staphylococcus aureus* in a neonatal nursery. Am J Infect Control 1995; 23: 200–208. A variety of aggressive efforts were unsuccessful in eradicating an outbreak of MRSA in a neonatal nursing. Implementation of handwashing and baby bathing with 0.3% triclosan soap was associated with immediate termination of the outbreak, with no additional cases occurring in 3.5 years of follow-up.

10
Pathogenesis of Dermatophytosis

Azer Rashid
Khyber Medical College, Peshawar, Pakistan

M. D. Richardson
University of Glasgow, Glasgow, Scotland

The infection caused by dermatophyte fungi in the keratinized tissue such as hair, nails and stratum corneum of the skin is known as dermatophytosis. It is among the most prevalent mycotic infections in the world (1). Its incidence is highest in hot, humid climates or in crowded environments where a high standard of hygiene is difficult to maintain. An important characteristic of the dermatophytes as parasites is their restriction to the dead keratinized tissue. Dermatophytes fail to invade the deeper layers of the skin because they cannot survive in the presence of serum; only in the keratinized tissue are they protected from a serum inhibitory factor (2).

The inflammatory response of ringworm infection involves the dermis and stratum malpighi of the epidermis, but the fungus itself is found growing only within the stratum corneum, within and around the fully keratinized hair and in the nail plate and keratinized nail bed. While all dermatophytes invade the stratum corneum, different species vary widely in their capacity to invade hair and nail. *Trichophyton rubrum* rarely invades the hair but frequently invades nail. *Epidermophyton floccosum* never invades the hair and only occasionally the nail. *T. mentagrophytes var. interdigitale* is commonly associated with tinea pedis (1). The clinical appearance of the various forms of ringworm infection depends largely on the body sites affected. The lesion results as a combination of direct damage to the keratinized tissue by the fungus (mainly in hair and nail infections) and the inflammatory manifestations. Destruction and disorganization of hair and nail occur with various degrees of intensity whenever they are involved. Various factors modify the basic type of lesion, including site of infection. Classically, the lesions of ringworm infection are scaly, erythematovesicular with peripheral extension and central clearing, which may occur anywhere on the trunk and limbs. The fungal hyphae are present at the periphery of the lesion in the active or inflammatory border and the annular lesions usually described are thought to be due to increased epidermal turnover at the periphery of the lesion (3).

Dermatophyte lesions cease to grow after they have attained a certain size, and spontaneous resolution of these lesions is not uncommon. Clinical symptoms often disappear even if left untreated (4). This most probably occurs because of the development of cell-mediated immunity. In some cases, however, the lesions do not heal and the infection becomes chronic (5). Dermatophytosis is not a debilitating or life-threatening infection, and serious invasive disease has been reported, but only in patients who are immunosuppressed (6). It is transmissile from person to person directly by means of contact or indirectly via formites contaminated with infected skin scales or hairs, and it can be acquired by humans from infected animals and by direct exposure to infected soil. Essentially, all humans come into contact with dermatophyte fungi during their lives, but only a small percentage of people manifest clinical symptoms of disease. Some people, therefore, feel that dermatophytosis is not a contagious disease (1).

HOST-PARASITE INTERACTIONS IN DERMATOPHYTOSIS

Mediators of Disease Transmission in Dermatophytosis

Dermatophytosis is unique among mycotic infections because of the communicable nature of the infection. There have been many outbreaks of dermatophytosis in schools, orphanages, chronic care institutions, dormitories, and other places (7). Disease transmission is mediated by two distinctly different types of propagules depending on the source of infection. From saprophytic sources such as soil or shed scales of animals, the disease is transmitted to others by saprophytic conidia, macroconidia, or microconidia, whereas from humans the disease is transmitted to others by parasitic conidia, arthroconidia (7). All these conidia possess the property of dormancy and resistance (7–10). No saprophytic conidia are produced by dermatophytes undergoing parasitization, and possibly the mechanism controlling saprophytic conidiogenesis in the dermatophytes is suppressed under the state of parasitization (7). Arthroconidia are the only infective conidia produced under parasitic conditions, the natural pathogenic elements of the dermatophytes, the major mediator of disease transmission in dermatophytosis (11, 12), and the only form of conidia found in tissues (7,13). Kilgman (14) suggested that arthroconidia were the main source of transmission of dermatophytes from one person to another, being present or surviving in fallen hair, and loosened squames. It is further supported by the fact that arthroconidia are the only resistant morphologies produced by the dermatophytes during parasitization and that viable dermatophytes can be recovered from clinical specimens of skin, hair, and nails stored for extended period of time under adverse conditions (15). Many surveys have shown that dermatophytes can be isolated from combs, brushes, the back of theatre seats, caps, bed linen, towels, undergarments, and jockstraps. Locker rooms, shower floors, and communal shower rooms are often contaminated with skin debris containing infective arthroconidia (7).

Aljabre et al. (12) demonstrated that germination of arthroconidia and hyphal penetration were important factors in the pathogenicity of *Trichophyton*. Further convincing evidence that dermatophyte arthroconidia are infective and capable of transmitting infections was obtained by experimental induction of tinea pedis in guinea pigs by inoculating *T. mentagropytes* arthroconidia. The lesions produced were clinically and histopathologically similar to human infection (16).

The infectious arthroconidia are very resistant to environmental extremes and are able to survive up to 20 months in a viable state in skin and hair (15). Therefore the original contact with the arthroconidia is usually indirect, and adherence of infected hair or skin scale carrying the arthroconidia is the major way by which dermatophyte fungi are transmitted from one source to another (17). The arthroconidia of *T. mentagrophytes* demonstrate an exogenous type of dormancy provided that the conditions are not lethal. Aljabre et al. (10) have shown that dormant arthroconidia can germinate when conditions become suitable. As arthroconidia are formed by fragmentation of hyphae, these dermatophyte spores are most suitable for the growth of dermatophytes in the stratum corneum, unlike macroconidia or microconidia, which are formed laterally on the hyphae, thus requiring a space for their expansive growth (7). The precise mechanisms involved in the formation of arthroconidia in the tissues are not clear. King et al. (18) suggested that arthroconidial formation in lesions may be stimulated by the diffusion of carbon dioxide through the skin. Allen and King (19) demonstrated that occlusion of the skin rendered it more susceptible to dermatophyte infection by raising the carbon dioxide tension on the skin surface. Hashimoto (7) suggested that elevated temperature, high humidity, high carbon dioxide tension, and some stimulatory metabolites may all contribute to arthroconidiation of the dermatophytes in the skin.

In vitro formation of arthroconidia has been studied extensively (7,20,21). Emmons (22) described arthroconidia in dermatophyte culture growing in vitro, although generally the formation of parasitic arthroconidia requires a living host. The most critical factor affecting arthroconidiogenesis in dermatophytes appears to be the incubation temperature. Temperatures between 32°C and 39°C (37°C optimal) strongly favor arthroconidiation of T. mentagrophytes in Sabouraud dextrose broth (21). Other factors important for arthroconidia formation in dermatophytes include medium pH, high humidity, carbon dioxide concentration, and certain stimulatory metabolites (7). In vitro conditions for arthroconidia formation bear some resemblance to factors present physiologically in the skin. It is possible that as yet unidentified cutaneous factors may be involved with predisposing physiological conditions in arthroconidia formation in vivo (17). It is possible, that, like in plants, some form of chemical signal or topographical signal along with temperature signals may be involved. Fungi respond morphologically to a varied array of physical and chemical signals, including touch, light, pheromones and nutrients (23). Signalling processes have been elucidated in mammalian cell systems and the major signal transduction pathways are active in keratinocytes (24). Cyclic AMP cascade is involved in the control of dormancy and induction of germination in fungal spores (25). The presence of transmembrane signalling systems and receptors in dermatophytes has not yet been elucidated.

Mechanism of Disease Initiation in Dermatophytosis

Dissemination of dermatophyte fungi depends on direct or indirect contact between infected and uninfected hosts. The first step in the infection process is colonization of the cornified surface of the stratum corneum. The initial contact between arthroconidia and stratum corneum seems to be the important event in the establishment and initiation of skin, hair, and nail infection (17). With the exception of white superficial onychomycosis in which the nail is invaded directly on its surface, nail and hair are infected from the adjacent stratum corneum. Zurita and Hay (26) and Aljabre et al. (27) have demonstrated the interaction between dermatophyte arthroconidia and corneocytes, and the importance of close adherence in initiation of infection. Arthroconidia seem to be able to adhere to all body surfaces including face, back of hand, palm, leg and sole (27). Adherence of arthroconidia to corneocytes occurs by 6 hours and increases with time. Aljabre et al. (27) showed that the number of corneocytes with adherent arthroconidia and number of arthroconidia adhering per corneocyte increases with time. Experimental tinea pedis has been incited in guinea pigs with a relatively small number of arthroconidia (16). Once an arthroconidium has made contact with stratum corneum, it becomes firmly adherent, possibly by some form of physical or chemical binding taking place between the arthroconidia and corneocyte. Ultrastructurally, there is close contact between dermatophyte arthroconidia and corneocyte with the presence of a fibrillar-floccular material in the space between the arthroconidial outer wall and corneocyte membrane (27,28). The nature and origin of this material, whether from the arthroconidial wall, the corneocyte, or both are not clear. Arthroconidia of dermatophytes undergo swelling before emergence of a germ tube (29), and the crenated surface of corneocytes flatten forming a hollow where arthroconidia adhere (28). The significance of these changes on arthroconidial adherence to corneocytes is not understood.

It is clear that arthroconidial adherence to human corneocytes is an early stage in colonization of the skin by dermatophytes. Adherence prevents arthroconidial detachment from host surfaces and enables them to remain on the stratum corneum and develop into the hyphal form and establish infection. Aljabre et al. (12) showed that germination of arthroconidia and hyphal penetration of stratum corneum are important factors in the pathogenicity of *T. mentagrophytes*. The arthroconidia must germinate very rapidly and penetrate the body surface. If not they will be lost by continuous desquamation of epithelium (17). Germination of arthroconidia occurs very rapidly, usually in 4 to 6 hours (12) and is the first step in the development of fungal mycelium from arthroconidia. By 7 days a well-formed mycelium is observed on stratum corneum (12). The corneocytes express soluble factors, which when added to isolated arthroconidia, induce germination. Factors isolated and characterized from corneocytes of human skin promote germination of arthroconidia (17). Moisture in the skin appears to break the dormancy of arthroconidia and encourage germination (17). Desquamated skin scales are normally dry, but if there is an increase in the moisture content, as in a shower cubicle or swimming pool, the state of dormancy is broken, and germination and penetration of host surface can then commence (30). Arthroconidia invading corneocytes demonstrate prolonged survival, which suggests that the stratum corneum confers some form of protection to arthroconidia and is epidemiologically significant as by increasing the longevity and thereby the infectivity of arthroconidia (30).

The next phase of infection is the penetration of the stratum corneum by the invasive germlings. This process has been studied by stripping layers of stratum corneum from body surfaces with adhesives (31), and then inoculating with arthroconidia (12). The penetration of the stratum corneum starts with the emergence of germ tubes from arthroconidia, which are lying extracellularly. Germ tubes invade corneocytes and grow transversely, between the layers, and through the thickness of the stratum corneum. The horizontal extension results in the clinically observable sign of peripheral expansion of lesion in dermatophytosis. Microcolonies develop, and the developing hyphae disarticulate into arthroconidia completing the cycle (12). The penetration of germ tubes into deeper layers of the stratum corneum has been seen in experimentally induced dermatophytosis (16). Intracellular location of dermatophytes has been seen (32). The mechanism by which germ tubes rupture the corneocyte membrane is not clear, although it is thought to be a combination of chemical and mechanical forces (17).

Dermatophytes produce enzymes capable of keratin digestion. Keratinases have been detected in lesions of experimental dermatophytosis in guinea pigs using fluorescent antibody probes (33).

Some of the extracellular hydrolytic enzymes produced by dermatophytes include proteases, lipases, phosphatases, nucleases, and glucosidases. Among these, proteolytic enzymes, keratinase, collagenase, and elastase are most frequently implicated in the pathogenesis of dermatophytosis (7). Some of these enzymes are involved in facilitating the penetration of germ tubes or hyphae into keratinous epidermal tissues, securing nutrients for fungal growth, and eliciting local inflammatory immune responses. It is not yet clear whether these enzymes play any significant role in disease initiation in dermatophytosis (34). From the pathogenic point of view, adherence of arthroconidia to corneocytes, along with their germination and penetration of the stratum corneum, can be regarded as mechanisms operative in the establishment of dermatophytosis.

HOST DEFENSE MECHANISMS AGAINST DERMATOPHYTOSIS

The mechanisms that defend the host against dermatophyte infections can be arbitrarily divided into local defenses such as the skin and systemic defenses such as the nonspecific and specific immune systems.

The skin is a tough, resistant, multilayered structure whose main function is protection. The epidermis is constantly proliferating, and hence corneocytes are shed from its surface. For dermatophytes to establish an infection, the arthroconidia must adhere and then rapidly germinate, and the growth of the fungus must keep pace with the rate of epidermiopioeosis and exfoliation (17). Increased susceptibility to dermatophyte infection of the palms occurs in patients with palmo-plantar keratoderma where there is excessive retention of stratum corneum (35). In psoriasis, which is characterized by hyperproliferation of the epidermis, the incidence of dermatophyte infection is low (36). Dry intact stratum corneum acts as a barrier against infection (37), and moist areas between toes in shoe wearing people and the groin in males are particularly susceptible. Macerated skin appears to provide an excellent environment for germination of infective arthroconidia (17).

The stratum corneum is covered with a film made up of the products of keratinization (desquamated cornecocytes), sweat and products of sebaceous glands (surface lipids), and a unique microbial flora. Unsaturated fatty acids found in sebum inhibit some dermatophytes in vitro. Resistance of adult scalp to tinea capitis and the spontaneous clearing of tinea capitis in children at puberty at a time when greater quantities of sebum begin to be formed has been attributed to the presence of fatty acids. Another factor to be considered is sweat, which is thought to be inhibitory to the growth of dermatophytes, possibly because of vitamin K-like substances (17). Human serum has been reported to have a factor inhibitory to dermatophytes which is possibly involved in limiting the growth of the dermatophyte fungi to the stratum corneum. King et al. (38) identified this factor as unsaturated transferrin. In inhibits growth of dermatophytes by binding to iron, which organisms need for growth. Transferrin in serum is thought to diffuse through the epidermis to the stratum corneum and inhibit fungal growth (4). Dermatophytes grow poorly at 37°C, which may explain why deep infections with dermatophytes are almost unknown. Failure of immunity in persistent infections and its relationship with chronicity are not understood, but there seems to be an association between atopy and chronic dermatophytosis. For example, Kaaman (40) found a decreased proportion of T-helper cells and increased number of T-suppressor cells in patients with chronic infections.

Antibody response occurs in the inflammatory and noninflammatory type of infection. The cell-mediated immune response as indicated by delayed type hypersensitivity occurs more readily in the inflammatory type of infection (41). Antibodies appear to have no protective effect in dermatophytosis. Dermatophyte infections mostly occur in perfectly healthy people, but can be more frequent and severe in immunodeficient patients. Another factor important in the susceptibility and resistance to infection is malnutrition, where fungal infections are more common. Increased susceptibility to ringworm occurs in patients with Cushing's syndrome and possibly diabetes. There are age and sex related factors and similarly genetic and racial factors. There seems to be an increased incidence of dermatophytosis in the elderly. Tinea cruris (groin ringworm) is unheard of in females; tinea pedis, tinea cruris and tinea unguium are more common in males. Tinea capitis is more common in boys. Negroid skin seems to be relatively less susceptible to dermatophyte infection than Caucasoid. In Negroid skin, there is less inflammation to infection than skin of other races. Tinea corporis caused by *T. rubrum* is particularly intractable in blacks. Susceptibility to tinea imbricata is inherited as an autosomal recessive characteristic (42).

Systematic immunological responses induced by dermatophytes are both antibody and cell mediated. The noninflammatory system is the primary defense of the nonimmune host because it does not require previous exposure to the invading organism for activation and can respond immediately to protect the host against invading fungus. Acquired immunoresistance mechanisms appear after adequate exposure to the organisms.

A very early event in the host reaction to invasion by dermatophytes includes infiltration of neutrophils and epidermal oedema (43). To a lesser extent, monocytes accumulate in the epidermal infiltrate, probably in response to chemotactic components of the dermatophyte cells such as C5a anaphylatoxin via the alternative complement pathway (4). Dermatophytes are damaged by toxic oxidative products produced by neutrophils and are destroyed by neutrophils extracellularly. Dermatophyte arthroconidia do not need an opsonin for ingestion by neutrophils to take place and can be readily ingested by neutrophils (30). The precise role played by the chemotactic epidermal cytokines, particularly interleukin 8, in the accumulation of neutrophils at the site of dermatophyte infections is not clear (44).

From dermatophyte experimental infection studies in animals and humans, and in natural human infections, T-cell responses such as the development of delayed hypersensitivity to dermatophyte antigens correlates not only with the development of inflammation in ringworm, but also with spontaneous recovery. Chronic infections are associated with poor T-lymphocyte-mediated immune response to specific fungal antigens. The ultimate establishment of dermatophytosis and the subsequent course of the infection are influenced by other host factors such as innate immune state, previous exposure to dermatophytes, or inherent genetic predisposition.

Other experimental systems, such as organ culture of hair follicles (45), a living skin equivalent (46), and a nail model (47) have been used to study further the pathogenesis of dermatophyte growth in specific micro-environments.

ACKNOWLEDGMENTS

The authors would like to thank the staff of the Department of Dermatology, University of Glasgow, UK, for their assistance in carrying out this work.

REFERENCES

1. Rippon JW. Dermatophytosis and dermatomycosis. In: Rippon JW, ed. Medical Mycology. The Pathogenic Fungi and the Pathogenic Actinomycetes. 3d ed. Philadelphia: WB Saunders, 1988: 169–275.
2. Carlisle DH, Inouye JC, King RD, Jones HE. Significance of serum fungal inhibitory factor in dermatophytosis. J Invest Dermatol 1974; 63: 239–241.
3. Berk SH, Penneys NS, Weinstein GD. Epidermal activity in annular dermato-phytosis. Arch Dermatol 1976; 112: 485–488.
4. Jones HE, Reinhardt JH, Rinaldi MG. Acquired immunity to dermatophytes. Arch Dermatol 1974; 109: 840–848.
5. Hay RJ. Chronic dermatophyte infections. I. Clinical and mycological features. Br J Dermatol 1982; 106: 1–7.
6. Ashmed AR. Immunology of human dermatophyte infections. Arch Dermatol 1982; 118: 521–525.
7. Hashimoto T. Infectious propagules of dermatophytes. In Cole GT, Hoch HC, eds. The Fungal Spore and Disease Initiation in Plants and Animals. New York: Plenum Press. 1991: 181–202.
8. Hashimoto T, Blumenthal HJ, Survival and resistance of *Trichophyton mentagro-phytes* arthrospores. Appl Environ Microbiol 1978; 35: 274–277.
9. Aljabre SHM, Scott EM, Shankland GS, Richardson MD. In vitro susceptibility of *Trichophyton mentagrophytes* arthroconidia to clotrimazole and griseofulvin in human corneocyte suspensions. Mycoses 1991; 34: 479–482.
10. Aljabre SHM, Richardson MD, Scott EM, Shankland GS. Dormancy of *Tricho-phyton mentagrophyes* arthroconidia. J Med Vet Mycol 1992; 30: 409–412.
11. Hashimoto T, Blumenthal HJ. Factors affecting germination of *Trichophyton mentagrophytes* arthrospores. Infect Immun 1977; 18: 479–486.
12. Aljabre SHM, Richardson MD, Scott EM, Shankland GS. Germination of *Tricho-phyton mentagrophytes* on human stratum corneum in vitro. J Med Vet Mycol 1992; 30: 145–152.

13. Gotz H. Zur morphologie der pilzelemente im stratum comeum beitinea (Epidermophytia) pedis, manus et Inguinalis. Mycopathol Mycol Appl 1959; 12: 124–140.
14. Kligman AM. Tinea capitis due to *M. audouini* and *M. canis*. II. Dynamics of the hostparasite relationship. Arch Dermatol 1955; 71: 313–337.
15. Dvorak J, Hubalek Z, Otcenasek M. Survival of dermatophytes in human skin scales. Arch Dermatol 1968; 98: 540–542.
16. Fujita S, Matsuyama T. Experimental tinea pedis induced by non-abrasive inoculation of *Trichophyton mentagrophytes* arthrospores on the plantar part of a guinea pig foot. J Med Vet Mycol 1987; 25: 203–213.
17. Richardson MD, Aljabre SHM. Pathogenesis of dermatophytosis. In: Borgers M, Hay RJ, Rinaldi MG, eds. Current Topics in Medical Mycology, Vol. 5. Barcelona: J Prous, 1993: 49–77.
18. King AD, Dillavou CL, Greenberg JH, et al. Identification of carbon dioxide as a dermatophyte inhibitory factor produced by *Candida albicans*. Can J Microbiol 1976; 2: 1720–1727.
19. Allen AM, King AD. Occlusion, carbon dioxide and fungal skin infections. Lancet 1978; 8060: 360–362.
20. Bibel DJ, Crumrine KY, King RD. Development of arthrospores of *Trychophyton mentagrophytes*. Infect Human 1977; 16: 958–971.
21. Emyanitoff AG, Hashimoto T. The effects of temperature, incubation atmosphere and medium composition on arthrospore formation in the fungus *Trichophyton mentagrophytes*. Can J Microbiol 1979; 25: 362–366.
22. Emmons CW. Dermatophyte: natural grouping based on the forms of the spores and accessory organs. Arch Dermatol Syphilol 1934; 30: 337–362.
23. Hoch HC, Staples RC, Staples RC. Signaling for infection structures formation in fungi. In: Cole GT, Hoch HC, eds. The Fungal Spore and Disease Initiation in Plants and Animals. New York: Plenum Press, 1881: 25–46.
24. Rosenbach T, Czarnetzki B. Signal transduction pathways in keratinocytes. Exp Dermatol 1992; 1: 59–66.
25. Thevelein JM. Activation of trehalase by membrane-depolarizing agent in yeast vegetative cells and ascospores. J Bacteriol 1984; 158: 337–339.
26. Zurita J, Hay RJ. Adherence of dermatophyte microconidia and arthroconidia to human keratinocytes in vitro. J Invest Dermatol 1987; 89: 529–534.
27. Aljabre SMH, Richardson MD, Scott EM, et al. Adherence of arthroconidia and germlings of anthropophilic and zoophilic varieties of *Trichophyton mentagrophytes* to human corneocytes as an early event in the pathogenesis of dermatophytosis. Clin Exp Dermatol 1993; 18: 231–235.
28. Rashid A, Scott EM, Richardson MD. Effect of terbinafine exposure on the ultrastructure of *Trichophyton interdigitale*. J Med Vet Mycol 1993; 31: 305–315.
29. Scott EM, Gorman SP, Wright LP. The effect of imidazoles on germination of arthrospores and microconidia to *Trichophyton metagrophytes*. J Antimicrob Chemother 1984; 13: 101–110.
30. Richardson MD. Diagnosis and pathogenesis of dermatophyte infection. Br J Clin Pract 1990; 71: 98–102.

31. Knight AG. Culture of dermatophytes upon stratum corneum. J Invest Dermatol 1973; 59: 427–431.
32. Miyazaki H, Seiji M, Takaki Y. Electron microscopic study on fungi in horny layer. Jpn J Dermatol 1966; 76: 265–271.
33. Koga M, Sei Y, Higuchi D, Takiuchi I. Partial purification and the localization of keratinase in plantar horny layer infected with tinea pedis. Jpn J Med Mycol 1986; 27: 107–112.
34. Odds FC. Potential for penetration of passive barriers to fungal invasions in humans. In: Cole GT, Hoch CT, eds. The Fungal Spore and Disease Initiation in Plants and Animals. New York: Plenum Press, 1981: 287–295.
35. Neilson PG. Immunological aspects of dermatophyte infections in hereditary palmoplantar keratoderma. Act Derm Venereol (Stockh) 1984; 64: 296–301.
36. Fransson J, Storgards K, Hammar H. Palmoplantar lesions in psoriatic patients and their relation to inverse psoriasis, tinea infection and contact allergy. Acta Derm Venereol (Stockh) 1985; 65: 218–223.
37. Richardson MD. Newly-recognised fungal infections originating from cutaneous sites in immunocomprised patients. Rev Med Microbiol 1991; 2: 61–67.
38. King RD, Khan HA, Faye JC, et al. Transferrin, iron and dermatophytes. I. Serum dermatophyte inhibitory component definitively identified as unsaturated transferrin. Lab Clin Med 1975; 86: 204–212.
39. Jones HE. The atopic-chronic-dermatophytosis syndrome. Acta Derm Venereol (Stockh) 1980; 92: 81–85.
40. Kaaman T. Dermatophyte antigens and cell-mediated immunity in dermatophytosis. In: McGinnis MR, ed. Current Topics in Medical Mycology, Vol. 1. Berlin: Springer-Verlag, 1985: 117–134.
41. Svejgaard E. Immunologic investigations of dermatophytes and dermatophytosis. Semin Dermatol 1985; 4: 201–221.
42. Hay RJ, Roberts SOB, Mackenzie DWR. Mycology. In: Champion RH, Buton JL, Ebling F, eds. Textbook of Dermatology, 5th Ed. Oxford: Blackwell Scientific Publications, 1992: 1134–1170.
43. Ackeman AB. Subtle cues to diagnosis by conventional microscopy. Neutrophils within the cornified layer as clues to infection by superficial fungi. Am J Dermatopathol 1979; 1: 69–75.
44. Schroder JM. Chemotactic cytokines in the epidermis. Exp Dermatol 1992; 1: 12–19.
45. Rashid A, Hodgins MB, Richardson MD. An *in vitro* model of dermatophyte invasion of the human hair follicle. J Med Vet Mycol 1996; 34, 37–42.
46. Rashid A, Edward M, Richardson MD. Growth of dermatophyte fungi on a human living skin equivalent. Br J Dermatol 1993; 129: 495.
47. Rashid A, Scott EM, Richardson MD. Early events in the invasion of the human nail plate by *Trichophyton mentagrophytes*. Br J Dermatol 1995; 133: 932–940.

11

Tinea Pedis: Epidemiology, Clinical Manifestations, Pathophysiology, and Therapy

Raza Aly
University of California School of Medicine, San Francisco, California

INTRODUCTION

Tinea pedis refers to dermatophytosis that includes several clinically distinctive infections of the foot. Dermatophytes are primarily involved for these infections. Some nondermatophytes such as *Scytalidium* are also implicated in patients living in tropical and subtropical areas. Tinea pedis is the most common fungus infection, having passed tinea capitis, formerly the most common infection. As the incidence of tinea capitis diminished, the incidence of tinea pedis increased. The style of wearing closed shoes and sneakers probably contributes to the increasing frequency of the disease

EPIDEMIOLOGY

Infection of the feet is the most common form of superficial fungal infection. Up to 70% of the population has had this infection (1). Tinea pedis is common in adult men and less so in women and children. Although tinea pedis is a common disease, it did not exist as a separate entity until the 1940s and 1950s. The incidence of tinea pedis increased in the late nineteenth century with the introduction of *Trichophyton rubrum* into Europe and the Americas as a result of worldwide travel. It is speculated that the

Table 1 Frequency of Organisms Isolated in Tinea Pedis

Patients	Dermato-phytes	Candida	Others	Dermatophyte percentages
171	92%	6%	2%	Trichophyton rubrum 79%
				Trichophyton mentagrophytes 11%
				Epidermophyton floccosum 9%
				Trichophyton tonsurans 1%

original endemic area of *T. rubrum* was Southeast Asia. However, this organism did not cause tinea pedis in this population because the people generally do not wear shoes. It is generally agreed that tinea pedis is more common among people frequenting swimming pools or using community washing facilities such as army camps, boarding schools, or prisons. The high frequency of *Trichophyton rubrum, Trichophyton mentagrophytes* and *Epidermophyton floccosum* found in swimming pools during the summer months testifies to the effective spread of tinea pedis. Tinea pedis occurs mostly among people who wear shoes. There is a maxim that "tinea pedis follows in the footsteps of shoe-wearing nations." The single most important factor that regulates the incidence, prevalence, and severity of tinea pedis is occlusion (2). Taplin was able to reproduce the severe inflammatory type of tinea pedis by inoculating socks with zoophilic strains of *T. mentagrophytes* (3). The socks were worn under occlusive boots. A severe, persistent tinea pedis was produced.

Frequency of organisms isolated from tinea pedis in the San Francisco Bay Area is shown in Table 1. *T. rubrum* was the major etiological agent (79%), followed by *T. mentagrophytes* (11%). *Scytalidium* was not noted in this population.

CLINICAL TYPES OF TINEA PEDIS

There are three general clinical types of tinea pedis (Table 2): (a) interdigital type, (b) "moccasin" or chronic hyperkeratotic type, and (c) highly inflammatory vesiculobullous type.

Interdigital Type of Tinea Pedis

The interdigital form of tinea pedis is the most common type (Figure 1). The clinical spectrum ranges from relatively asymptomatic mild scaling to

Table 2 Causative Agents of Tinea Pedis

Pattern	Causative organism
Interdigital type	*Trichophyton rubrum* *Trichophyton mentagrophytes var. interdigitale* (downy) *Epidermophyton floccosum* *Candida albicans* *Scytalidium dimidiatum* *Scytalidium hyalinum*
Moccasin type	*T. rubrum* *T. mentagrophytes var. interdigitale* *E. floccosum* *C. albicans* *S. dimidiatum* *S. hyalinum*
Inflammatory	*T. mentagrophytes var. mentagrophytes* (granular)

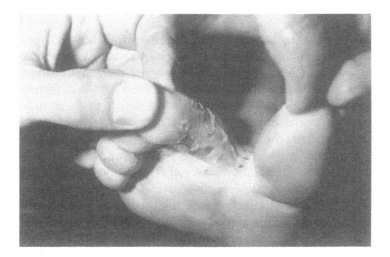

Figure 1 Interdigital type of tinea pedis: exudative, macerated lesions, *T. rubrum* infection.

exudative, macerated, malodorous conditions. The recovery of dermato-phytes from exudative, macerated toe web infections has been low. This mystery has been at least partially explained by new insights with the microbial ecology of interdigital space after invasion by a dermatophyte (4,5).

In macerated, malodorous, highly symptomatic infected interspaces, there is an overgrowth of various bacterial species, including *Brevibacterium epidermidis*, *Corynebacterium minutissimum*, *Micrococcus sedentarius*, *Pseudomonas* and *Proteus* species, and *Staphylococcus aureus*. Many of these bacteria are resistant to penicillin and penicillin derivatives, and their proliferation may be caused by the production of penicillin- and streptomycin-like antibiotics by dermatophytes (6). In the presence of a stratum corneum damaged by dermatophyte invasion, these ecologically advantaged bacteria proliferate and induce inflammation. *M. sedentarius* and *B. epidermidis* also produce a variety of thioesters, which have an extremely pungent malodor and are fungicidal. This ecological interaction explains the transition from a simple scaling process (dermatophytosis simplex) in which fungi are readily recovered, into a macerated, malodorous, symptomatic process (dermatophytosis complex) in which fungus is recovered in only a small percentage of cases.

Plantar Moccasin Type of Tinea Pedis

This type of tinea pedis is a minimally inflammatory infection, characterized by a dull erythema, dryness, scaling, and hyperkeratosis affecting the entire plantar skin of both feet in sandal or moccasin distribution (Figure 2). At times, one hand will be similarly involved with this diffuse scaling condition. These patients seem to have a defect in their cell-mediated immunity and are unable to mount a delayed-type hypersensitivity response, which is the host mechanism by which fungi are eliminated. Many patients are atopics or have a history of family or personal atopy. These patients do not show delayed response to *Trichophyton* antigen. Patients with moccasin type of tinea pedis often have onychomycosis (Figure 3). This type of infection is recalcitrant to ordinary treatments. The resistance could be due to the fact that stratum corneum of the plantar surface is too thick for drugs to penetrate. For successful treatment of this type of tinea pedis, toe nail infection should also be dealt with. *T. rubrum*, which is frequently associated with moccasin tinea pedis, is less efficient in eliciting T-cell response.

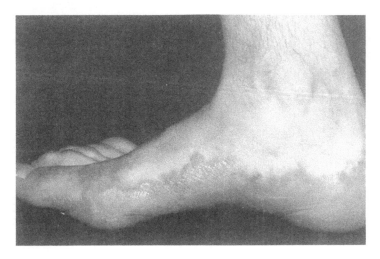

Figure 2 Plantar moccasin type of tinea pedis: *T. rubrum* infection.

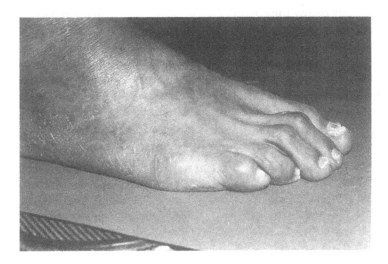

Figure 3 Moccasin type of tinea pedis associated with onychomycosis.

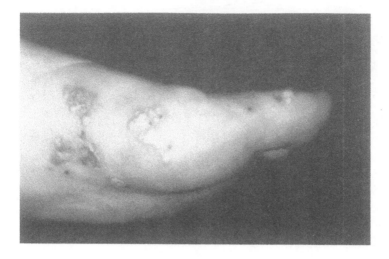

Figure 4 Vesiculobullous type of tinea pedis, *T. mentagrophytes* infection.

Vesiculobullous Type of Tinea Pedis

Intense inflammatory vesicular infections occur anywhere on the foot. The eruptions occur typically with vesicles and bullae in clusters (Figure 4). During primary infection, sensitized T cells appear in the living layers of the skin immediately below fungus-infected stratum corneum (7). In cases where the T-effector cell response to fungal antigen is vigorous, an inflammatory reaction starts, and the skin becomes intensely inflamed; that is, an allergic contact dermatitis occurs. At times the inflammatory response is so acute that cellulitis, lymphangitis, and adenopathy may occur and is incapacitating. *T. mentagrophytes* is usually associated with these lesions.

During the Vietnam War, in addition to toe web and plantar surface infection, severe infections of the dorsal surfaces of the feet and ankles were often present under the wet boots. This condition caused a major difficulty in walking. Secondary bacterial pyodermas or cellulitis often complicated these infections (8).

TREATMENT

Two parameters should be considered in determining care of a fungal infection: clinical cure with reduction in erythema and scaling and mycological cure evaluated by potassium hydroxide (KOH) preparations and cultures. Total cure can be achieved only when both of these criteria are met. In recent years, there has been a rapid increase in the number of topical and systemic fungal agents. These agents (imidazoles, triazoles, and allylamines) inhibit the synthesis of ergosterol, the main sterol constituent of fungal cell walls, which is vital to cell growth. Unlike imidazoles and triazoles, allylamines do not interact with cytochrome-P450 mammalian enzymes (9). The azoles and allylamines work differently than griseofulvin, which inhibits microtubule formation and blocks mitosis. Terbinafine seems to have an additional advantage in that this agent is fungicidal in vitro. The rapid response and high cure rate without relapse after a brief course of therapy suggest in vivo fungicidal activity.

With large numbers of antifungal agents both topical and oral, the clinician has an extensive menu from which to choose a treatment (Table 3). Long-term experience with topical imidazole derivatives and ciclopirox olamine has confirmed their safety, clinical efficacy, and reliability in controlling fungal infections.

Table 3 Prescription and Over-the-Counter Topical Antifungal Products

Generic name	Drug class
Prescription products	
Griseofulvin	
Ciclopirox	
Haloprogin	
Clotrimazole	
Miconazole	
Econazole	Imidazole derivatives
Ketoconazole	
Oxiconazole	
Sulconazole	
Itraconazole	Triazoles
Fluconazole	
Naftifine	Allylamines
Terbinafine	
Over-the-counter products	
Tolnaftate	
Miconazole	
Clotrimazole	
Undecylenic acid	
Gentian violet	
Whitfield's ointment	
Selenium sulfide	
Hydroxyquinolones	

Treatment of Interdigital Toe Web Infections

Topical agents such as allylamines, imidazoles, and ciclopirox olamine are beneficial (10). The imidazoles and ciclopirox have an additional advantage because of anticandidal and antibacterial activity (11). Because bacteria are often involved in macerated and erosive type of tinea pedis, broad-spectrum topical antifungal agents should be the first line of therapy. Tolnaftate has little effect on *Candida* and bacteria (11).

Plantar Moccasin Type of Infection

Treatment of this type of infection is complicated by the thickness of the stratum corneum, the relatively low immunogenicity of *T. rubrum*, and involvement of the nails. Combined systemic and topical therapy followed by long-term use of topical therapy can contain the process. Itraconazole and oral terbinafine in the treatment for recalcitrant tinea pedis seems promising (12,13).

Vesiculobullous Type of Tinea Pedis

Acute vesicular lesions should be treated as any acute dermatitis. Compresses such as Burow's solution and topical corticosteroids coupled with systemic antifungal therapy are sufficient for acute attacks. The allylamines, which are fungicidal, appear to be the best choice.

NONDERMATOPHYTES AND TINEA PEDIS

Several nondermatophytes have been implicated in foot and nail infections, but it is often difficult to establish their etiology. In recent years, *Scytalidium dimidiatum* (Hendersonula toruloidea) and *Scytalidium hyalinum* have been reported as agents of recalcitrant foot and nail infections (14–16).

Today, *S. dimidiatum* is one of the most frequently isolated fungi from patients with tinea pedis and/or onychomycosis in Great Britain. Hay and Moore (14) described the clinical appearance of infection caused by *S. dimidiatum* and *S. hyalinum* in 128 patients. The clinical features noted with *Scytalidium* were mostly those that are seen in *T. rubrum* infection of the feet. Another distinctive feature noted with this type of tinea pedis was the absence of dorsal infection of the feet.

S. dimidiatum is a recognized plant pathogen and most likely is a soil organism. *S. hyalinum*, on the other hand, has never been isolated from the environment. In reviewing the geographical distribution of *Scytalidium*, Moore (18) found that all the patients originated from the tropics or subtropics of the Caribbean or West Africa. Frankel and Rippon (15) reported 40 cases of infection related to *Scytalidium* in the Chicago area. The largest contributor to this patient population was the Indian subcontinent, accounting for 40%. In direct microscopic examination of infected scales, hyphae of *Scytalidium* are scarcely distinguishable from dermatophytic hyphae. Greer and Guitierrez (16) reported typical dermatophyte type of hyphae associated with the above fungus when examined directly under the microscope. Cultures of *S. dimidiatum* should show a white colored, velvety to cottony, rapidly growing colony, which often darkens with age, developing a gray or brown pigment. *S. hyalinum* is white colored with cottony growth. In culturing a suspected infection of tinea pedis, it is important to remember that *Scytalidium* is sensitive to the presence of cyclohexmide; therefore, many cases related to this type of tinea pedis may be misdiagnosed as recalcitrant dermatophytosis. Confirming the diagnosis of *Scytalidium* can be made by the findings when KOH is positive but there is no growth on cycloheximide-containing agar.

Infections caused by *Scytalidium* do not respond to griseofulvin and oral ketoconazole treatment (14). Therapy with topical bifonazole, clotrimazole, or econazole for 4 weeks was not effective. A single case of mycotic verrucose dermatitis caused by *Scytalidium* was cleared with amphotericin B (17). Half-strength Whitfield's ointment showed very limited success; only 2 of 93 patients were cured (18). Newer drugs, itraconazole and terbinafine, are being investigated for nondermatophyte infections.

REFERENCES

1. Rippon JW. Cutaneous infections. Dermatophytosis and dermatomycosis. In: Medical Mycology. The Pathogenic Fungi and the Pathogenic Actinomycetes. 3d ed. Philadelphia: Saunders, 1988: 169–275.
2. Taplin D. Superficial mycoses. J Invest Dermatol 1976; 67: 177–180.
3. Blank HD, Taplin D et al. Cutaneous *Trichophyton mentagrophytes* infection in Vietnam. Arch Dermatol 1969; 99: 135–144.
4. Leyden JJ, Kligman AM. Interdigital athlete's foot: the interaction of dermatophytes and resident bacteria. Arch Dermatol 1978; 114: 1466–1472.
5. Leyden JJ, Aly R. Tinea pedis. Semin Dermatol 1993; 12: 280–284.

6. Youssef N, Wayborn CHE, Holt G, et al. Antibiotic production by dermatophyte fungi. J Gen Microbiol 1978; 105: 105–111.

7. Jones HE, Reinhardt JH, Rinaldi MG. Model dermatophytosis in naturally infected subjects. Arch Dermatol 1974; 110: 369–379.

8. Allen AM, Skin diseases in Vietnam, 1965-1972. In: Ogibene AJ, ed. Internal Medicine in Vietnam. Vol. 1. Washington: Medical Department, US Army, Office of the Surgeon General and Center of Military History, 1977.

9. Birnbaum JE. Pharmacology of the allylamines. J Am Acad Dermatol 1990; 23: 783–785.

10. Gupta AK, Sander DN, Shear NH. Antifungal agents: an overview. Part II. J Am Acad Dermatol 1994; 30: 911–933.

11. Lesher JL Jr, Smith JG Jr. Antifungal agents in dermatology. J Am Acad Dermatol 1987; 17: 383–396.

12. Hay RJ, Clayton YM, Moore MK, Midgeley G. Itraconazole in the treatment of chronic dermatophytosis. J Am Acad Dermatol 1990; 23: 561–564.

13. Savin RC. Oral terbinafine vs. griseofulvin in the treatment of moccasin type of tinea pedis. J Am Acad Dermatol 1990; 23: 807–809.

14. Hay RJ, Moore MK. Clinical features of superficial fungal infections caused by *Hendersonula toruloidea* and *Scytalidium*. Br J Dermatol 1984; 110: 677–683.

15. Frankel DH, Rippon J. *Hendersonula toruloidea* infection in man. Mycopathologia 1989; 105: 175–186.

16. Greer DL, Guitierrez M. Tinea pedis caused by *Hendersonula toruloidea*. J Am Acad Dermatol 1987; 16: 1111–1115.

17. Mariat F, Liautaud B, Liautaud M, et al. *Hendersonula toruloidea* agent d'une dermatitis verrugeuse observee en Algerie. Sabouraudia 1978; 16: 133–140.

18. Moore MK. Morphological and physiological studies from human skin and nail samples. J Med Vet Mycolol 1988; 26: 25–39.

12
Diagnosis and New Treatments in the Management of Onychomycosis

Robert L. Baran
Nail Disease Center, Cannes, France

Raza Aly
University of California School of Medicine, San Francisco, California

ETIOLOGY

Onychomycosis is primarily caused by a narrow group of dermatophytes; however, nondermatophytic molds and some yeasts can induce disease that is clinically indistinguishable from tinea unguium (nail infection due to dermatophytes only). The common causative agents of onychomycosis are listed in Table 1. Dermatophytes are the most common pathogen, accounting for more than 90% of nail infections. *Trichophyton rubrum* is isolated with greatest frequency. The prevalence of nail disease caused by molds depends on geographical region. Scytalidium infection has been reported as a major etiological factor in onychomycosis in tropical and subtropical countries. Nondermatophytes, such as *Scapulariopsis, Fusarium, Aspergillus,* and *Acremonium,* which have a worldwide distribution, are agents of infection in previously damaged nail. *Candida* species, particularly *C. albicans,* can affect nail by causing distal or lateral onycholysis, paronychia, and, in rare cases of chronic mucocutaneous candidiasis, total nail dystrophy.

Table 1 Major Organisms of Onychomycosis

Dermatophytes
  Trichophyton rubrum
  Trichophyton mentagrophytes (var. interdigitale)
  Epidermophyton floccosum
Nondermatophytes
  Aspergillus spp
  Scopulariopsis brevicaulis
  Fusarium spp
  Acremonium spp
  Scytalidium dimidiatum
  Scytalidium hyalinum
Yeast
  Candida albicans

DIAGNOSIS OF ONYCHOMYCOSIS

Not all patients with dystrophic nails have onychomycosis; therefore, it is important to make a correct diagnosis to select appropriate treatments. The diagnosis of nail infections is confirmed by the demonstration of fungal elements in nail materials and then by isolation and identification of the microorganism on culture.

Specimen Collection

In patients with distal subungual onychomycosis, fungi invade the hypo-nichial region of the nail bed. The specimen is obtained from the nail bed with a small, 1 ml curet. The specimen should be obtained from the onychomycotic border where the highest number of viable hyphae exist. In superficial white onychomycosis, scraping with a No. 15 blade from affected areas is satisfactory to obtain suitable material. This infection is a result of direct mycotic invasion of the dorsal nail plate. The surface of the infected nail is roughened and the consistency is softer than the normal plate. Proximal white subungual onychomycosis is rarely found in the normal population, but it can occur in patients with AIDS. A No. 15 blade scalpel is used to remove the superficial layers of the nail. Samples from the infected area are then removed with a curet.

Direct Examination

The diagnosis of fungal infections is most easily confirmed by direct microscopic examination of nail materials on a potassium hydroxide slide mount. The use of 15% to 20% KOH in dimethyl sulfoxide will hasten the process. Chlorazol E stain specific for fungus cell walls is useful for nail specimens.

Culture Method

Although the microscopic features seen in infected nails may be characteristic of dermatophyte infection, the accurate identification can be made only by culture. The standard medium for growing dermatophytes in Sabouraud's dextrose agar containing chloramphenicol and cycloheximide, which inhibit bacteria and saprophytic fungi, respectively. These selective media are commercially available as Mycobiotic agar or Mycosel agar. Media containing a pH indicator, such as DTM, are also found commercially. Dermatophytes release alkaline metabolites into the medium, which results in an increase in pH, thus changing the color of the medium. For best results, however, it is essential to include media with and without cycloheximide if *Scytalidium* or other nondermatophytic fungi are suspected. Media without cycloheximide will encourage isolation of nail pathogens that are sensitive to this antibiotics, such as *Scytalidium dimidiatum, Scytalidium hyalinum, Scopulariopsis brevicaulis* and *Aspergillus* sp.

THERAPY

Onychomycosis therapy has been unsatisfactory because of the site of fungal involvement in the nail keratin, the organisms identity, inefficacy of conventional topical therapy, long duration of systemic treatment, drug interactions, need for continuous monitoring, high rates of relapses, and cost. A fungus enters into the nail by three main routes, resulting in different clinical patterns of infection: (a) via the lateral nail groove and distal subungual area, leading to distal lateral subungual onychomycosis (DLSO); (b) via the dorsal surface of the nail plate, producing superficial white onychomycosis (SWO); or (c) via the undersurface of the proximal nail fold, which remains normal in proximal white subungual onychomycosis, but is inflamed in chronic paronychia with secondary nail involvement.

Total dystrophic onychomycosis may result either from the progression of any of these forms of infection or appear primarily in patients with chronic mucocutaneous candidiasis. Despite the advent of new improved oral and topical antifungal drugs, no patient with dystrophic nails and suspected onychomycosis should be treated without establishing a precise diagnosis.

Unfortunately, the clinical patterns of change in fungal nail disease provide only a clue to the type of infection. The diagnosis of onychomycosis, therefore, must be confirmed in the laboratory using an appropriate technique. Nevertheless, it may be difficult to isolate fungi in culture even from nails positive on direct microscopy. Infection may be presumed if invasion of nail keratin by fungus can be proven histologically.

With the new systemic antifungal drugs, the rationale for treating onychomycosis has changed. The newer triazoles, fluconazole and itraconazole, and the oral allylamine, terbinafine, differ from the traditional antifungal drugs by their mode of rapid penetration into the nail via the nail bed and their strong incorporation into matrix tissue, allowing drug retention in the nail plate after discontinuation of therapy. This produces a continuous improvement permitting short duration treatment or pulse therapy management. Taking the pharmacokinetics and the potential adverse effects and drug interactions into account, age, health, and ease of compliance of the patient, as well as cost, are the factors to consider in selecting therapy.

Itraconazole (3,4)

Itraconazole has the broadest spectrum of all oral antifungal drugs. It is effective against dermatophytes, *Candida*, and some nondermatophyte molds. Because of its pharmacokinetic profile, illustrated by its biphasic mechanisms of penetration into the nail (5), the recommended schedule is 200 mg twice a day given without food, for 1 week a month (6) in an à la carte treatment strategy 1 to 2 months for fingernail infection and 3 to 4 months for toenails infection. Although the nail will not be normal when therapy is discontinued, improvement continues, sometimes slower than during the treatment period when an increase in linear nail growth may be observed (7).

Potential Drug Interactions (3)

Rifampin, isoniazid, phenobarbitone, carbamazepine, and phenytoin may induce hepatic drug metabolizing enzymes, with a resultant decrease in itraconazole blood levels and subsequent antifungal treatment failure. Conversely, inhibiting drug-metabolizing enzymes by cimetidine may elevate itraconazole levels. Itraconazole can slow hepatic drug metabolism and thereby potentiate the effect of phenytoin, oral hypoglycemic agents, warfarin, digoxin, terfenadine, astemizole, and cyclosporin A.

Potential Adverse Effects (3)

Embryotoxicity, gastrointestinal disturbance, rash, pruritus, hypokalemia, reversible telogen effluvium, and very rarely hepatotoxicity have been recorded with itraconazole use.

Fluconazole (3,4)

Fluconazole, which is active against *Candida* and other yeasts, has received much acclaim in HIV-infected patients. As with griseofulvin and keto-conazole, long-term therapy is usually required. However 150 mg administered once a week may be a useful intermittent regimen (8) in patients taking multiple medications.

Potential Adverse Effects (3)

Most side effects are related to gastrointestinal disturbances. Hepato-toxicity is extremely rare.

Terbinafine (3,49)

Terbinafine is the only in vitro fungicidal oral antifungal with activity against the dermatophytes, some species of *Candida*, and even some molds. It is detectable in the nail plate in 1 to 3 weeks and persists for up to 4 months after therapy is discontinued. A 12-week course of 250 mg once a day is effective in toenail infections (10), and 6 weeks of therapy is sufficient for fingernail disease. As with itraconazole, the nail will not be clinically normal when the drug is discontinued, but because terbinafine is retained in its keratin, the nail plate grows out health.

Potential Adverse Effects (3)

Most adverse effects with terbinafine have been noted during the first few weeks of therapy. Approximately half are related to the gastrointestinal system. Taste disturbances resolve on completion of treatment. Ter-binafine may rarely cause varying degrees of hepatobiliary dysfunction.

If a progressive cutaneous reaction appears, the drug should be discontinued.

A double-blind study, comparing itraconazole and terbinafine (11) in a small group of patients demonstrated that the cure rates are identical (i.e., less than 65%).

Interestingly, in our own patient population who did not respond to, or relapsed on, oral itraconazole or terbinafine, we often found lateral nail disease (12). A review of the normal histology of this nail region convinces us that this lateral nail disease results from poor penetration of the antifungal agent into the lateral edge of the nail via the lateral nail groove, because the nail does not adhere to the subungual tissue in that region. Diffusion of the drug into the lateral nail area probably results mainly from take-up of the antifungal within the newly formed nail via the matrix. To test our hypothesis, we took 400 mg itraconazole daily for 1 week. On the eighth day, we cut 56 mg of the distal margin and 23 mg of the lateral edges of the fingernails (Janssen Research, unpublished data). The concentrations of itraconazole was 1013 ng/g in the distal margin, but only 677 ng/g in the lateral edges. This difference supports our premise and could also explain some treatment failures when the nail has lost its adherence to the nail bed.

Because the highest cure rate obtained with these oral antifungals is only 82%, there is still a need for the development of alternative therapeutic strategies. Moreover, some patients are unable or unwilling to take oral drugs and, where appropriate, it may be best to offer an alternative treatment regimen.

Because conventional topical antifungal therapy is ineffective since its formulation is inadequate and prevents diffusion of the chemical into the nail keratin, improved topical antifungal formulations have been tested.

Transungual Antifungal Delivery Systems

Because a proposed alcoholic solution containing 28% tioconazole and undecylenic acid has had rather poor results (13), nail laquers offer a better option. They have improved results, provided the lunula is spared. Because their formulation is close to that of a cosmetic nail lacquer, they maintain the active agent in a polymer film reservoir on the nail surface from which the antifungal evenly diffuses through the nail keratin to reach the nail bed. In addition, after evaporation of the solvent, the concentration of the antifungal in the film increases, which enhances penetration and diffusion. Two chemicals, 5% amorolfine (14) and 8% ciclopirox (15), are currently used in this formulation in Europe.

Therapeutic Combinations

Transungual drug delivery systems have opened a new era in topical antifungal therapies, but despite interesting results in monotherapy, the future probably consists of using the modern systemic antifungal drugs in combination with an antifungal nail lacquer and/or nonsurgical avulsion with bifonazole–urea (which eradicates the pathogens) in an *à la carte* treatment strategy. Use of a combination of systemic and topical treatment or nail avulsion will eliminate mycotic lunular involvement, which topical agents cannot do. Additionally the new systemic antimycotic agents and transungual drug delivery systems act on different targets on the fungal cell, which is a giant step toward cured nails.

LONG-TERM MANAGEMENT

Long-term management such as intermittent application of topical antifungals to the plantar surface and toe webs should prevent reestablishment of tinea pedis and limit the possibility of reinfection. Transungual antifungal delivery systems could be used periodically to prevent recurrences.

REFERENCES

1. Kotrajaras R, Chongsathien S, Rojanavanich V, et al. *Hendersonula toruloidea* infection in Thailand. Int J Dermatol 1988; 27:391–395.
2. Summerbell RC, Kane J, Krajden S. Onychomycosis, tinea pedis, and tinea manuum caused by nondermatophytic filamentous fungi. Mycoses 1989; 32: 609–619.
3. Gupta AK, Sauder DN, Shear NH. Antifungal agents. Part II. J Am Acad Dermatol 1994; 30: 911–933.
4. Elewski BE. Onychomycosis. Fitzpatrick's J Clin Dermatol 1994: 48–54.
5. Matthieu L, De Doncker P, Cauwenbergh G, et al. Itraconazole penetrates the nail via the nail matrix and the nail bed: an investigation in onychomycosis. Clin Exp Dermatol 1991; 16: 374–376.
6. Roseew D, De Doncker P. New approaches to the treatment of onychomycosis. J Am Acad Dermatol 1993; 29: 545–550.
7. De Doncker P, Pierard G. Acquired nail beading in patients on itraconazole: an indicator of faster nail growth? Clin Exp Dermatol 1994; 19: 404–406.
8. Suchil P, Montero-Gei F, Robles M, et al. Once-weekly oral doses of fluconazole 150. Clin Exp Dermatol 1992; 17: 397–401.

9. Shear NH, Gupta AK. Terbinafine for the treatment of pedal onychomycosis. A foot closer to the promised land of cured nails. Arch Dermatol 1995; 131: 937–942.

10. Goodfield MJ. Short-duration therapy with terbinafine for dermatophyte onychomycosis. A multicentre trial. Br J Dermatol 1992; 126: 33–35.

11. Arenas R, Dominguez-Cherit J, Fernandez LM. Open randomized comparison of itraconazole versus terbinafine in onychomycosis. Int J. Dermatol 1995; 34: 138–143.

12. Baran R, De Doncker P. Lateral edge nail involvement indicates poor prognosis for treating onychomycosis with the new systemic antifungals. Act Derm Venereol 1996; 76: 82–83.

13. Degreef H. Onychomycosis. Br J Clin Pract 1990; 44:(suppl 9): 91–97.

14. Marty JPL. Amorolfine nail lacquer: a novel formulation. J Eur Acad Derm Vener 1995; 4(suppl 1): 517–521.

15. Meisel CW, Nietsch P. Ein neues Therapiekonzept bie Onychomykosen. Dtsch Dermatol 1992; 7: 1038–1053.

13

Pharmacokinetics in Onychomycosis

Piet De Doncker
Janssen Research Foundation, Beerse, Belgium

INTRODUCTION

As the incidence of onychomycosis increases, the choice of an appropriate antifungal therapy becomes even more important. The ideal antifungal drug must be specific against the causative organism, have a high affinity for the nails and infected tissues, remain at the affected site in amounts sufficient to produce an antifungal effect, have a low retention in serum and other organs, and be safe and efficacious. This combination of drug attributes permits shorter treatment regimens and fewer side effects.

Investigative studies have traditionally focused on the in vitro spectrum of an antifungal agent to determine against which species and genera the drug is active. Although in vitro analysis is important, it does not address the drug's action against the organism in vivo. Moreover, no matter how efficacious an antifungal agent is in vitro, if it does not reach the site of infection in therapeutic concentrations, the in vivo results will be disappointing. Pharmacokinetics play an important role in the therapeutic outcome of onychomycosis because of the physical characteristics of the nail, which preclude easy delivery and absorption of topical drugs, and because of the slow growth of nails, which makes it difficult to assess therapeutic effectiveness.

Because the mechanisms of drug failure in onychomycosis were not well understood, several nail kinetic studies were undertaken in

This study was made possible through an unrestricted grant from Janssen Pharmaceutica.

157

hopes of linking the presence of bioactive antifungal in nail plate with the clinical response. This may be a more accurate interpretation of the problem in onychomycosis because the infection is located in the hard keratin structures of the nail. Pharmacokinetics are consequently important in the evaluation of antifungal drugs in onychomycosis in the sense that concentrations of the antifungal agent in the stratum corneum or the nail plate are more relevant than blood levels in cutaneous antifungal therapy.

DISTRIBUTION OF ORAL ANTIFUNGALS IN THE NAIL

In dermatology, an oral antifungal drug should be absorbed before it is distributed to all organs of the body and can reach the infection site. In the case of onychomycosis, the antifungal should penetrate the different cell layers, including the cell membranes of the fungal pathogens. Even if the drug is well absorbed, however, adequate concentrations in the infected tissue are not certain.

For onychomycosis, this biophase includes the keratin tissues, as well as the fungal organisms (dermatophytes, yeasts, and molds) that may invade the nail. Therefore, the drug availability at the infection site (the nail plate/nail bed) is not necessarily related to the free concentration of drug in plasma and body fluids, but rather to its tissue concentration. Because of the different physicochemical properties of antifungal drugs, the pharmacokinetic profiles may be different. These variances offer clues to potential efficacy, as well as the different delivery and excretion properties.

These processes of release into the plasma, transport to the site of infection, and activity is called the pharmacokinetic/pharmacodynamic activity phase of a drug. To obtain a good effect, a minimal quantity of the drug should be present at the site of action. The quantity necessary (i.e., the minimal inhibitory concentration [MIC] value for the different fungal organisms) is not measurable in most diseases. In onychomycosis, however, drug concentrations can be measured in the keratinized nail plate during treatment and then correlated with the clinical outcome. This correlation may be an advantage in drug development.

In contrast to skin, the nail plate is a slow-growing structure and is composed of layers of flattened keratinocytes. It takes several months to 1 year before toenail outgrowth is obtained. This slow renewal of the nail influences the ability of drugs to reach the site of action. If a systemic drug was taken up only in the newly formed nail, it would take a long time for the nail to become fully impregnated with the drug (this was one of the reasons why griseofulvin or ketoconazole was administered until complete cure was obtained). During our first studies, it was clear that there were penetration routes other than the nail matrix. If drugs have the ability to accumulate the nail matrix, then the drug would be eliminated with renewal of the nail. This elimination is an important factor in developing a rational strategy for treatment. In addition, differences in growth speed between fingernails and toenails also influence drug penetration into the nail, as will other factors that delay or increase the speed of the nail growth (e.g., age, psoriasis, medications).

Because of the slow growth of the nail, the final outcome of drug therapy cannot be determined for months, sometimes a year later, even when the disease process has effectively been stopped. This is in contrast to most infections in which drug therapy is needed only to destroy the organism. In this case, a rapid clinical response is more or less in parallel with the action of the drug. This response provides immediate feedback about the efficacy of the therapy. Therefore, to predict the effectiveness of an antifungal drug in onychomycosis, the final mycological and clinical outcome of therapy must be evaluated after a sufficiently long follow-up period and correlated to the tissue levels observed during and after treatment.

The nail plate is a difficult environment for oral drugs to penetrate. It is now known that effective drug therapy requires uptake of the drug into the nail unit. Because of this fact, drug pharmacokinetics have been recognized as an essential tool to identify and support the strengths of pharmaceutical agents. Pharmacokinetic studies of griseofulvin were elementary, but the available data demonstrate griseofulvin's limitations, for example in toenail onychomycosis. Ketoconazole kinetics were somewhat better studied and understood, but it was not until the mid-1980s that kinetic studies with itraconazole in skin and nails linked the presence of bioactive antifungal in tissue with the clinical response. Similar studies with fluconazole and terbinafine rapidly followed.

The ultimate goal for an antifungal drug is to find the optimal treatment regimen in terms of efficacy, safety, patient compliance, and cost of treatment. Because the mechanisms of drug therapy failure in onychomycosis were often not understood, several nail kinetic studies were undertaken to elucidate the behavior of these drugs in the nail. Today, pharmacokinetic/pharmacodynamic studies are crucial to reach this goal.

Terbinafine

Terbinafine is an allylamine agent. In vitro data indicate that terbinafine is fungicidal for dermatophytes and for some *Candida* species. When terbinafine comes in contact with serum or proteins, however, this activity is decreased and leads to a reduced bioavailability (1,2). Therefore, the term *fungitoxic* better describes the activity of terbinafine in the clinical situation (3). Extensive studies of the skin and nail pharmacokinetics of terbinafine have been performed. Terbinafine has a slow elimination, probably because of its strong lipophilic nature, with good distribution in skin, adipose tissue, and nails (4–6). Terbinafine is well absorbed within 2 hours after ingestion, with plasma concentrations varying between 2.09 ± 0.78 μg/ml. Urinary excretion is above 70% after 48 hours. Plasma elimination half-life results vary, with one study showing +26 hours and other studies showing 100 hours (6). Low plasma levels can be measured for several weeks after discontinuation of therapy.

Terbinafine is a lipophilic and keratophilic compound. The drug is delivered to the stratum corneum by a positive diffusion from the blood stream through the dermis–epidermis. It is also excreted extensively through the sebum, but the drug is undetectable in eccrine sweat. It was shown in skin kinetic studies that tissue levels persist up to 7 weeks after discontinuation of therapy (7–9). In an ex vivo model using skin strippings, the lingering antifungal effect of terbinafine in human stratum corneum lasted for 2 to 3 weeks after cessation of therapy (3).

Several studies by Finlay et al. (10,11) have explored the nail kinetics of terbinafine. They have shown that the pharmacokinetics in the normal nail are analogous to those of the infected nail. In an initial kinetic study, terbinafine levels of 250 to 550 ng/g appeared in distal nails within 7.8 weeks, with a range of 3 to 18 weeks (10). These levels were well within the therapeutic range. Early detection of terbinafine in the distal portion of the nail led to the conclusion that the diffusion of terbinafine is faster than the rate of nail growth and must also occur via the nail bed. A subsequent study by Finlay et al. (12) showed that when terbinafine reaches the nail, a fast diffusion occurs, resulting in a steady state. During treatment, the levels of terbinafine in the nail did not increase with time. This finding suggests that the mechanism of penetration is probably through both the nail matrix and nail bed, and not by incorporation into the matrix cells. They also found that terbinafine drug concentration declines in parallel with the plasma level after 3 months of therapy.

Finlay et al. (12) also investigated the relationships between an oral dose of terbinafine, nail plate levels during therapy, and posttreatment levels. Twenty-four patients with onychomycosis were treated in a double-blind study with either 125, 250, or 500 mg/day for 16 weeks, with a follow-up at 32 weeks. Toenail levels of terbinafine reached a maximum at 8 weeks, whereas distal levels reached a maximum at 12 weeks. Nail levels in the 125 and 250 mg group were lower, demonstrating a correlation between dosage and drug levels in the nail. After discontinuation of therapy, terbinafine persisted in distal nail clippings in a steady state for at least 4 weeks, but was not detectable after 8 weeks. Effendy et al. (13) presented results that differ somewhat from Finlay's. Although diffusion into the nail was still evident, terbinafine continued to accumulate in the toenail after a 3-month treatment, after which drug levels persisted for several months. Although these findings need to be confirmed, they suggest that terbinafine penetrates the nail by diffusion from the matrix and the nail bed and that terbinafine is incorporated to a certain extent into the nail matrix.

The value of a short, single-pulse course of therapy with terbinafine for fingernail and toenail onychomycosis was determined by Shuster and Munro (14). Although no kinetic data are available from this limited study, outcome of therapy was determined by adequacy of dosage rather than by duration of treatment. Work by Faergemann et al. (15) supports the theory that the length of therapy necessary to affect cure is less than the currently recommended 12 weeks. Therapeutic concentrations of terbinafine persisted in distal nail clippings for 2 to 3 months after the medication was stopped after 1 week of treatment (16). Consequently, 1 week pulse therapy is being studied in onychomycosis.

Fluconazole

Fluconazole is a hydrosoluble bistriazole whose pharmacokinetic profile differs from that of other azole derivatives. The low molecular weight and relatively higher water solubility compared with the other azoles contribute to its high bioavailability, which exceeds 90%. Fluconazole is not extensively bound to tissue, protein, or fat; the apparent volume of distribution is approximately that of total body water (17). The unmetabolized drug is extensively absorbed. Serum concentrations of 1.0 µg/ml are obtained after a single oral dose of 50 mg (18). The peak plasma concentrations achieved in healthy volunteers after single doses of fluconazole, 100 mg and 400 mg, are 1.9 µg/ml and 6.7 µg/ml, respectively. Continued administration leads to an increase in peak plasma concentrations of 2.5 times that achieved after a single dose. Half-life is sufficiently long (> 30 hours) to permit once daily dosing. Fluconazole is metabolically stable and is excreted almost unchanged (91%) in the urine (19).

Fluconazole penetrates well into body fluids and tissue, including skin and nails (19). Tissue affinity is limited and keratin adherence is weak. Sweat is the most important route of delivery of fluconazole to the skin followed by excretion in sebum. Uptake or excretion in the basal layer is limited (20).

Two fluconazole nail kinetic studies have been reported. In a first study by Hay (21), nine male volunteers were treated with 50 mg fluconazole daily for 2 weeks. Mean plasma concentrations of fluconazole on days 1 and 14 of treatment were 760 and 2120 ng/ml, respectively. Mean nail concentrations were 1300 and 1800 ng/g, respectively (21). The fast diffusion into the distal portion of nails within 48 hours of treatment onset suggests that diffusion from the nail bed is a key route of penetration in the nail.

In a second study of nail kinetics, Fraki et al. (22) administered 150 mg fluconazole on a once-a-week pulse dosing regimen for a minimum of 6 months. They found that fluconazole concentrations in the nail increased monthly and that the concentrations increased more quickly in healthy than in diseased nails. At the 6-month interval, both healthy and diseased nails achieved similar concentrations of 2000 ng/g. They also found that pretreatment of the affected nails with urea increased the cure rate. Long-term posttreatment data were not reported in this study, nor was there any available data with regard to how long fluconazole remained in the nail. A recent study by Faergemann suggests that fluconazole is detectable in the nail for 5 months after therapy cessation (Faergemann, personal communication).

Other studies using a once-a-week dose of fluconazole for onychomycosis suggest that pulse regimens be continued until there is mycological and clinical cure (22,23). Dose response studies are ongoing to establish the optimal dosage and duration for this regimen.

Itraconazole

Itraconazole is a broad-spectrum triazole derivative with high lipophilicity, good oral absorption, extensive tissue distribution, and a high affinity for keratinous tissue (24,25). Because it is almost totally insoluble in water, it is currently available only as a capsule. Its bioavailability is enhanced in an acid environment and in the presence of food (26).

Itraconazole's strong affinity for keratinized tissues results in high concentrations of the drug in nails and explains its effectiveness in the treatment of onychomycosis. Skin kinetic studies indicate that the major routes of itraconazole to the skin are probably through passive diffusion from the blood in the keratinocytes, with strong adherence to keratin, incorporation into the basal layers, and excretion by sebaceous glands. In contrast to ketoconazole, griseofulvin, and fluconazole, excretion of itraconazole in sweat is limited (25). Redistribution of itraconazole from the skin and appendages into the plasma appears negligible, and renewal of the stratum corneum or growth of the hair and nails accounts for the disappearance of itraconazole from these tissues.

Several studies have been conducted to define and elucidate the kinetics of itraconazole in the nail. Itraconazole concentrations were determined by using a specific high performance liquid chromatographic (HPLC) method of assay analysis (27). In one of the first nail pharmacokinetic studies conducted, itraconazole was detectable by day 7 of the treatment schedule, even though it had disappeared almost completely from the plasma (28). These results demonstrate two pharmacokinetic properties of itraconazole that may explain why itraconazole treatment is so effective in onychomycosis. The early detection of itraconazole in the nail clippings after 7 days shows that itraconazole may act rapidly on the fungus in the nail plate not only by incorporating itself in the nail matrix, but also by diffusion from the nail bed into the nail plate. The fact that itraconazole could be detected in the nail plate with no evidence of the drug in the plasma demonstrates its affinity for keratinous material.

The potential for shorter treatment schedules was investigated in a study that compared the results of treatment in 39 patients given either 100 mg or 200 mg of itraconazole daily for 3 months (28). Itraconazole concentrations in the toenail and fingernails were also measured for up to 6 months after completion of therapy. Throughout the 6-month follow-up period, the 200 mg group yielded higher concentrations of itraconazole in the distal nail plate of both toenails and fingernails than the 100 mg group. In the toenail, mean itraconazole levels ranged from 84 to 149 ng/g of tissue for the 100 mg dosage group, with a mean maximum of 149 ng/g at the fifth month. In the 200 mg dosage group, mean itraconazole levels ranged from 490 to 990 ng/g, with a mean maximum of 990 ng/g at the fifth month. Almost half the patients in the 200 mg dosage group had concentrations of more than 1000 ng/g in their toenails. The toenail concentrations remained high throughout the 6-month follow-up period, while concentrations in fingernails declined faster. Mean itraconazole concentrations persisted unchanged in both groups for 6 months after therapy, with a mean of 149 ng/g in the 100 mg dose group and a mean of 670 ng/g in the 200 mg dose group.

In the fingernails, similar posttreatment inhibitory levels of itraconazole were found for each dosage group, but they declined in each dosage group from 3 months after discontinuation of treatment onward (29).

The better cure rate of 79% in the 200 mg dosage group versus the 26% cure rate in the 100 mg dosage group suggests that the drug level in the nail is a good indicator of efficacy in onychomycosis (28). In addition, itraconazole levels achieved in the cured patients treated with 200 mg itraconazole daily were significantly higher compared to the noncured patients in the 200 mg group (29).

The therapeutic concentration of itraconazole found in the distal nail ends of fingernails and toenails within both dosage groups shows that the drug reaches the nail via passive diffusion from the nail bed into the nail plate, as well as via incorporation into the nail matrix as generally presumed.

Clinical studies to support the diffusion of itraconazole from the nail bed into the nail plate are limited because of the invasive procedures required to measure drug levels in this area. De Doncker (30) reported that drug concentrations in the nail bed in this sample were more than double the drug concentrations in the distal nail clippings; 547 ng/g versus 240 ng/g, respectively. Considering the kinetics of the nail bed, which may contribute to nail formation and subsequent growth of the nail plate, it can be expected that any drug found in the subungual material located within the nail bed will be actively delivered at a slow rate from the nail bed into the nail plate.

Based on these pharmacokinetics, the potential of itraconazole given as a pulse-dose regimen was explored. In a pharmacodynamic investigation of monthly cycles of 400 mg daily for 1 week pulse therapy with itraconazole (31), the group of patients receiving three pulses had mean toenail drug levels that ranged from 67 ng/g 1 month after starting therapy to a peak concentration of 471 ng/g 6 months after therapy. Toenail drug levels persisted in the three-pulse group to the eleventh month, with remaining concentrations of 186 ng/g. In fingernails, similar drug concentrations were found, but itraconazole decreased faster in the distal nail and the drug became undetectable from the ninth month on.

In contrast to the persistent level of drug in the nail, drug plasma levels decreased after 1 week and were completely eliminated before the initiation of another pulse dose. Plasma kinetics between pulse dosing and continuous dosing show that the total drug exposure for the patient, as expressed in AUC, is three times less in the pulse therapy than in the continuous dose therapy; 743 µg/ml versus 1785 µg/ml, respectively (31). This reduction in total exposure contributes to the favorable safety profile of itraconazole.

Results of clinical studies in 909 patients with toenail onychomycosis demonstrated a clinical and mycological cure of 79% and 85% for the three-pulse regimen, and 76% and 77%, respectively, for the four-pulse dose group at the end of a 12-month treatment period (32). Further studies are required to confirm these results. Development in intermittent therapy is ongoing and is focusing on adaptation of dosing and/or frequency of pulses.

DISCUSSION AND CONCLUSION

The nail plate is a difficult environment for oral drugs to penetrate. Effective oral drug therapy requires uptake of the drug into the nail unit. Pharmacokinetics has long been recognized as an essential tool to identify and support the strengths of antifungal agents.

Although some drugs are lipophilic and have a strong affinity for keratin, they exhibit different pharmacokinetic profiles, offering clues to the mechanisms of altered efficacy in terms of their inherent pharmacological activity, as well as the different delivery and excretion properties. The different studies with itraconazole suggest an almost ideal pharmacokinetic profile for the treatment of onychomycosis. Itraconazole is detected within 7 to 14 days in the nail, suggesting penetration via the nail bed. Additionally, although itraconazole plasma levels fall rapidly once therapy has ended, reaching zero within 1 week to 10 days, its strong affinity for keratin and incorporation into matrix cells allows itraconazole to persist in the nail for 6 to 9 months posttherapy.

The drug levels are a good indicator for the therapeutic activity as shown in the study where the 10-fold higher content in the nail reached with 200 mg itraconazole for 3 months resulted in a higher mycological cure as compared to the 100 mg regimen (29). The persistence of drug levels was for both dosages quite similar but with a faster decline in fingernails (correlates with the faster nail growth).

The presently reported pharmacokinetic findings with itraconazole illustrate a unique biphasic sequence of itraconazole penetration into the nail: diffusion via nail bed and matrix and incorporation into the matrix cells. This dual phenomenon of penetration and incorporation in a unique biphasic sequence is the key to itraconazole's efficacy in both short-duration and intermittent therapy. Both phenomena were clearly demonstrated in a study where 1 week itraconazole was administered at a dosage of 200 mg or 400 mg for 1 week (data on file, Janssen Pharmaceutica). Drug levels were determined in fingernails from day 7 to month 6 (> 5 months posttreatment). Two distinct waves were seen; the first wave, starting at day 7 and decreasing by month 2, was followed by a second wave that appeared at month 4, contributing to the higher drug levels still detectable at month 6. Drug levels with pulses of 400 mg were two to four times higher as compared to the pulses of 200 mg group. For toenails, the biphasic sequence of itraconazole penetration into the nail could not be evidenced, most probably because of the slower rate of nail growth.

The pharmacokinetic findings are the keys to therapeutic improvement and have led to rational refinement in dosing strategy, from long-term use to the 3-month therapy and finally to the intermittent treatment of this disease.

REFERENCES

1. Ryder N, Frank I. Interaction of terbinafine with human serum and serum proteins. J Med Vet Mycol 1992; 30: 451–460.
2. Van Cutsem J. An investigation of the in vitro activity and antifungal spectrum of itraconazole and terbinafine in relation to in vivo efficacy in dermatophytosis. Mycologie Medicale 1994; 4: 137–144.
3. Pierard G, Arrese J, De Doncker P. Antifungal activity of itraconazole and terbinafine in human stratum corneum: a comparative study. J Am Acad Dermatol 1995; 32: 429–435.
4. Jenssen J. Pharmacokinetics in humans. J Dermatol Treat 1990; 1(suppl 2): 15–18.
5. Kovarik J, Kirkesseli S, Humbert H, et al. Dose-proportional pharmacokinetics of terbinafine and its N-demethylated metabolite in healthy volunteers. Br J Dermatol 1992; 126(suppl 2): 15–18.
6. Samsoen M. Terbinafine (Lamisil). The first oral fungistatic and fungicidal allylamine. Nouv Dermatol 1992; 11: 743–762.
7. Lever L, Dykes P, Thomas R, et al. How orally administered terbinafine reaches the stratum corneum. J Dermatol Treat 1990; 1(suppl 2):23–26.
8. Faergemann J, Zehender H, Jones T, et al. Terbinafine levels in serum, stratum corneum, dermis-epidermis (without stratum corneum), hair, sebum and eccrine sweat. Acta Derm Venereol 1990; 71: 322–326.
9. Faergemann J, Zehender H, Millerioux L. Levels of terbinafine in plasma, stratum corneum, dermis-epidermis (without stratum corneum), sebum, hair and nails during and after 250 mg terbinafine orally once daily for 7 and 14 days. Clin Infect Dis 1994; 19: 121–126.
10. Finlay A, Lever L, Thomas R, et al. Nail matrix kinetics of oral terbinafine in onychomycosis and normal nails. J Dermatol Treat 1990; 1(suppl 2): 51–54.
11. Finlay A. Pharmacokinetics of terbinafine in the nail. Br J Dermatol 1992; 126(suppl 39): 28–32.
12. Finlay A, Thomas R, Chawla M. Does the oral dosage of terbinafine influence its concentration in nail? Dermatology 2000, Vienna. May 18–21, 1991. Abstract No. 40.
13. Effendy I, Mensing H, Schatz M, et al. Preliminary results of nail kinetics of terbinafine (abstr). International Summit on Cutaneous Antifungal Therapy. San Francisco, October 21, 1993.

14. Shuster S, Munro C. Single dose treatment of fungal nail disease. Lancet 1992; 339: 1066.

15. Faergemann J, Zehender H, Millerioux L. Terbinafine levels in plasma, stratum corneum, dermis-epidermis (without stratum corneum), hair and nails during and after 250 mg terbinafine orally once per day for 7 and 14 days. Dermatology 2000, Vienna. May 18–21, 1991. Abstract No. 37.

16. Tosti A, Stinchi C, Morelli R, Columbo MD. Terbinafine versus itraconazole in the treatment of dermatophyte nail infection. Poster presented at the 53rd Annual AAD meeting. February 1995, New Orleans.

17. Humphrey M, Jevons S, Tarbit M. Pharmacokinetic evaluation of UK-49858, a metabolically stable triazole antifungal drug in animals and humans. Antimicrob Agents Chemother 1985; 28: 648–653.

18. Brammer K, Tarbit M. A review of the pharmacokinetics of fluconazole (UK-49858) in laboratory animals and in man. In: Fromtling R, ed. Recent trends in the discovery, development and evaluation of antifungal agents. Barcelona, Spain: JR Prous, 1987; 12(suppl 3): 318–326.

19. Grant S, Clissold S. Fluconazole: a review of its pharmacodynamic and pharmacokinetic properties and therapeutic potential in superficial and systemic mycoses. Drugs 1990; 39: 877–916.

20. Faergemann J, Laufen H. Levels of fluconazole in serum, stratum corneum, epidermis-dermis (without stratum corneum) and eccrine sweat. Clin Exp Dermatol 1993, 18: 102–106.

21. Hay R. Pharmacodynamic and pharmacokinetic evaluation of fluconazole in skin and nails. Int J Dermatol 1992; 31(suppl 2): 6–7.

22. Fraki J, Heikkila H, Kero M, et al. Fluconazole in the treatment of onychomycosis: an open non-comparative study with oral 150 mg fluconazole once weekly. Dermatology 2000, Vienna. May 18–21, 1991. Abstract No. 14.

23. Monterro-Gei, Melendez M, Siles L. Fluconazole in the treatment of onychomycosis. XI Congress International Society Human Animal Mycology, Montreal, Canada. June 24–28, 1991 Abstract No. 3.84.

24. Van Cutsem J, Van Gerven F, Janssen P. Activity of orally, topically and parenterally administered itraconazole in the treatment of superficial and deep mycoses: animal models. Rev Infect Dis 1987; 9(suppl 1): 15–32.

25. Heykants J, Van Peer A, Van de Velve V et al. The clinical pharmacokinetics of itraconazole: an overview. Mycoses 1989; 32(suppl 1): 67–87.

26. Bodey G. Azole antifungal agents. Clin Infect Dis 1992; 14(suppl 1): S161–S169.

27. Woestenborghs R, Lorreyne W, Heykants J. Determination of itraconazole in plasma and animal tissues by high performance liquid chromatography. J Chromatogr Biomed Appl 1987; 413: 332–337.

28. Cauwenbergh G, Degreef H, Heykants J, et al. Pharmacokinetic profile of orally administered itraconazole in human skin. J Am Acad Dermatol 1988; 18: 263–268.

29. Willemsen M, De Doncker P, Willems J, et al. Post-treatment itraconazole levels in the nail. J Am Acad Dermatol 1992; 26: 731–735.

30. De Doncker P. Pharmacokinetics: Basis for research in fungal nail disease. Issues in the modern management of onychomycosis: New approaches to diagnosis and management, Monaco. April, 1993. Symposium.
31. De Doncker P, DeCroix J, Pierard G, et al. Antifungal pulse therapy in onychomycosis: a pharmacokinetic/pharmacodynamic investigation of monthly cycles of 1 week pulse with itraconazole. Arch Dermatol 1996; 132: 34–41.
32. Andre J, De Doncker P, Ginter G, et al. Intermittent pulse therapy with itraconazole in toenail onychomycosis: an update. EADV. Brussels. October 11, 1995. Poster.

14
Tinea Capitis

Ilona J. Frieden
University of California School of Medicine, San Francisco, California

INTRODUCTION

Tinea capitis is a relatively common infection in preschool and school-aged children, but the condition can occur at any age from the neonatal period (1) to adulthood (2–4). Although the diagnosis and management of most cases are straightforward, in some cases tinea capitis can be difficult to diagnose or treat. The specter of both asymptomatic carriage in the scalp and the presence of viable fungi on fomites also complicate diagnosis and management.

EPIDEMIOLOGY

After epidemics in the 1940s and 1950s, infection in the United States decreased until the 1970s, when increasing cases caused by *Trichophyton tonsurans* were noted (5–14). Widespread infection caused by *T. tonsurans* has continued to increase, particularly among African-American children (13,16). Moreover, several other nations including Trinidad, Australia, and Taiwan have also noted increased cases caused by *T. tonsurans* (17–19). In Belgium, the Netherlands, and South Wales, increasing numbers of infections caused by *Trichophyton violaceum* have been reported (20,21).

The shift away from fluorescent organisms has made tinea capitis more difficult to detect; Woods light examination is not useful for screening large numbers of individuals. Nevertheless, *Microsporum canis* is the second most common cause of tinea capitis in the United States, and the examination can be helpful, particularly in cases with exposure to cats or dogs. The reason(s) for the prevalence of this infection in African-American children is not known. Contiguous spread within predominantly African-American communities almost certainly plays a role. Although some have speculated that certain hair care practices, such as the use of pomades, tight-braiding, and infrequent hair washing, may play a role, this hypothesis has never been proven (22,23).

Infection is most common in preschool and school-aged children, particularly those between 4 and 6 years of age (24,25). Infection becomes increasingly rare after puberty, possibly because of the antifungal properties of sebum (26). Boys and girls are equally affected (7,9).

CLINICAL MANIFESTATIONS

The most common clinical presentation of T. tonsurans infection is seborrheic dermatitis-like scaling, with little or no alopecia (Figure 1) (27,28). Another common appearance is honey-crusting and/or pustules, resembling a scalp pyoderma. The more classic presentations, black-dot tinea, with large areas of noninflammatory alopecia and the so-called kerion, with tender boggy areas of alopecia, are less common, and together probably constitute approximately 20% to 30% of cases (Figure 2). Cases caused by M. canis usually present with alopecia and inflamed scalp, often in association with tinea corporis. Tinea corporis, particularly in the head and neck area, can also occur as a result of T. tonsurans infection (Figure 3). Occasionally, the presenting complaint is enlarged occipital lymph nodes, and only a focused history and/or examination reveals the presence of subtle scalp changes (28,29).

DIFFERENTIAL DIAGNOSIS

The differential diagnosis of tinea capitis includes alopecia areata, atopic dermatitis, traction alopecia, bacterial infection, psoriasis, seborrheic dermatitis, pityriasis amiantacea (30), trichotillomania, lupus erythematosus (31), and Langerhans' cell histiocytosis (32). Because of the large number of conditions that can mimic tinea capitis (and vice versa), direct confirmation of infection with potassium hydroxide (KOH) preparation and/or fungal culture should be obtained whenever possible.

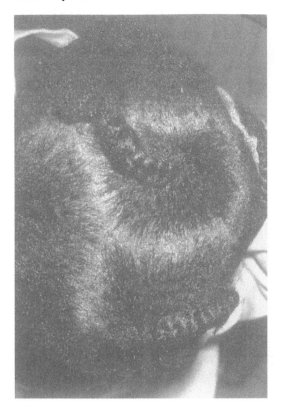

Figure 1 Tinea capitis: Diffuse scaling without significant alopecia is typical.

DIAGNOSIS

Potassium hydroxide is a helpful means of diagnosis if alopecia and scales are present, but is rarely positive with kerion or in cases in which there is no alopecia. The "brush culture" technique, in which toothbrushes or Pap smear cytology brushes are used for sampling, is probably the best diagnostic method in symptomatic and asymptomatic individuals because it is painless, quick, and nonthreatening and permits the evaluation of large areas of scalp. A recent study comparing the diagnostic accuracy of samples taken using #15 surgical blades and toothbrushes indicates that there is a good correlation between the results obtained with the two methods (33). An alternative method is the use of a cotton swab, rubbed

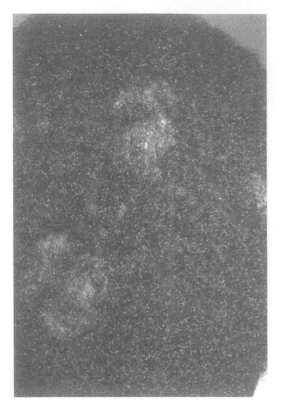

Figure 2 Kerion: Boggy areas of alopecia may contain pustules and significant bacterial overgrowth.

vigorously over the affected area, then smeared across the fungal media. Although this method has not been compared directly to toothbrush culturing, it is as effective as using a #15 blade (34).

COMPLICATIONS OF TINEA CAPITIS

Although tinea capitis is generally considered to be a benign disease, several complications have been described. Pomeranz and Fairley (35) recently described 10 children in whom tinea capitis was the primary reason for hospital admission. Most of these children had kerions and were presumed to have secondary bacterial infections. Occasionally,

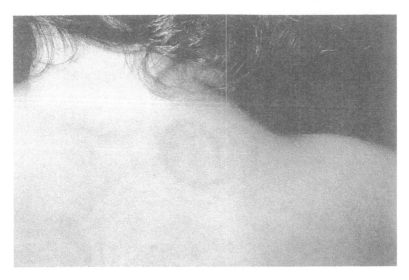

Figure 3 Tinea corporis: The location on the upper back should suggest the possibility of concomitant tinea capitis.

secondary bacterial infection results in the spread of bacterial infection to other areas of the body. Sahn and Gerscovich (36) described a generalized ichthyosiform rash and fever in a young girl with tinea capitis and widespread tinea corporis.

Scarring alopecia is a feared but fortunately rare complication of tinea capitis. Lymphadenitis is common even in patients with subtle scalp infection. Erythema nodosum has also been reported (37). The so-called "id" reaction is a relatively frequent complication, noted in a recent report in 10 of 30 patients with scalp kerions (38). "Id" reactions often begin after the initiation of therapy and are frequently confused with a drug eruption, but their distribution and morphology may help in differentiating them from a true drug allergy. The lesions of the "id" reaction to tinea capitis are usually more profuse on the face and upper torso, and they usually consist of either minute papules, or scaling papules and plaques (Figure 4), rather than the urticarial, morbilliform, or targetlike lesions more typical of true drug eruptions. If the morphology and distribution of the lesions are typical, the antifungal medication can generally be continued even in the presence of the rash, which gradually fades over time. Occasionally symptomatic therapy, including topical corticosteroids and antihistamines, is necessary.

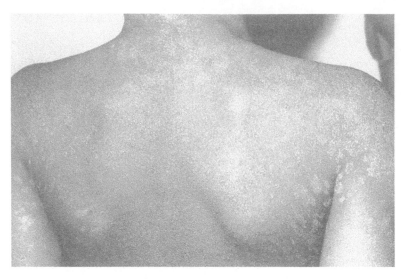

Figure 4 "Id" reaction: The papulosquamous nature of the condition and location on the face and upper torso usually help distinguish it from a true allergic drug eruption.

Tinea corporis is a frequent complication, in both patients and family members. Sharply demarcated pityriasis albalike lesions on the face should suggest the possibility of tinea capitis in populations where tinea capitis is endemic (39).

TREATMENT

Systemic therapy is always required for the treatment of tinea capitis, because topical therapy does not adequately penetrate into the half follicle. The duration of therapy varies depending on the clinical response to therapy and which medication is used, but a minimum of 4 weeks and often up to several months of treatment may be required to adequately eradicate infection. This need for prolonged therapy may result in poor compliance, which is probably a major cause of treatment failure. Treatment failure may also be caused by reinfection from other family members, impaired host immune response, and drug resistance (22).

Griseofulvin

Griseofulvin is the most frequently prescribed therapy for tinea capitis in the United States. The usual initial starting dose is 15 mg/kg per day micronized or 10 mg/kg per day ultramicronized griseofulvin, taken as a single dose with fat-containing food (40), but in our experience doses as high as 20 to 25 mg/kg per day are often necessary to clear infection. A minimum of 6 weeks of therapy is given. Ideally, patients should be rechecked and recultured monthly. The routine monitoring of laboratory parameters such as complete blood count or liver function tests is controversial, but is probably unnecessary in otherwise healthy children taking griseofulvin for less than 3 or 4 months. "Id" reactions to griseofulvin are relatively common, whereas true drug hypersensitivity to griseofulvin is rare. Thus, patients developing a rash shortly after beginning therapy should be examined to determine its cause before being labeled as griseofulvin-allergic.

Although relatively high doses of griseofulvin are often necessary for therapy, absolute resistance of *T. tonsurans* to griseofulvin is probably rare. Howard et al. (41) used a screening assay to evaluate the sensitivity of *T. tonsurans* to griseofulvin dissolved in acetone at concentrations of 4, 8, 16, and 32 μg/ml. Most of the 43 isolates tested were sensitive, but six were inhibited only at a concentration of 32 μg/ml, and one grew at a concentration >32 μg/ml, suggesting intermediate and possibly absolute resistance. Additional studies will be needed to establish standardized methods of in vitro antimycotic susceptibility testing and to determine whether such tests can be helpful in guiding therapy (42).

Other Systemic Agents

Gan et al. (25) found that the administration of griseofulvin, 15 mg/kg per day, resulted in more rapid clearing of tinea capitis than did ketoconazole, 5 mg/kg per day. At week 4, one-third of the patients treated with griseofulvin and two-thirds of those treated with ketoconazole had positive cultures (25).

Itraconazole also has been used for treating tinea capitis. In an open-label study, itraconazole, 100 mg, was administered daily for 5 weeks to 50 patients, most of whom had tinea capitis caused by *T. tonsurans* or *M. canis.* At the end of the study, 93% of the study participants had negative cultures, and only 7% had positive cultures (43). More recently, a double-blind study compared itraconazole, 100 mg daily, to griseofulvin, 500 mg daily, both given for 6 weeks in 34 children and 1 adult, nearly all of whom had *M. canis* infection. At 8 weeks, 88% of both groups were cured. All tolerated the treatment well except two 2-year-olds given 500 mg of griseofulvin, both of whom had significant gastrointestinal upset (44).

Terbinafine, an allyamine oral antifungal agent also has been used in the treatment of tinea capitis. A small study of children with *Trichophyton violaceum* infection revealed good results using 125 mg a day for at least 6 weeks. Seven of 12 children had a negative culture at 3 weeks; all were cured at the end of the study (45,46). A recent meta-analysis of the efficacy and tolerance of terbinafine in children in several different studies showed it to be effective and well tolerated in children, with approximately 93% cured in 4 weeks. Recommended pediatric dosages were 62.5 mg/day for children weighing <20 kg, 125 mg/day for children weighing 20 to 40 kg, and 250 mg for those weighing >40 kg (47).

Adjunctive Therapy

A recent study of the microbiology of kerions isolated *Staphylococcus aureus* from the pus of kerions in 48% of cases. Gram-negative organisms (*Pseudomonus, Proteus,* and *Klebsiella*) were found in 18% of cases (48). Despite these findings, a concomitant study of treatment of kerions found no difference between treatment with griseofulvin and treatment with griseofulvin plus erythromycin and/or prednisone, but the number of patients in each group (7 or 8) may have been too small to demonstrate a significant effect (38). I rarely find oral antibiotics necessary in patients who are receiving antifungal therapy, even when positive bacterial cultures or pustules are present, unless fever or skin lesions away from the scalp are present. I treat those kerions with significant elevation and tenderness with prednisone 1 mg/kg per day for 1 to 2 weeks both to decrease symptoms and in the hopes of minimizing the potential for scarring alopecia.

Selenium sulfide shampoo, 2.5% used twice a week, decreases spore shedding (49). More recently, this shampoo in a 1% concentration (available over the counter) has been shown to be equally effective to the 2.5% concentration (50).

THE CARRIER STATE OF TINEA CAPITIS

Mounting evidence suggests that a large reservoir of asymptomatic infection may play a role in the spread of tinea capitis. In certain parts of Africa, where tinea capitis is usually caused by *T. violaceum*, up to 41% of asymptomatic school-aged children are carriers (51). Adults are affected as well:

In one survey, 29% of asymptomatic mothers of children with tinea capitis had positive scalp cultures (52).

An analogous situation may exist with *T. tonsurans* in the United States. Babel and Baughman (53) recovered fungus from the scalps of 14 of 46 (30%) asymptomatic adult contacts of children with tinea capitis. Most of the adults available for culture were women, and all were African American. Random culturing of 200 asymptomatic children in a pediatric clinic in Kansas City found *T. tonsurans* in eight (4%), but the rate in African-American girls was 12.7% (23). A study by Vargo and Cohen (54) demonstrated positive cultures in 15% of a control group of African-American children visiting an urban outpatient clinic for nondermatological problems.

Williams et al. (24) reported a study of all children attending an all-black parochial school, in which 14% of children were asymptomatic carriers. Interestingly, 50% of positive cultures came from children in kindergarten and first grade. More than half of untreated carriers remained culture-positive after 2 months. Semiquantitative assessment of spore loads demonstrated that carriers had lower spore counts than symptomatic individuals, but that asymptomatic carriers with higher spore counts were more likely to remain carriers after 2 months than those with lower counts. One of 38 carriers became overtly symptomatic during the study.

To my knowledge, the only published study treating the carrier state was on patients infected with *T. violaceum*. The study compared econazole, selenium sulfide, povidone–iodine, and baby shampoos and found 50% clearing in all groups except povidone–iodine, where 94% of carriers became culture-negative (51). A study that evaluates topical therapy of asymptomatic *T. tonsurans* infection is needed.

FOMITE SPREAD OF INFECTION

Most tinea capitis is probably spread through close interpersonal contact, but fomites may also play a role. MacKenzie isolated *T. tonsurans* from combs, brushes, and bed linens at a residential school and demonstrated aerial spread of organisms (55,56). Hebert et al. (57) cultured *T. tonsurans* from a telephone receiver, combs and brushes, furniture, and even the hair of a doll in the household where many family members were affected. A recent report implicated a used car as a source of *M. canis* tinea capitis in a child who had no contact with animals (58). Similarly, fomites from tinea capitis can also cause tinea corporis. In a hospital outbreak, two workers, whose only contact with a patient with tinea capitis case came indirectly through changing bed sheets, developed tinea corporis (59). Fomite spread may represent a greater source of infection than has been previously appreciated, but reliable methods for ridding the environment of viable fungi are not well established.

CONCLUSION

Tinea capitis continues to a common childhood infection. Its clinical presentation may be subtle and mimic a variety of other scalp diseases. Although griseofulvin remains a mainstay of therapy, newer antifungal agents such as itraconazole and terbinafine may be effective alternatives. Comparative trials are necessary to determine whether they are even more efficacious and cost-effective than griseofulvin. The potential spread of disease by asymptomatic carriage and fomites raises new issues in the management of tinea capitis.

REFERENCES

1. Manglani PR, Ramanan C, Durairaj P. *Trichophyton tonsurans* infection in a 9-day-old infant. Int J Dermatol 1988; 27: 128.
2. Moberg S. Tinea capitis in the elderly, a report on two cases caused by *Trichophyton tonsurans*. Dermatologica 1984; 169: 36–40.
3. Conerly SL, Greer DL. Tinea capitis in adults over fifty years of age. Cutis 1988; 41: 251–252.
4. Pursley TV. Tinea capitis in the elderly. Int J Dermatol 1980; 19: 220.
5. Prevost E. The rise and fall of fluorescent tinea capitis. Pediatr Dermatol 1983; 1: 127–133.
6. Laude TA, Shah BR, Lynfield Y. Tinea capitis in Brooklyn. Am J Dis Child 1982; 136: 1047–1050.
7. Ravits MS, Himmelstein R. Tinea capitis in the New York City area. Arch Dermatol 1983; 119: 532–533.
8. Bronson DM, Desai DR, Barsky S. An epidemic of infection with *Trichophyton tonsurans* revealed in a 20-year survey of fungal infections in Chicago. J Am Acad Dermatol 1983; 8: 322–330.
9. Prevost E. Nonfluorescent tinea capitis in Charleston, SC: a diagnostic problem. JAMA 1979; 242: 1765–1767.
10. Shockman J, Urbach F. Tinea capitis in Philadelphia. Int J Dermatol 1983; 22: 521–524.
11. McLean T, Levy H, Lue YA. Ecology of dermatophyte infections in South Bronx, New York, 1969 to 1981. J Am Acad Dermatol 1987; 16: 336–340.

12. Babel DE, Rogers AL, Beneke ES. Dermatophytosis of the scalp: incidence, immune response, and epidemiology. Mycopathologia 1990; 109: 69–73.
13. Sinski JT, Flouras K. A survey of dermatophytes isolated from human patients in the United States from 1979 to 1981 with chronological listings of worldwide incidence of five dermatophytes often isolated in the United States. Mycopathologia 1984; 85: 97–120.
14. Aly R. Incidence of dermatophytes in the San Francisco Bay Area. Dermatologica 1980; 161: 97–100.
15. Lobato MN, Vugia DJ, Frieden IJ. Tinea capitis in California children: a growing epidemic (Abstract K195). Interscience Conference on Antimicrobial Agents and Chemotherapy. American Society of Microbiology, San Francisco, September, 1995.
16. Wilmington MR, Aly R, Frieden IJ. Tinea capitis in the San Francisco Bay Area: evolution of an epidemic due to *Trichophyton tonsurans*. J Med Vet Mycol In Press.
17. Chao S-C, Hsu MM-L. *Trichophyton tonsurans* infection in Tainan area. J Formos Med Assoc 1994; 93: 697–701.
18. Moore MK, Suite M. Tinea capitis in Trinidad. J Tropic Med Hyg 1993; 96: 346–348.
19. Rogers M, Muir D, Pritchard R. The pattern of childhood tinea in New South Wales, Australia 1979–1988: the emergence of *Trichophyton tonsurans* as an important pathogen in tinea capitis in white children. Australas J Dermatol 1993; 34: 5–8.
20. Korstanje MJ, Staats CCG. Tinea capitis in Northwestern Europe 1963–1993: etiologic agents and their changing prevalence. Int J Dermatol 1994; 33: 548–549.
21. Mills CM, Philpot CM. Tinea capitis in South Wales—observations in change of causative fungi. Clin Exp Dermatol 1994; 19: 473–475.
22. Howard R, Frieden IJ. Tinea capitis: new perspectives on an old disease. Semin Dermatol 1995; 14: 2–8.
23. Sharma V, Hall JC, Knapp JF, et al. Scalp colonization by *Trichophyton tonsurans* in an urban pediatric clinic: Asymptomatic carrier state. Arch Dermatol 1988; 124: 1511–1513.
24. Williams JV, Honig PJ, McGinley KJ, Leyden JJ. Semiquantitative study of tinea capitis and the asymptomatic carrier state in inner-city school children. Pediatrics 1995; 96: 265–267.
25. Gan VN, Petruska M, Ginsburg CM. Epidemiology and treatment of tinea capitis: ketoconazole vs. griseofulvin. Pediatr Infect Dis J 1987; 6: 46–49.
26. Rothman S, Smiljanic BS, Shapiro AL. The spontaneous cure of tinea capitis in puberty. J Invest Dermatol 1947; 8: 81–98.
27. Honig PJ, Smith RS. Tinea capitis masquerading as atopic or seborrheic dermatitis. JAMA 1979; 94: 604–605.
28. Krowchuk DP. Current status of the identification and management of tinea capitis. Pediatrics 1983; 72: 625–631.
29. Frieden IJ. Diagnosis and management of tinea capitis. Pediatr Ann 1987; 16: 39–48.

30. Ring DS, Kaplan DL. Pityriasis amiantacea: a report of 10 cases. Arch Dermatol 1993; 129: 913–914.
31. Kamalam A, Thambiah AS. Lupus erythematosus like tinea capitis caused by *Trichophyton tonsurans*. Mykosen 1983; 27: 316–318.
32. Pakula AS, Paller AS. Langerhans cell histiocytosis and dermatophytosis. J Am Acad Dermatol 1993; 29: 340–343.
33. Hubbard TW, deTriquet JM. Brush-culture method for diagnosing tinea capitis. Pediatrics 1992; 90: 416–418.
34. Head ES, Henry JC, Macdonald EM. The cotton swab technique for the culture of dermatophyte infections—its efficacy and merit. J Am Acad Dermatol 1984; 11: 797–801.
35. Pomeranz AJ, Fairley JA. Management errors leading to unnecessary hospitalization for kerion. Pediatrics 1994; 93: 986–988.
36. Sahn EE, Gerscovich MJ. Ichthyosiform rash and fever in a child. Arch Dermatol 1993; 129: 1189, 1192.
37. Martinez-Roig A, Llorens-Terol J, Torres J. Erythema nodosum and kerion of the scalp. Am J Dis Child 1982; 136: 440–442.
38. Honig PJ, Caputo GL, Leyden JJ, et al. Treatment of kerions. Pediatr Dermatol 1994; 11: 69–71.
39. duToit MJ. Pigmenting pityriasis alba. Pediatr Dermatol 1993; 10: 1–5.
40. Ginsburg CM. Effect of feeding on bioavailability of griseofulvin in children. J Pediatr 1983; 102: 309–311.
41. Howard R, Aly R, Frieden I. Analysis of *Trichophyton tonsurans* sensitivity to griseofulvin in vitro (abstr.). J Invest Dermatol 1993; 100: 519.
42. Rinaldi ME. In vitro susceptibility of dermatophytes to antifungal drugs (editorial). Int J Dermatol 1993; 32: 502–503.
43. Legendre R, Eola-Macre J. Itraconazole in the treatment of tinea capitis. J Am Acad Dermatol. 1990; 23: 559–560.
44. Lopez-Gomez S, Del Palacio A, Van Cutsem J, et al. Itraconazole versus griseofulvin in the treatment of tinea capitis: a double-blind randomized study in children. Int J Dermatol 1994; 33: 743–744.
45. Haroon TS, Hussain I, Aman S, et al. A randomized, double-blind, comparative study of terbinafine vs griseofulvin in tinea capitis. J Dermatol Treat 1992; 3: 25–27.
46. Nejjam F, Zagula M, Cabiac MD, et al. Pilot study of terbinafine in children suffering from tinea capitis: evaluation of efficacy, safety, and pharmacokinetics. Br J Dermatol 1995; 132: 98–105.
47. Jones TC. Overview of the use of terbinafine (Lamisil) in children. Br J Dermatol 1995; 132: 683–689.
48. Honig PJ, Caputo GL, Leyden JJ, et al. Microbiology of kerions. J Pediatr 1993; 123: 422–424.
49. Allen HB, Honig PJ, Leyden JJ, et al. Selenium sulfide: adjunctive therapy for tinea capitis. Pediatrics 1982; 69: 81–83.
50. Givens TG, Murray MM, Baker RC. Comparison of 1% and 2.5% selenium sulfide in the treatment of tinea capitis. Arch Pediatr Adolesc Med 1995; 149: 808–811.

51. Neil G, Hanslo D. Control of the carrier state of scalp dermatophytes. Pediatr Infect Dis J 1990; 9: 57–58.
52. Barlow D, Saxe N. Tinea capitis in adults. Int J Dermatol 1988; 27: 388–390.
53. Babel DE, Baughman SA. Evaluation of the adult carrier state in juvenile tinea capitis caused by *Trichophyton tonsurans*. J Am Acad Dermatol 1989; 21: 1209–1212.
54. Vargo K, Cohen B. Prevalence of undetected tinea capitis in household members of children with disease. Pediatrics 1993; 92: 155–156.
55. MacKenzie DWR, Burrows D, Walby AL. *Trichophyton sulphureum* in a residential school. Br Med J 1960; 2: 1055–1058.
56. MacKenzie DWR. The extra-human occurrence of *Trichophyton tonsurans* var. *sulfureum* in a residential school. Sabouraudia 1961; 1: 58–64.
57. Hebert AA, Head ES, Macdonald EM. Tinea capitis caused by *Trichophyton tonsurans*. Pediatr Dermatol 1985; 2: 219–223.
58. Thomas P, Korting HC, Strassl W, Ruzicka T. *Microsporum canis* infection in a 5-year-old boy: transmission from the interior of a second-hand car. Mycoses 1994; 37: 141–142.
59. Arnow PM, Houchins SG, Pugliese G. An outbreak of tinea corporis in hospital personnel caused by a patient with *Trichophyton tonsurans* infection. Pediatr Infect Dis 1991; 10: 355–359.

15

The Risk/Benefit Ratio of Modern Antifungal Pharmacological Agents

David T. Roberts
Southern General Hospital, Glasgow, Scotland

INTRODUCTION

The increasing incidence of both systemic and superficial fungal infections in immunocompromised patients, together the advent of newer, more effective drugs for preexisting disease, suggests that use of antifungal drugs will increase over the coming years. It is appropriate, therefore, to review both the risks and benefits that may accrue from their use. Clearly the risk/benefit ratio of any drug is not fixed and will alter according to the severity of the disease; it is permissible to run a greater degree of risk in the treatment of life-threatening systemic infection than it is when treating relatively trivial but possibly chronic superficial disease. This chapter concentrates on the risk/benefit ratio related to the treatment of superficial fungal infection.

Initially one should examine the outcome if the disease is left untreated. Most fungal infections tend to run a chronic course and do not resolve spontaneously. Infections that induce a profound inflammatory response, such as a kerion, are exceptions in that secondary bacterial infection together with an enhanced immune response tends toward spontaneous resolution. A good deal of scarring, however, is likely to result from this process, and if scarring occurs on the scalp, alopecia will ensue. Dermatophyte infection of the skin (tinea corporis) will slowly spread and produce significant morbidity. The most common dermatophyte infection is tinea pedis or athlete's foot, which may in some circumstances remain confined to the toe clefts for many years and produce little in the way of symptoms. However, secondary infection and inflammation and even cellulitis and lymphangitis can occur, and a strong case can be made for treatment of this condition given the extremely low risk of topical anti-fungal medication. Fungal nail infection or onychomycosis is a disease of insidious onset and relentless progression that ultimately destroys the nail plate. A recent survey suggests that 2.71% of the population of the United Kingdom has dermatophyte onychomycosis. The same survey suggests that about 50% of this group seeks no medical advice, and fewer than 20% are treated with systemic agents, which is the only method of treatment likely to be successful. More than 80% of the same population, however, stated that they would wish treatment if the diagnosis were known to them and if effective treatment were available (1). Therefore, both from the point of view of the likely course of the disease and the wishes of the affected population, there is a strong case to treat superficial infection, providing that the risk of drug therapy is acceptable. It is reasonable to examine the risks and benefits of systemic antifungal therapy with reference to onychomycosis because the nail is pharmacokinetically difficult tissue in which to achieve adequate drug concentration, and therapy has to be prescribed in adequate doses over longer periods than for any other area of skin. Experience suggests that drugs that are effective in fungal infection of nails in a high percentage of cases would certainly be effective elsewhere over a much shorter treatment period. In addition, both toxic and allergic drug effects and drug interactions are always more likely to surface in patients treated for a long period.

BENEFITS OF ANTIFUNGAL DRUGS

Data relating to drug efficacy are almost always obtained during the course of controlled clinical trials with strict entry and exclusion criteria. At least in such studies the diagnosis is confirmed both clinically and by laboratory investigation, which is not always the case in general use. Care should be taken, however, to examine the results of such studies to ensure that not only "easy" cases are selected for treatment. It is well recognized that onychomycosis affecting only the distal portion of nail will respond better to treatment than cases in which the whole of the nail plate is involved, and cure rates will be correspondingly higher in studies where only distal nail disease is treated. Patients with many intercurrent diseases are often excluded from clinical studies, as are patients on some other drugs, so it is possible that data relating to toxic effects and drug interactions will be falsely low in patients in clinical trials. The incidence of such effects in general use is likely to be a more accurate guide, but such data are rarely published and come to light only via experience, reporting schemes for adverse events, and in some cases after marketing surveillance studies. Although some drug interactions may be predicted pharmacologically, others emerge only when the drug is released for general use.

Onychomycosis was untreatable medically until the advent of the drug griseofulvin in the late 1950s. This drug is a weakly fungistatic agent that requires a duration of therapy equivalent to keratin turnover at the affected site. It has proved reasonably effective for infections of glabrous skin in which the keratin turnover time is about 28 days.

Scalp infections often require longer periods of treatment, but there is no doubt that griseofulvin has radically altered the prognosis of anthropophilic dermatophyte infections of the scalp, and many previously common species have been virtually eradicated. However, in slow growing nails when treatment periods of at least 6 to 12 months for fingernails and toenails, respectively, are necessary, the drug has proved disappointing, particularly in toenail infection. Cure rates are rarely better than 30% to 40%, and the use of the drug was curtailed for this reason. Ketoconazole became available in the early 1980s and was the first agent active against yeasts and dermatophytes that was available for long-term oral use. However, it was not much more effective than griseofulvin in toenail onychomycosis, and serious side effects have emerged.

Recently, the allylamine terbinafine and the oral triazole itraconazole have become available for the treatment of superficial infection including nail infection. Cure rates of 70% to 90% in various studies can be achieved with these drugs with treatment as short as 6 weeks for fingernails and 3 months for toenails. The oral triazole fluconazole is likely to be effective in nail infections, but thus far its use is concentrated on systemic disease and vaginal candidosis. Comparatively far fewer studies are available examining its efficacy in onychomycosis. Recently, novel treatment regimens using intermittent or pulse therapy have been examined, particularly using itraconazole. These new regions await full evaluation. All of these drugs are as effective or more so than griseofulvin over shorter treatment durations in infections of the skin, hair, and nail (2).

ADVERSE EFFECTS AND DRUG INTERACTIONS

In most countries drug manufacturers must list reported adverse events and drug interactions in the data sheet. In the United Kingdom, the

Association of the British Pharmaceutical Industry (ABPI) publishes an annual compendium of all data sheets of drugs licensed for use in the UK (3). This useful publication allows easy access to lists of adverse events and drug interactions and has the advantage of being relatively up-to-date. Physicians must keep both drug companies and regulatory authorities informed of any new effects, either directly or through publications in the literature, although the latter method inevitably causes delay.

All antifungal drugs are reported to cause minor gastrointestinal (GI) upset and occasional skin rashes. Many are also reported to cause headache. These three effects seem to occur in virtually all classes of drug and, indeed, GI upset is seen in about 2% of all patients treated with placebo. These effects, therefore, have to be accepted, providing they are not too severe or too frequent. Griseofulvin is notable for causing quite severe headache on occasion and in addition may cause photosensitivity (Table 1). It should not be used in patients with porphyria or systemic lupus erythematosus, but may also precipitate such diseases where they were not previously overt. Drug interactions that affect the level of other drugs and griseofulvin itself do occur and are listed in Table 2. Keto-conazole occasionally produces hormonal effects such as gynecomastia and oligospermia, but the drug has largely fallen out of use for long-term therapy because of the risk of hepatitis, which is said to occur in 1:10,000 treated cases and may be even more common in those treated long-term. There have been several fatalities from drug-induced hepatitis with keto-conazole and thus the risk/benefit ratio has become unacceptable in cases requiring relatively lengthy treatment. Ketoconazole and all other azole derivatives acts by interfering with the enzyme 14-α demethylase, thus preventing the conversion of lanosterol to ergosterol within the fungal cell. Ergosterol is essential for fungal cells to be produced, and thus these

Table 1 Adverse Effects

Griseofulvin	Ketoconazole	Itraconazole	Fluconazole	Terbinafine
Headache	GI upset	GI upset	GI upset	GI upset
GI upset	CNS effects	CNS effects	Rashes	Rashes
Urticaria	Rashes	Rashes	Hepatitis in	TEN/EM
CNS effects	Gynecomastia	Menstrual	patients with	Taste distortion
TEN/EM	Oligospermia	disturbance	underlying	Hepatitis/
	Hepatitis	Hepatitis/	disease	cholestasis
		cholestasis		

Table 2 Drug Interactions with Antifungal Agents

Griseofulvin	Ketoconazole	Itraconazole	Fluconazole	Terbinafine
Coumarins	Terfenedine	Rifampicin	Warfarin	Rifampicin
Oral	Astemizole	Phenytoin	Hypoglycemics	H₂ blockers
contraceptives	H₂ blockers	Terfenedine	Thiazides	
Phenobarbitone	Cyclosporin	Astemizole	Phenytoin	
Phenylbutazone	Anticoagu-	Midazolam	Rifampicin	
Hypnotics	lants	Triazolam	Cyclosporin	
	Steroids	Digoxin	Theophylline	
	Alcohol	Dihydro-		
	Isoniazid	pyridine		
	Rifampicin	Quinidine		
		H₂ blockers		

drugs are quite potent fungistatic agents, which may become fungicidal in increasing concentrations. Because 14-α demethylase is a cytochrome P-450 enzyme, all azole drugs interfere potentially with other drugs that use this enzyme system either by competitive inhibition or by other means. Ketoconazole, therefore, potentially interacts adversely with several other drugs shown in Table 2. The triazoles itraconazole and fluconazole act via the same enzyme system, and a significant number of drug interactions are listed for these agents. However, they do not appear to have the capacity to cause hepatitis with the same frequency as ketoconazole and are now generally accepted to be safe for long-term use.

Terbinafine is an allylamine that also inhibits the production of ergosterol, but it acts via a different enzyme, squalene epoxidase, inhibiting the conversion of squalene to squalene epoxide. This leads to a buildup as squalene, as well as to depletion of ergosterol. This buildup of squalene is considered to be responsible for the drug's fungicidal effect and, because squalene epoxidase is not a cytochrome P-450 enzyme, this drug gives rise to relatively few drug interactions. Hepatic reactions, mainly cholestasis, can occur with terbinafine in about 1:50,000 cases. This reaction may give rise to cholestatic jaundice, but thus far has always proved reversible on cessation of therapy. Taste disturbance is a curious and unique side effect of terbinafine and its mechanism is unknown. It occurs in about 0.25% of cases and thus far has always been reversible on cessation of treatment (4).

Skin rashes occur in 2% to 5% of cases with nearly all drugs, and antifungal drugs are no exception. Almost all of these cases are minor, often not requiring interruption of therapy. Most drug-induced allergic rashes are either morbiliform or urticarial and are not too significant. Erythema multiforme and particularly toxic epidermal necrolysis however, are serious allergic reactions that are difficult to treat and occasionally may prove fatal. Only one or two such cases have been identified during therapy with antifungal drugs among many millions of patients who have been treated, and the risk, therefore, is no greater than with many other commonly used agents.

Hepatotoxicity or drug-induced hepatic injury is always likely to be the most worrisome effect, partly because of their metabolism and partly because of the fatalities that have occurred during ketoconazole treatment. It is important, therefore, that the frequency of such reactions is acceptably low and that they are reversible. The known incidence of hepatic reactions following the use of fluconazole, itraconazole, and terbinafine fits both criteria and has to be set within the context of the lengthy list of other drugs in common use that may cause both hepatitis and cholestasis Tables 3 and 4 (5). The most important variable is probably early identification of such reactions so that the drug may be stopped. Patients should be instructed to consult their physician immediately if they develop any evidence of liver injury such as darkening of the urine, jaundice, or prolonged nausea and malaise so that any drug therapy likely to be responsible may be stopped. The majority of cases of drug-induced hepatic injury will most likely resolve if this criterion is met.

It would be best to be able to predict such injury before it occurs, either by identification of patients in an at-risk group or by identifying the reaction before it becomes symptomatic. This raises the question of monitoring liver function. Although it would appear to be worthwhile to

Table 3 Drugs Associated with Hepatocellular Necrosis

Allopurinol	Halothane	Phenacemide
Chloroform	Hydralazine	Phenytoin
Cytarabine	Isoniazid	Salicylates
Clindamycin	Mepacrine	Sulfa
Clotrimazole	Methoxypsoralen	Valproate
Dapsone	Methyldopa	Verapamil
Etretinate	Paracetamol	Vincristine
Frusemide	PAS	Vinyl ether

Table 4 Drugs Associated with Cholestasis

Amitriptyline	Diazepam	Phenobarbitone
Azathioprine	Erythromycin	Quinidine
Captopril	Fenbufen	Quinine
Chlorambucil	Gold salts	Rifampin
Cimetidine	Haloperidol	Spironolactone
Cloxacillin	Imipramine	Sulfa
Colchicine	Indomethacin	Tolbutamide
Cyclosporin	Istoretinoin	Warfarin

identify patients with abnormal liver function before therapy is begun, it is well recognized that even patients who have abnormal liver function may be treated with impunity with antifungal drugs because hepatic reactions are likely to be idiosyncratic rather than toxic. Excluding such patients may deny them treatment unnecessarily. A significant percentage of the population have asymptomatic liver function test abnormalities. About 6% of the population of the United Kingdom have an abnormal gamma-glutamyl transferase level, a particularly sensitive indicator of liver function (6). Monitoring patients during treatment may sound worthwhile, but allergic reactions can occur at any time and tend to develop suddenly. One could argue, therefore, that such monitoring would almost have to be carried out daily to be foolproof, which is clearly not feasible. Monitoring should be carried out on the basis of frequency of reaction. Currently in the United Kingdom, monitoring of liver function is only suggested for itraconazole therapy that is continued for longer than 1 month and for all drugs in which the patient may be considered at risk because of preexisting liver disease (7).

CONCLUSION

The risk/benefit ratio of ketoconazole is unacceptable for long-term use because of potentially fatal hepatitis. Although griseofulvin has been used for superficial fungal infection for many years and has proven acceptable in terms of its side effect profile, the risk/benefit ratio has become much less acceptable with this drug when its efficacy is compared with the newer agents terbinafine and itraconazole, which provide much higher cure rates over shorter treatment durations. The risk/benefit ratio of fluconazole would also likely be acceptable, but comparatively much less data are available with regard to its efficacy in superficial fungal infections, particularly onychomycosis where long-term treatment is indicated.

Modern antifungal pharmacological agents have a positive risk/benefit ratio and will prove to be a significant advance in treatment of common diseases.

REFERENCES

1. Roberts DT. Prevalence of dermatophyte onychomycosis in the United Kingdom: results of an omnibus survey. Br J Dermatol 1992; 126(suppl 39): 23–27.
2. Roberts DT. Oral therapeutic agents in fungal nail disease. J Am Acad Dermatol 1994; 32: (Part 2): 578–581.
3. Association of British Pharmaceutical Industry. Data Sheet Compendium. London: Datapharm Publications, 1995.
4. Needham CA, Bangs AJ, Atkin K, O'Sullivan DP. Repeat of UK post marketing surveillance study of oral Lamisil (terbinafine). Br J Dermatol 1995; 133(suppl 45): 27.
5. Pessayre D, Larrey D. Drug induced liver injury. In: McIntyre N, Benhamou JP, Bircher J, et al, eds. Textbook of Clinical Hepatology. Oxford: Oxford University Press, 1991: 873–902.
6. Penn R, Worthington DJ. Is serum gamma glutamyl transferase a misleading test? Br Med J 1983; 286: 531–536.
7. Hay RJ. Risk/benefit ratio of modern antifungal therapy: focus on hepatic reactions. J Am Acad Dermatol 1992; 29: 1: 50–54.

16

Dermatophytes and Nondermatophytes: Their Role in Cutaneous Mycoses

Dennis E. Babel
Michigan State University, East Lansing, Michigan

Fungal infection of the keratinized tissues of the body (tinea or ringworm) is attributed to colonization and subsequent invasion by any one of a number of dermatophyte species. These hyaline molds, which are contracted from species-specific environmental sources, involve hair, skin, and nail. Yeasts and nondermatophytic molds may cause similar mycoses. On occasion these later organisms may be secondary invaders to the primary tineal process. Unlike the opportunistic mycoses caused by saprophytic molds, dissemination of dermatophyte infections in the immunocompromised patients is rarely observed. Antifungal therapy must be designed to impact on all organisms thought to be responsible for the mycosis.

TINEA CAPITIS

Tinea capitis includes dermatophyte infections of the hair follicles of the scalp and eyebrows. It can be caused by fungal species in the genera *Trichophyton* and *Microsporum*, but not *Epidermophyton*. Species that normally reside in the soil are referred to as geophilic, those that have a specific animal host are called zoophilic, and those that are obligate parasites of humans are described as anthropophilic (1,2). The geophilic and zoophilic species usually result in a much more inflammatory human tinea.

"Gray patch" ringworm is characterized by areas of well-defined alopecia containing short, lusterless hair stubs. The use of a wood's lamp may demonstrate a bright blue-green fluorescence because of the ultraviolet light activation of the fungal metabolite, pteridine. This form of disease was epidemic among school-aged children from the 1930s through the mid-1960s. The responsible dermatophyte, *Microsporum audouinii*, an anthropophilic pathogen, has virtually disappeared from North America and along with it this gray patch form of ringworm.

Trichophyton tonsurans, another anthropophilic species, has filled the resulting void, gradually moving into this country from Central America. In this form of infection, the hyphae are retained within the hair shaft (endothrix) where they separate into arthroconidia, elaborate keratinases, and disrupt the keratin fibrils. The resulting weakened hair curls and breaks at the follicular orifice, giving the appearance of black dots on the scalp surface within the area of alopecia. This "black dot" tinea capitis will not fluoresce and is demonstrated most frequently in Black and Hispanic patients. The mycosis is usually chronic and noninflammatory, with only 15% to 20% evolving into the pustular to kerion type of host response (3). In urban areas, it can comprise approximately 90% of dermatophytosis of the scalp. It can be transferred by direct human-to-human contact or indirectly through certain fomites including brushes, combs, hats, pillowcases, furniture, carpeting, stuffed animals, and telephone receivers. *T. tonsurans* ringworm of the scalp has become a problematic source of tinea gladiatorum among high school wrestlers. These athletes are usually prevented from competing when their fungal lesions of the skin become apparent.

Tinea capitis caused by the zoophilic pathogen *Microsporum canis* can result in an inflammatory process that will usually fluoresce. This infection is most frequently contracted from infected household pets such as cats and dogs. Attention must be directed to the elimination of the mycosis in the animal source, as well as in the patient. *M. canis* infections can be recalcitrant and may require multiple courses of antifungal therapy.

Management of dermatophyte infection of the hair requires systemic antifungal therapy, as topical antimycotics will not penetrate deeply enough to be curative (4). The use of the fungistatic agent griseofulvin will usually result in a clinical response within 4 to 6 weeks. Unresponsive disease occasionally needs to be managed with a triazole antimycotic such as itraconazole. The adjunct use of a topical antifungal shampoo such as 2.5% selenium sulfide or ketoconazole will help prevent the transmission of this mycosis during the prolonged healing process.

Nondermatophytic fungal infections of the hair are relatively uncommon and would include the granulomas of the scalp associated with chronic mucocutaneous candidiasis, as well as the formation of hard stony nodules on the hair shaft that are seen in black piedra. The former is caused by the yeast *Candida albicans* and the later by the monomorphic, dematiaceous mold, *Piedraia hortae.*

TINEA CORPORIS

Dermatophytosis of the glabrous skin can manifest itself in a variety of presentations, depending on the anatomical site, fungal species, patient predisposition, etc. The classical tinea corporis lesion is described as "doughnut-shaped," being annular and having a clearing center. Viable organism is recovered only from the advancing edge of the lesion, not from the center. Infections acquired from zoophilic or geophilic sources can be quite inflammatory, presenting with erythematous, vesiculobullous lesions. In the elderly, tinea corporis lesions may be viewed as a diffuse, superficial follicular process and may be attributed mistakenly to a bacterial etiology. Dermatophytic granulomas of the skin occur when superficial fungi are encouraged to grow more deeply down a hair follicle, erode into the dermis, and elicit a strong host response. This may be associated with occlusion of a skin site. In the immunosuppressed, cutaneous dermatophytosis may present as a noninflammatory, diffuse, scaly process without any lesion delineation. The total body surface may become covered with this infection. All species of dermatophytes may contribute to tinea corporis.

TINEA CRURIS

Tinea cruris is a dermatophytic infection of the glabrous skin of the thigh, crural fold, abdomen, and buttocks. It is characterized by the formation of well-defined, annular to serpiginous, moderately inflammatory lesions of the glabrous skin. This mycosis is usually caused by the anthropophilic species *T. rubrum, T. mentagrophytes,* and *Epidermophyton floccosum* (5). Concurrent tinea pedis and onchomycosis of the toenails are common and possible provide the pathogen source for this crural eruption.

Nondermatophytic infections of the crural fold can include candidiasis and erythrasma. *C. albicans* infections of the groin present with a "beefy-red" erythema, satellite pustules and a lack of well-defined lesion edge. Erythrasma is caused by the filamentous bacterium, *C. minutissimum.*

Lesions are red-brown and scaly and demonstrate a coral-red fluorescence when illuminated with a Wood's lamp.

TINEA MANUUM

"Dorsal" tinea manuum can involve the dorsum of the hand and fingers and is frequently attributed to one of the zoophilic species of dermatophytes such as *T. mentagrophytes, T. verrucosum,* or *M. canis*. This infection can be seen in animal handlers such as veterinarians, pet shop owners, laboratory workers, dog or horse groomers, and so forth. Fungal lesions can be quite inflammatory, demonstrating erythema and vesiculation.

"Palmar" tinea manuum usually involves the palms and palmar aspects of the fingers and wrists. It tends to be a chronic, noninflammatory, dry scaling process with variable pruritis. It is seldom seen bilaterally, most frequently involving only one palm along with a concurrent, bilateral tinea pedis. This "one hand, two foot syndrome" is attributed to the anthropophilic dermatophyte, *T. rubrum*.

Nondermatophytic fungal infections of the hands can be caused by the molds, *Scytalidium hyalinum* and *S. dimidiatum* (*Hendersonula toruloidea*). This dry, scaly mycosis can be misdiagnosed as a tinea, but is usually bilateral and more extensive. It does not respond to oral griseofulvin or many of the topical antimycotics.

TINEA PEDIS

Dermatophyte infection of the feet can present as an inflammatory scaling process of the toewebs ("interdigital" tinea pedis). The resulting masceration and disruption of the stratum corneum barrier can provide a portal of entry for pathogenic bacteria and formation of subsequent pyodermas.

"Plantar" tinea pedis is a dry scaling infection of the sole of the foot, which may or may not demonstrate inflammation. This form tends to be chronic, resolving or exacerbating with the change of seasons or physical activity of the patient. It can be bilateral and, when associated with unilateral tinea manuum, forms the "one hand, two foot syndrome" as mentioned previously.

"Moccasin-type" tinea pedis involves the interdigital, plantar, lateral, and dorsal aspects of the foot, effectively covering that appendage like a scaly shoe. It can be recalcitrant to antifungal management and remain a reservoir of infectious material for the development of new mycoses.

These three forms of tinea pedis—interdigital, plantar and moccasin—can be caused by the anthropophilic dermatophytes, *T. rubrum*, *T. mentagrophytes var. interdigitale*, and *E. floccosum*, *T. rubrum* however, is responsible for the greatest share of disease worldwide.

"Vesicular" tinea pedis is an inflammatory, vesiculobullous infection of the plantar and lateral aspect of the foot. Its cause is the granular form of *T. mentagrophytes*, which is usually considered to be animal in origin. Frequent recurrence of this form of disease might lead one to consider a zoophilic environmental source initiating reinfection. Various strains of *T. mentagrophytes* can be carried by birds, primates, dogs, cats, and furry rodents including mice and rats.

Nondermatophytic fungal infection can present as an extensive, dry, scaly process of the foot caused by the saprophytic molds, *S. hyalinum* and *S. dimidiatum*. This mycosis can be virtually indistinguishable from its tinea counterpart, but will not respond to most antidermatophyte therapies. Also, unlike the dermatophytes, these fungal pathogens cannot be isolated on an inhibitory medium such as Sabouraud's dextrose agar with chloramphenicol and cyclohexamide.

TINEA UNGUIUM

Dermatophytosis of the nail unit can involve both the fingers and toes, with the toenails being infected with the greatest frequency. "Distal subungual" onychomycosis is initiated by the introduction of an organism underneath the distal nail plate. The mycelia begin to grow through the hyponychium and distal nail bed, resulting in hyperkeratosis and subsequent onycholysis. Eventual invasion of the nail plate results in thickening, discoloration, and onychodystrophy. The infection progresses from the distal toward the proximal nailfold with the viable pathogen being found at the advancing edge rather than at the distal fold. The anthropophilic dermatophytes responsible include *T. rubrum*, *T. mentagrophytes*, and *E. floccosum*, with *T. rubrum* being the most commonly isolated species. This mycosis is seen more frequently in the elderly. Trauma, tinea pedis, and immunocompromise may be predisposing factors.

"Proximal subungual" onychomycosis is thought to be initiated by the introduction of a dermatophyte underneath the proximal nailfold, with subsequent involvement of the nail matrix. All new nail plate, which is manufactured by the matrix, will by mycotic, and this process will progress from the proximal toward the distal nailfold. This form of disease is seen in immunocompromised individuals, especially those who are HIV-positive. The fungal pathogen that is usually isolated is *T. rubrum*.

"White superficial" onychomycosis (leukonychia mycotica) presents as a superficial "chalking" or colonization of the surface of the nail plate. The causative dermatophyte is *T. mentagrophytes* or occasionally *T. rubrum*.

Nondermatophytic onychomycosis can present in a distal subungual form and may be caused by a variety of saprophytic molds including species of *Fusarium, Scopulariopsis, Trichosporon,* and *Scytalidium* (6). These invaders may be primary, especially in a nail unit whose anatomy has been altered by trauma, or they may be secondary to an initial dermatophyte infection. More than one organism may coexist within the same infected nail unit. Proximal subungual onychomycosis has been attributed to saprophytic molds such as *Fusarium* sp. A much more erosive form of white superficial onychomycosis has been demonstrated by saprophytic molds such as *Aspergillus* and *Fusarium* spp.

Yeast onychomycoses have included infections of the nail unit associated with chronic mucocutaneous candidiasis, candidal paronychia, and *Candida* colonization of the distal nail plate as a result of a preexisting onycholysis.

DISCUSSION

The dermatophytes are the most common cause of mycoses of cutaneous tissue. Consideration of the source of the dermatophytic pathogen may be necessary to help prevent infection. Nondermatophytic molds and yeast may occasionally be the primary pathogen, especially in the predisposed patient. The presence of more than one fungal pathogen within the same mycotic infection should be a consideration and the physician's therapeutic strategy adjusted accordingly. In most situations dermatophytoses of the skin can be managed with topical antifungal agents. Mycoses of hair follicles, or the nail unit require systemic antimycotic therapy because of poor penetration by the topical antimicrobials. Selection of the appropriate antifungal agent requires a knowledge of the identity and susceptibility of the offending pathogens (7,8).

REFERENCES

1. Babel DE, Rogers AL. Dermatophytes: their contribution to infectious disease in North America. Clin Microbiol Rev 1983; 5: 81–85.

2. Svejgaard EL. Epidemiology of dermatophytes in Europe. Int J Dermatol 1995; 34: 525–528.
3. Babel DE, Rogers AL, Beneke ES. Dermatophytosis of the scalp: incidence, immune response, and epidemiology. Mycopathologia 1988; 109: 69–73.
4. Drake LA, Dinehart SM, Farmer ER, et al. Guidelines of care for superficial mycotic infections of the skin: tinea capitis and tinea barbae. J Am Acad Dermatol 1996; 34: 290–294.
5. Weitzman I, Summerbell RC. The dermatophytes. Clin Microbiol Rev 1995; 8: 240–259.
6. Greer DL. Evolving role of nondermatophytes in onychomycosis. Int J Dermatol 1995; 34: 521–524.
7. Drake LA, Dinehart SM, Farmer ER, et al. Guidelines of care for superficial mycotic infections of the skin: onychomycosis. J Am Acad Dermatol 1996; 34: 116–121.
8. Drake LA, Dinehart SM, Farmer ER, et al. Guidelines of care for superficial mycotic infections of the skin: tinea corporis, tinea cruris, tinea faciei, tinea manuum, and tinea pedis. J Am Acad Dermatol 1996; 34: 282–286.

17

Superficial and Cutaneous Phaeohyphomycosis in Immunocompetent Patients

Michael R. McGinnis
University of Texas Medical Branch, Galveston, Texas

Numerous fungi are capable of infecting hair, nail, and skin on the living host. In addition to the dermatophytes, several darkly colored fungi have been reported to have an ability to infect the cutaneous barrier of immunocompetent individuals (Table 1). Opportunistic infections caused by dematiaceous yeasts and molds can be difficult at times to diagnose owing to the fact that many of these fungi can be recovered from clinical specimens as contaminants. In some instances, their clinical presentation is identical to that of dermatophyte infections. To assess the importance of darkly colored fungi, criteria should be developed that will permit the separation of infection, colonization, and contamination.

DEMATIACEOUS

The term *dematiaceous* has been used classically in two senses. First, it describes a color range that encompasses olivaceous gray-to-black-to-brown, which is the result of melanin being present in the cell walls of fungi. Second, it is used taxonomically to classify hyphomycetes having darkly colored hyphae, conidia, conidiophores, or any combination of these structures within the family Dematiaceae of the Fungi Imperfecti. At times, these two concepts are used interchangeably by some investigators and clinicians.

199

Table 1 Molds and Yeasts Having Darkly Colored Colonies Associated with Hair, Nail, and Skin Infections in Immunocompetent Hosts

Fungus	Selected references		
	Hair	Nail	Skin
Alternaria alternata		1,2	2,3
A. chlamydospora			3
A. pluriseptata		4	
A. teniussima			5
Arthrinium phaeospermum			6
Aureobasidium pullulans		7	8
Bipolaris australiensis			9
Botryomyces caespitosus			10
Chaetomium globosum		11	12
Chmelia slovaca			13[a]
Cladophialophora carrionii		14	
Cladosporium cladosporioides		15[a]	16[a]
C. sphaerospermum		17[a]	17[a]
Curvularia sp.			18
C. clavata			19
Cyphellophora laciniata			20[a]
C. pluriseptata		21[a]	21a
Exophiala mansonii			22[a]
Exserohilum rostratum			18
Hormonema dermatioides			23
Lasiodiplodia theobromae		24,25[a]	
Moniliella suaveolens			26[a]
Onychocola canadensis		27,28	28
Phaeoannellomyces werneckii			29,30
Phialophora parasitica			31
Phoma eupyrena		32	
P. hibernica			33
P. sorghina			34[a]
Piedraia hortae	35		
Pyrenochaeta unguis-hominis		36,37	
Sarcinomyces phaeomuriformis			38,39
Scopulariopsis brumptii		40	41[a]
S. fusca		42	
S. koningii		42	
Scytalidium dimidiatum		43	43[b]
Stenella araguata			44,45
Wangiella dermatitidis			46,47

[a]Inadequately documented case report.
[b]Synanamorph of *Nattrassia mangiferae*.

Pappagianis and Ajello (48) researched the epistemology of the term *dematiaceous* and concluded that Saccardo modified the meaning of the word by including the character of dark color in its definition. The Greek term *dema* or its diminutive form refers to bundle, band, or bunch. Because of this problem, these investigators recommend that dematiaceous should be used only in a taxonomic sense to describe hyphomycetes classified in the family Dematiaceae. A term such as *phaeoid* should be used to describe the color range of gray-to-olivaceous-to-black-to-brown exhibited by these fungi.

In this chapter, dematiaceous is used to describe both color and taxonomic classification. The term *dematiaceous* has been used consistently for more than 100 years to describe both color and the family Dematiaceae. Change in the meaning of the word dematiaceous, its wide acceptance, and consistent usage by the mycological community are examples of the evolution of language. Because dematiaceous is a universally accepted term, having both descriptive and taxonomic importance, there is little need to disrupt its nomenclatural stability at this time.

The dematiaceous fungi are darkly colored because they possess melanin in their cell walls. Melanins are dark brown to black pigments of high molecular weight that are not essential for growth or development, but they enhance the survival and competitive abilities of dematiaceous fungi when they grow in certain environments (49). Fungi having melanin in their cell walls are more resistant to the effects of ultraviolet radiation, x-rays, gamma radiation, heat, and desiccation in comparison to non-dematiaceous fungi.

Some fungi like *Cryptococcus neoformans*, a basidiomycetous yeast, can synthesize melanin from tyrosine via 3,4-dihydroxyphenylalanine (DOPA) when it is incorporated into culture media. Gamma-glutaminyl-3,4-dihydroxybenzene or catechol is an immediate phenolic precursor of the melanin polymer found in the cell walls of basidiomycetes. In asco-mycetes and ascomycetous imperfecti fungi 1,8-dihydroxynaphthalene (DHN) is the precursor for the melanin polymer found in their cell walls (50,51). Because essentially all of the darkly colored etiological agents of phaeohyphomycosis are ascomycetes or related imperfect fungi, DHN melanin is of special importance. In fungi such as *Wangiella dermatitidis*, DHN melanin has been shown to be an important virulence factor (51).

PHAEOHYPHOMYCOSIS

Melanized fungi may cause chromoblastomycosis, mycetoma, and phaeohyphomycosis. Only a few species such as *Exophiala jeanselmei* and

Phialophora verrucosa are known to cause all three types of infections. *Phaeohyphomycosis* (52,53) is a term that encompasses superficial, cutaneous, subcutaneous, systemic, and allergic diseases caused by dematiaceous fungi. Constitutive DHN melanin can be detected in the cell walls of the etiological agents of phaeohyphomycoses by direct microscopy or when necessary, in tissue, by use of the Fontana–Masson stain (54).

Dermatomycosis refers to an infection involving hair, nail, or skin that is caused by a fungus other than a dermatophyte. A dermatophyte, which causes dermatophytosis, is a hyphomycete classified in either the genus *Epidermophyton, Microsporum,* or *Trichophyton* which infects hair, nail, or skin on the living host. This definition of dermatophyte excludes keratino-philic members of these three genera as dermatophytes if they are unable to use keratin on the living host. Dematiaceous and nondematiaceous fungi may cause dermatomycosis. Dermatomycosis caused by dematiaceous fungi are referable to either superficial or cutaneous phaeo-hyphomycosis depending on the tissue affected, the host response, and the degree of tissue damage. As an example, tinea nigra caused by *Phaeoannel-lomyces werneckii* is referred to as superficial phaeohyphomycosis.

Onychomycosis includes nail infections (Figure 1) caused by either yeasts such as *Candida albicans,* molds, dermatophytes, or various com-binations of these fungi (15,55–57). Onychomycosis involves either the healthy nail unit, nails with preexisting disease, or both. When dermato-phytes cause onychomycosis, they are always considered primary pathogens. In contrast, molds are typically thought of as secondary invaders when they cause onychomycosis. Of course, some molds such as *Scytalidium dimidiatum* (synonym *Scytalidium* synanamorph of *Hendersonula*

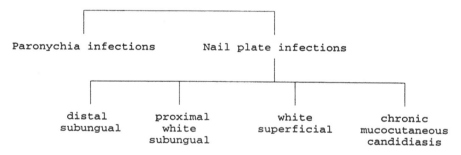

Figure 1 Onychomycosis.

toruloidea) or its corresponding pycnidial form *Nattrassia mangiferae* (synonym *H. toruloidea*) can be primary pathogens (58). Nail infections caused by dermatophytes are known clinically as tinea unguium. Onychomycosis caused by dematiaceous fungi fall under the umbrella of cutaneous phaeohyphomycosis.

Dematiaceous fungi have not been reported to cause hair invasion such as endothrix and ectothrix. *Piedraia hortae*, a loculoascomycete, forms its sexual fruiting body around hair shafts. These structures are black, hard, and difficult to separate from the hair shaft. Clinically, such infections are known as black piedra. As in the situation of tinea nigra, black piedra is placed under the umbrella of superficial phaeohyphomycosis.

DIAGNOSIS

Infection is the invasion and replication of an organism in tissues of the host with or without disease being present. Disease occurs when there is functional or structural harm in the host, which is accompanied by signs and symptoms. Subclinical infectious diseases occur when infection is present without clinical manifestations, even though there is some harm to the host. Colonization occurs when fungi replicate either in or on host tissue and can be seen in the microscopic examination of clinical specimens. In addition, they are typically isolated in culture. In contrast, contamination involves the presence of fungi on the surface of the patient without invasion of tissue. A diagnostic problem involves determining whether or not a particular fungus is causing an infection.

A challenge often exists in differentiating lesions caused by dermatophytes from those caused by dematiaceous fungi. *Scytalidium dimidiatum* infections of nails, feet, and hands are clinically indistinguishable from those caused by dermatophytes (57,59). In endemic areas such as Thailand, one study of 68 cases of tinea pedis revealed that dermatophytes caused 5.5% of the infections, whereas *S. dimidiatum* caused 39% of the infections (60). In another study, approximately 95% of the *S. dimidiatum* infections contained hyaline hyphae like that of dermatophytes in the infected tissue (61). Thus, in some instances, infections caused by dematiaceous fungi are essentially identical to infections caused by dermatophytes.

Different investigators have suggested criteria that can be used to determine the role, if any, a particular fungus may have in an infection. Nail infections are frequently difficult to access because many of the dematiaceous pathogens can also be recovered as contaminants of hair, nail, and skin. English (62) suggested for nails that the isolation of a dermatophyte should always be treated as the etiological agent of the infection. If molds and yeasts are detected in the direct microscopy of the specimen, she feels that they may be significant. For a mold to be considered a pathogen, English believes no dermatophyte should be isolated and at least 5 or more of 20 inocula must yield the same mold. Rosenthal et al. (63) feel that the fungus must be visualized in the clinical specimen when examined microscopically, the isolated fungus must be morphologically compatible with what was seen in the tissue, the same fungus must be repeatedly seen while the infection persists, a traditional pathogen was not isolated, and the mold disappears when the infection is resolved. Some useful diagnostic criteria are included in Table 2 in the form of several questions.

The diagnosis of infections involving hair, nail, and skin is made by a combination of direct microscopic examination of clinical specimens and their culture. Davies (64) reported that in 3955 nail collections, a fungal diagnosis would have been missed in 15% if cultures were not done. Fifty-three percent of the infections would have been missed if direct microscopic examinations were not done on the specimens. Clayton (56) reported that in her study of toe and fingernails, 19% and 11%, respectively, were culture negative even when the etiological agent could be seen in the clinical specimens. In another study of 2113 nails, 19% of the toenails and 11% of the fingernails that were potassium–hydroxide–positive had negative cultures (56).

Direct microscopic examination of clinical material is needed as a means to distinguish yeasts, dermatophytes, and nondermatophytes. Specimen collection is obviously an important consideration (65–68). Dermatophytes typically form hyaline, septate, branched, delicate hyphae, with or without arthroconidia. Dematiaceous fungi typically form hyphae that are variable in diameter, smooth, distorted, irregular, nodulose, or

Table 2 Criteria for the Diagnosis of Mycoses

1. Could the process be caused by a fungus?
2. Was a fungus seen in clinical specimens submitted for laboratory examination?
3. Was a fungus isolated?
4. Was the same fungus isolated more than once?
5. Was the isolated fungus compatible with the morphology of the fungus seen in the clinical specimens?

sinuous in appearance and that vary from hyaline to pale brown in color. Other diseases such as psoriasis, atopic eczema, seborrhaeic dermatitis, and contact dermatitis must be distinguished from fungal skin infections.

Culture of the suspected etiological agent is important because the identity of the fungus is determined after its isolation. Culture also confirms that a viable fungus is present in the clinical material. Because cycloheximide is used to eliminate fungi other than dermatophytes, isolation media with and without cycloheximide must be used together. Determining the significance of more than one isolated fungus can be difficult. Mixed infections involving dermatophytes and molds, dermatophytes and yeasts, molds and molds, and molds and yeasts are known to occur.

MANAGEMENT

Some infections such as those caused by *S. dimidiatum* are recalcitrant to antifungal chemotherapy. Antifungal agents such as clotrimazole (32,19), ketoconazole (5,23,30), miconazole (6,10), and oxyconazole (12), as well as surgical excision (24) have cured or improved infections caused by various fungi. Griseofulvin and amphotericin B do not appear to be effective in these types of cases. Itraconazole appears to be effective in some patients with phaeohyphomycosis (69,70). Its effectiveness against various dematiaceous fungi is enhanced by itraconazole's pharmacokinetic profile in skin and nails (70,71,72).

REFERENCES

1. Pritchard RC, Muir DB. Black fungi: a survey of dematiaceous hyphomycetes from clinical specimens identified over a five year period in a reference laboratory. Pathology 1987; 19: 281–284.
2. Singh SM, Naidu J, Pouranik M. Ungual and cutaneous phaeohyphomycosis caused by *Alternaria alternata* and *Alternaria chlamydospora*. J Med Vet Mycol 1990; 28: 275–278.
3. Galgóczy J, Simon G, Vályi-Nagy T. Case report: human cutaneous alternariosis. Mycophathologia 1985; 92: 77–80.
4. Wadhwani K, Srivastava AK. Some cases of onychomycosis from North India in different working environments. Mycophathologia 1985; 92: 149–155.
5. Badillet G, De Bièvre C, Maleville J, et al. Un cas d'alternariose cutanée chez un enfant. Bull Soc Fr Mycol Med 1985; 14: 67–72.
6. Rai MK. Mycosis in man due to *Arthrinium phaeospermum* var. *indicum*. First case report. Mycoses 1989; 32: 472–475.

7. Vieira JR. Onicomicose por *Auerobasidium pullulans* (de Bary) Arnaud. Proceedings of the 6th International Congress on Tropical Medicine and Malaria 1959; 4: 768–777.

8. Vermeil C, Gordeff A, Leroux MJ, et al. Blastomycose chelordienne à *Aureobasidium pullulans* (de Bary) Arnaud en bretagne. Mycopathol Mycol Appl 1971; 43: 35–39.

9. Chalet M, Howard DH, McGinnis MR, Zapatero I. Isolation of *Bipolaris australiensis* from a lesion of viral vesicular dermatitis on the scalp. J Med Vet Mycol 1986; 24: 461–465.

10. de Hoog GS, Rubio C. A new dematiaceous fungus from human skin. Sabouraudia 1982; 20: 15–20.

11. Naidu J, Singh SM, Pouranik M. Onychomycosis caused by *Chaetomium globosum* Kunze. Mycopathologia 1991; 113: 31–34.

12. Costa AR, Porto E, da S. Lacaz C, et al. Cutaneous and ungual phaeohyphomycosis caused by species of *Chaetomium* Kunze (1817) ex Fresenius, 1829. J Med Vet Mycol 1988; 26: 261–268.

13. Svobodová Y. *Chmelia slovaca* gen. nov. a dematiaceous fungus, pathogenic for man and humans. Biologia (Bratisl) 1966; 21: 81–88.

14. Barde AK, Singh SM. *Cladosporium carrionii* Trejos 1954 infection of human nail. Mykosen 1984; 27: 366–369.

15. Zaias N. Onychomycosis. Arch Dermatol 1972; 105: 263–274.

16. Otčenášek M, Hubálek Dvořak J, Sabatová M. Ein weiterer Chromomykose-Fall in der Tschechoslowakei? Mykosen 1968; 11: 719–724.

17. Badillet G, de Bièvre C, Spizajzen S. Isolement et dematiées à partir d'ongles et de squames. Bull Soc Fr Mycol Med 1982; 11: 69–72.

18. Lavoie SR, Espinel-Ingroff A, Kerkering T. Mixed cutaneous phaeohyphomycosis in a cocaine user. Clin Infect Dis 1993; 17: 114–116.

19. Gugnani HC, Okeke CN, Sivanesan A. *Curvularia clavata* as an aetiological agent of human skin infection. Lett Appl Microbiol 1990; 10: 47–49.

20. De Vries GA. *Cyphellophora laciniata* nov. gen., nov. sp. and *Dactylium fusarioides* Fragoso et Ciferri. Mycopathol Mycol Appl 1962; 16: 47–54.

21. De Vries GA, Elders MCC, Luykx MHF. Description of *Cyphellophora pluriseptata* sp. nov. Antonie van Leeuwenhoek 1986; 52: 141–143.

22. Listemann H, Sinner U, Meigel W. *Exophiala mansonii* als Erreger einer superfiziellen Phaeohyphomykose. Mykosen 1986; 29: 480–485.

23. Coldiron BM, Wiley EL, Rinaldi MG. Cutaneous phaeohyphomycosis caused by a rare fungal pathogen, *Hormonema dematioides*: successful treatment with ketoconazole. J Am Acad Dermatol 1990; 23: 363–367.

24. Restrep A, Arango M, Velez H, Uribe L. The isolation of *Botryodiplodia theobromae* from a nail lesion. Sabouraudia 1976; 14: 1–4.

25. Vélez H, Díaz F. Onychomycosis due to saprophytic fungi. Mycopathologia 1985; 91: 87–92.

26. Kocková-Kratochvílova A, Šimordová M, Šternbersky S. *Moniliella suaveolens* var. *nigra*. Mykosen 1987; 30: 544–547.

27. Sigler L, Congly H. Toenail infection caused by *Onychocola canadensis* gen et sp. nov. J Med Vet Mycol 1990; 28: 405–417.

28. Sigler L, Abbott SP, Woodgyer AJ. New records of nail and skin infection due to *Onychocola canadensis* and description of its teleomorph *Arachnomyces nodosetosus* sp. nov. J Med Vet Mycol 1994; 32: 275–285.

29. Miegeville M. Tinea nigra plantaris. Bull Soc Fr Mycol Med 1986; 15: 413–416.

30. Pereiro Ferreirós M, Pereiro M, Alvarez J, Toribio J. Tinea nigra palmaris. J Mycol Med 1992; 2: 113–114.

31. Porto E, Silva Lacaz C, Utiyama Y, et al. Feo-hifomicose do couro cabeludo por *Phialophora parasitica*. Registro de um caso. An Bras Dermatol 1986; 61: 91–96.

32. Bakerspigel A, Lowe D, Rostas A. The isolation of *Phoma eupyrena* from a human lesion. Arch Dermatol 1981; 117: 362–363.

33. Bakerspigel A. The isolation of *Phoma hibernica* from a lesion on a leg. Sabouraudia 1970; 7: 261–264.

34. Rai MK. *Phoma sorghina* infection in human being. Mycopathologia 1989; 105: 167–170.

35. Molero B, Volcán GS, Medrano CE. Differences in the prevalence of piedra between the mixed population of a city in Bolivar State, Venezuela and the Indian population of that region. Pan American Health Organization Sci Pub 1980; 396: 77–81.

36. English MP, Atkinson R. Onychomycosis in elderly chiropody patients. Br J Dermatol 1974; 91: 67–72.

37. Punithalingam E, English MP. *Pyrenochaeta unguis-hominis* sp. nov. on human toe-nails. Trans Br Mycol Soc 1975; 64: 539–541.

38. Ide T, Eno T. A case of chromomycosis on the face spreading to conjunctiva. Jpn Rev Clin Ophthalmol 1972; 66: 255–257.

39. Take M. A case of chromomycosis. Jpn J Dermatol 1980; 90: 1039.

40. Naidu J, Singh SM, Pouranik M. Onychomycosis caused by *Scopulariopsis brumptii*. A case report and sensitivity studies. Mycopathologia 1991; 113: 159–164.

41. Piontelli E, Alicia Toro LM. Comentarios biomorfologicos y clinicos sobre el genero *Scopulariopsis* Bainier. Hialohifomicosis en uñas y piel. Bol Micol 1988; 3: 259–273.

42. Schönborn C, Schmoranzer H. Untersuchungen über schimmelpilzinfektionen der zehennägel. Mykosen 1970; 13: 253–272.

43. Frankel DH, Rippon JW. *Hendersonula toruloidea* infection in man. Index cases in the non-endemic North American host, and a review of the literature. Mycopathologia 1989; 105: 175–186.

44. Di Prisco J, Borelli D. Tinea nigra por *Cladosporium* species. Castellania 1973; 1: 97–100.

45. Reyes O, Borelli D. Caso de tina por cepa peculiar de *Cladosporium castellanii*. Dermatol Venezol 1974; 13: 21–28.

46. Kano K. Über die Chromoblastomykose durch einen noch nicht als pathogen beschriebenen Pilz: *Hormiscium dermatitidis* n. sp. Aichi Igakkai Zasshi 1934; 41: 1657–1674.

47. Saruta T, Nakamizo Y. A case of chromomycosis. Skin Res (Osaka) 1973; 35: 9–21.

48. Pappagianis D, Ajello L. Dematiaceous—a mycologic misnomer? J Med Vet Mycol 1994; 32: 319–321.

49. Bell AA, Wheeler MH. Biosynthesis and functions of fungal melanins. Annu Rev Phytopathol 1986; 24: 411–451.

50. Wheeler MH, Bell AA. Melanins and their importance in pathogenic fungi. In: McGinnis MR, ed. Current Topics in Medical Mycology. Vol. 2. New York: Springer-Verlag, 1988: 338–387.

51. Dixon DM, Szaniszlo PJ, Polak A. Dihydoxynaphthalene (DHN) melanin and its relationship with virulence in the early stages of phaeohyphomycosis. In: Cole GT, Hoch HC, eds. The Fungal Spore and Diseases Initiation in Plants and Animals. New York: Plenum, 1991: 297–318.

52. McGinnis MR. Chromoblastomycosis and phaeohyphomycosis: new concepts, diagnosis, and mycology. J Am Acad Dermatol 1983; 8: 1–16.

53. McGinnis MR. Black fungi: a model for understanding tropical mycosis: In: Walker DH, ed. Global Infectious Diseases. Prevention, Control and Eradication. New York: Springer-Verlag, 1992: 129–149.

54. Wood C, Russel-Bell B. Characterization of pigmented fungi by melanin staining. Am J Dermatopathol 1983; 5: 77–81.

55. Summerbell RC, Kane J, Krajden S. Onychomycosis, tinea pedis and tinea manuum caused by non-dermatophytic filamentous fungi. Mycoses 1989; 23: 609–619.

56. Clayton YM. Clinical and mycological diagnostic aspects of onychomycoses and dermatomycoses. Clin Exp Dermatol 1992; 17(suppl 1): 37–40.

57. Zaias N. Clinical manifestations of onychomycosis. Clin Exp Dermatol 1992; 17(suppl 1): 6–7.

58. Frankel DH, Rippon JW. *Hendersonula toruloidea* infection in man. Index cases in the non-endemic North American host and a review of the literature. Mycopathologia 1989; 105: 175–186.

59. Hay RJ, Moore MK. Clinical features of superficial fungal infections caused by *Hendersonula toruloidea* and *Scytalidium hyalinum*. Br J Dermatol 1984; 110: 677–683.

60. Kotrajaras R, Chongsathien S, Rojanavanich V, et al. *Hendersonula toruloidea* infection in Thailand. Int J Dermatol 1988; 27: 391–395.

61. Moore MK. *Hendersonula toruloidea* and *Scytalidium hyalinum* infections in London, England. J Med Vet Mycol 1986; 24: 219–230.

62. English M. Nails and fungi. Br J Dermatol 1976; 94: 697–701.

63. Rosenthal SA, Stritzler R, Villafane J. Onychomycosis caused by *Aspergillus fumigatus*. Arch Dermatol 1968; 97: 685–687.

64. Davies RR. Mycological tests and onychomycosis. J Clin Pathol 1968; 21: 729–730.

65. Elewski BE. Clinical pearl: diagnosis of onychomycosis. J Am Acad Dermatol 1995; 32: 500–501.
66. Luedemann GM, LeBreton E. Laboratory mill for pulverizing and homogenizing nail specimens as an aid to microscopy and culture confirmation of onychomycosis. Appl Microbiol 1972; 23: 814–818.
67. Zaias N. The longitudinal nail biopsy. J Invest Dermatol 1967; 49: 406–408.
68. English MP, Atkinson R. Onychomycosis in elderly chiropody patients. Br J Dermatol 1974; 91: 67–72.
69. Sharkey PK, Graybill JR, Rinaldi MG, et al. Itraconazole treatment of phaeohyphomycosis. J Am Acad Dermatol 1990; 23: 577–586.
70. Whittle D, Kominos S. Use of itraconazole for treating subcutaneous phaeohyphomycosis caused by *Exophiala jeanselmei*. Clin Infect Dis 1995; 21: 1068.
71. Cauwenbergh G, Degreef H, Heykants J, et al. Pharmacokinetic profile of orally administered itraconazole in human skin. J Am Acad Dermatol 1988; 18: 263–268.
72. Willemsen M, DeDoncker P, Willems J, et al. Posttreatment itraconazole levels in the nail. J Am Acad Dermatol 1992; 26: 731–735.

18
Pityriasis Versicolor: Current Treatments

Jan Faergemann
Sahlgrenska University Hospital, Gothenburg, Sweden

INTRODUCTION

Pityriasis versicolor is a superficial chronic fungal disease characterized by lesions varying in color from red to hypopigmentation to hyperpigmentation. The areas usually involved are the upper trunk, neck, or upper arms, although lesions may be found elsewhere on the skin, with the exception of soles and palms. Lesions may be papular, nummular, or confluent and are slightly scaly. Besides the main complaint of cosmetic disfigurement, about one-third of patients also have slight to moderately severe itching. The lipophilic yeast *Pityrosporum ovale* is seen microscopically in scales from lesions (1).

P. ovale, described in 1913 by Castellani and Chalmers (2), is lipophilic and requires the addition of lipids to the culture medium for optimal growth (3,4). It is a member of the normal human cutaneous flora and can be cultured from almost all body areas (5–10). The colonization starts during puberty and is uncommon on the skin of children (8). *P. ovale* is not only a saprophyte but is associated with several diseases such as pityriasis versicolor, *Pityrosporum* folliculitis, seborrhoeic dermatitis, some forms of atopic dermatitis, some forms of psoriasis, confluent and reticulate papillomatosis (Gougerot–Carteaud Syndrome); even systemic infections have been described (6–13).

Under the influence of predisposing factors, *P. ovale* changes in pityriasis versicolor from the round blastosphere form to the mycelial form. The most important exogenous factors are high temperatures and a

211

high relative humidity; the most important endogenous factors are greasy skin, hyperhidrosis, hereditary factors, corticosteroids, and immuno-deficiency. The presence of these factors explains the high rate of recurrence after treatment seen in this disease. Without treatment, the disease is chronic; after treatment the recurrence rate is high because of the presence of predisposing factors.

TREATMENT

There are numerous ways of treating pityriasis versicolor topically, with many different formulation alternatives (14–24). Patients should treat the whole trunk, neck, arms, and legs down to the knees, even when small areas are involved. A cheap, effective, and cosmetically elegant treatment is to use propylene glycol, 50%, in water (14). This is applied twice a day for 2 weeks with excellent results and with very little risk of skin irritation. Another treatment is to use ketoconazole as a cream (21) or more recently even in a foam solution (24). Topical application of bifonazole (20), clotri-mazole (15), econazole (17), or miconazole (16) once or twice a day for 2 weeks, is also effective. Another effective treatment is zinc pyrithione shampoo (18). It is applied on affected areas after showering, allowed to remain for approximately 5 minutes, and then rinsed off. This procedure should be repeated every evening for 2 weeks. Selenium sulfide is also effective (19), but patients sometimes complain about the offensive odor and stinging sensation on the skin after application.

   Ciclopiroxolamine 0.1% solution applied once a day for 4 weeks was effective in 86% of 90 treated patients at a follow-up visit 4 weeks after the last day of treatment (23). Terbinafine, a new orally and topically active allylamine antifungal derivative, is orally active primarily against der-matophytes. Topically, it has been effective in the treatment of pityriasis versicolor in a 1% cream formulation applied once a day for 4 weeks (22). In a single blind comparative study against bifonazole 1% cream, 100% were cleared in the terbinafine group after 4 weeks of treatment (22).

   Systemic therapy is primarily indicated for extensive lesions, for lesions resistant to topical treatment, and for frequent relapse. With short-term treatment, however, the risk of side effects with systemic therapy may be minimized, and oral antifungals may be used even for other indications. Ketoconazole is an effective oral drug, with a broad anti-mycotic spectrum (25). Overall, results have shown cure rates of 92%, with a mean treatment period of 4 weeks (25,26). With longer treatment periods, however, the risk for serious liver reactions seen with oral ketoconazole increases (27). Hay and Midgley (27) have treated patients successfully with 200 mg tablets once a day for 5 days (27). Rausch and Jacobs (28) have shown that even one single dose of 400 mg may be effective. The risk of side effects is minimized with short-term treatment.

Itraconazole, a triazole derivative developed by Janssen, Belgium, has been shown to be effective orally in several well-conducted, controlled trials (29,30). An effective treatment schedule is 200 mg/day for 5 to 7 days (29). The risk for serious side effects, especially liver toxicity, is much lower for itraconazole than for ketoconazole.

Fluconazole, a triazole derivative developed by Pfizer, Central Research, U.K., has also been used in the treatment of pityriasis versicolor in a single dose of 400 mg (31). Three weeks after treatment, 17 of 23 patients or 74% were cleared, indicating that this treatment is an effective and elegant alternative to other treatments. However, skin pharmaco-kinetic studies indicate that two doses given 1 week apart may be even more effective (32), and the patient compliance should still be high. The risk of side effects with fluconazole is low.

The high rate of recurrence, reaching 60% in 1 year and 80% after 2 years, is an outstanding problem in pityriasis versicolor. Recurrence is due to the presence of predisposing factors, which may be difficult to eradi-cate. A permanent cure, therefore, is difficult to achieve, which explains the chronicity. Consequently, a prophylactic treatment regimen is neces-sary to avoid recurrence. An effective prophylactic treatment is 200 mg ketoconazole on 3 consecutive days every month (26). Rausch and Jacobs (28) have used a single dose of 400 mg ketoconazole every month as an effective prophylaxis in pityriasis versicolor. Topical prophylactic treat-ment schedules also may be used, but patient compliance is much lower.

REFERENCES

1. Faergemann J. *Pityrosporum* infections. In: Elewski BE, ed. Cutaneous Fungal Infections. New York-Tokyo: Igaku-Shoin, 1992: 69–83.
2. Castellani A, Chalmers AJ. Manuel of Tropical Medicine. London: Ballieré Cox, 1913.
3. Porro MN, Passi S, Caprilli F, et al. Growth requirements and lipid metabolism of *Pityrosporum orbiculare*. J Invest Dermatol 1976; 66: 178–182.
4. Wilde PF, Stewart PS. A study of the fatty acid metabolism of the yeast *Pityrosporum ovale*. Biochem J 1968; 108: 225–231.
5. Gordon MA. The lipophilic mycoflora of the skin. Mycologica 1951; 43: 524–534.
6. Roberts SOB. *Pityrosporum orbiculare*: incidence and distribution on clinically normal skin. Br J Dermatol 1969; 81: 264–269.

7. Faergemann J, Aly R, Maibach HI. Quantitative variations in distribution of *Pityrosporum orbiculare* on clinically normal skin. Acta Derm Venereol (Stockh) 1983; 63: 346–348.

8. Faergemann J, Fredriksson T. Age incidence of *Pityrosporum orbiculare* on human skin. Acta Derm Venereol (Stockh) 1980; 60: 531–533.

9. Bergbrant IM. Seborrhoeic dermatitis and *Pityrosporum ovale*: Cultural, Immunological and Clinical Studies (thesis). Acta Derm Venereol (Stockh) Suppl 167, 1991.

10. Faergemann J, Fredriksson T. Experimental infections in rabbits and humans with *Pityrosporum orbiculare* and *P. ovale*. J Invest Dermatol 1981; 77: 314–318.

11. Faergemann J, Tjernlund U, Scheynius A, Bernander S. Antigenic similarities and differences in genus *Pityrosporum*. J Invest Dermatol 1982; 78: 28–31.

12. Faergemann J, Aly R, Maibach HI. Growth and filament production of *Pityrosporum orbiculare* and *P. ovale* on human stratum corneum in vitro. Acta Derm Venereol (Stockh) 1983; 63: 388–392.

13. Faergemann J. A new model for growth and filament production of *Pityrosporum ovale* (*orbiculare*) on human stratum corneum in vitro. J Invest Dermatol 1989; 92: 117–119.

14. Faergemann J, Fredriksson T. Propylene glycol in the treatment of tinea versicolor. Acta Derm Venereol (Stockh) 1980; 60: 92–93.

15. Fredriksson T. Topical treatment with BAY b 5097, a new broad spectrum antimycotic agent. Br J Dermatol 1972; 86:628–630.

16. Svejgaard E. Double-blind trial of miconazole in dermatomycosis. Acta Derm Venereol (Stockh) 1973; 53: 497–499.

17. Swartz KJ, Moch TH, Kenzelmann M. Poloklinische Prüfung von Econazole bei 594 Fallen von Hautmykosen. Dtsch Med Wochenschr 1975; 100: 1497–1500.

18. Faergemann J, Fredriksson T. An open trial of the effect of a zinc pyrithione shampoo in tinea versicolor. Cutis 1980; 25: 667–669.

19. Albright SD, Hitch JM. Rabbit treatment of tinea versicolor with selenium sulphide. Arch Dermatol 1966; 93: 460–461.

20. Hernandez-Perez E. A comparison between one and two week's treatment with bifonazole in pityriasis versicolor. J Am Acad Dermatol 1986; 14: 561–564.

21. Savin RC, Horwitz SN. Double-blind comparison of 2% ketoconazole cream and placebo in the treatment of tinea versicolor. J Am Acad Dermatol 1986; 15: 500–503.

22. Aste N, Pau M, Pinna AL, et al. Clinical efficacy and tolerability of terbinafine in patients with pityriasis versicolor. Mycoses 1991; 34: 353–357.

23. Corte M, Jung K, Linker U, et al. Topical application of a 0.1% ciclopiroxolamine solution for the treatment of pityriasis versicolor. Mycoses 1989; 32: 200–203.

24. Rekacewicz I, Guillaume JC, Benkhraba F, et al. A double-blind placebo-controlled study of a 2 percent foaming lotion of ketoconazole in a single application in the treatment of pityriasis versicolor. Ann Dermatol Venereol 1990; 117: 709–711.

25. Jones HE. Ketoconazole today. A review of clinical experience. Manchester, England, ADIS Press, 1987.

26. Faergemann J, Djärv L. Tinea versicolor: treatment and prophylaxis with ketoconazole. 1982; 30: 542–545.
27. Hay RJ, Midgley G. Short course ketoconazole therapy in pityriasis versicolor. Clin Exp Dermatol 1984; 9: 571–573.
28. Rausch LJ, Jacobs PH. Tinea versicolor: treatment and prophylaxis with monthly administration of ketoconazole. Cutis 1984; 34: 470–471.
29. Delesclusc J. Itraconazole in tinea versicolor. A review. J Am Acad Dermatol 1990; 23: 551–554.
30. Faergemann J. Treatment of pityriasis versicolor with itraconazole. A double-blind placebo-controlled study. Mykoses 1988; 31: 377–379.
31. Faergemann J. Treatment of pityriasis versicolor with a single dose of fluconazole. Acta Derm Venereol (Stockh) 1992; 72: 74–75.
32. Faergemann J, Laufen H. Levels of fluconazole in serum, stratum corneum, epidermis-dermis (without stratum corneum) and eccrine sweat. Clin Exp Dermatol 1992; 18: 102–106.

19

Lessons from the AIDS Epidemic

Marcus A. Conant
University of California School of Medicine, San Francisco, California

In the decade preceding the AIDS epidemic, medical science thought it had successfully conquered and contained infectious diseases. Public health measures and mass vaccination programs were eliminating diseases such as smallpox and polio. Plagues were a phenomenon of the past.

Suddenly in 1981, cases of rare opportunistic infections and malignancies, primarily *Pneumocystis* pneumonia and Kaposi's sarcoma suddenly appeared among sexually active gay men in major cities in the United States. The epidemic has now lasted for nearly two decades, and during that time we have had the unfortunate opportunity to watch the same pattern of inappropriate behavior, which has characterized epidemics of the past, play out on the social and political stages of the United States and other countries severely affected by AIDS.

For an epidemic to establish itself successfully in a population, many factors must come to play simultaneously. The Black Death of 1348, which killed 25% to 30% of the population of Europe within 2 years, would not have been possible 200 years earlier. In the twelfth century, Europe was primarily an agrarian society with populations concentrated in large feudal farms, with little travel and little contact between societies. Transmission and spread of an epidemic disease were difficult because of this isolation, and epidemics are virtually unrecorded during this period.

Two hundred years later, in 1348, population concentrations had shifted to large financial and industrial centers and ports, with Paris, London, and Amsterdam becoming major centers of population and commerce. When people moved to cities from the farm, they also took their constant companion, the rat, and the rat took its companion, the flea.

Sanitary conditions were abysmal, living quarters were cramped, and infection control procedures were unknown.

In 1348, a ship landed in Marseille, bringing fleas infected with the plague. The Black Death spread rapidly through the heavily populated centers in Europe and within 2 years the carnage was incalculable.

The hemorrhagic vesicles of the Black Death were characterized by an erythematous ring. The stench of death and dying was so great that survivors carried bouquets of flowers for their fragrance and the ashes of the dead were used as a talisman to ward off infection. These macabre facts are memorialized even today in the nursery rhyme:

Ring around the rosey
Pocket full of poseys
Ashes, ashes,
All fall down.

A retrospective review of the Black Death provides a vivid insight into the way societies react to cataclysmic epidemics; further, these reviews reveal the intellectual and philosophical weaknesses of societies incapable of dealing with the threat posed by an alien invader. Society's reaction to the Black Death can be characterized by four major stages. The first and earliest is *denial*. The second, which occurs almost simultaneously, is *scapegoating*. The third and fourth, which occur much later, are *inappropriate legislation* and *loss of faith in existing institutions*. Let us examine each of these reactions. When the Black Death began in Europe, there was an immediate outcry to seal the ports and close the city gates. In every instance, the leadership belittled such measures with the simplistic rationalization that this new disease was happening to someone else who was usually perceived as racially or socially inferior. The population was reassured "It cannot happen here," an unfortunate and clear example of classic denial. As the death toll mounted, an explanation of what was happening became essential. Jews were widely accused of poisoning the wells, and discrimination and persecution of the Jews became widespread. Nobody seems to have asked why Jewish citizens would poison the wells from which they themselves were drinking and cause a plague of which they themselves were dying.

Inappropriate laws were enacted forcing the Jews into ghettos and limiting travel and immigration. Two major institutions long revered by society were questioned and reshaped when it was realized that these venerable organizations could not do what they had promised by curing disease and preventing death. Before the Black Death, the physician was supreme in European medicine, and surgeons were relegated to a lesser role. Because physicians were unable to stop the carnage of the epidemic, their stock fell precipitously, and surgery ascended to a leadership role it has enjoyed since. The Church, the other major institution, which promised God's protection and benevolence for the faithful, was unable to save the faithful from the plague. Celibate monks were carried off in the same death carts as prostitutes, and a fissure was created in the foundation of the Church, which lead ultimately to the reformation 200 years later. These patterns of denial, scapegoating, inappropriate legislation, and loss of faith in institutions have repeated themselves with uncanny predictability as new plagues and pestilences were visited on humanity.

When Columbus returned from the New World, his sailors brought with them their newly contracted disease, syphilis. Syphilis was endemic in the New World and unknown in Europe. By the time these young sailors landed in Seville, many were in the secondary stages of syphilis and were highly contagious. They were welcomed as returning heroes, much as the American and Soviet space astronauts were welcomed in this century. Columbus and his crew traveled from Seville to Barcelona to the court of Isabel and Ferdinand and were showered with gifts and the favors of the young women of the court. Soon, syphilis, a far more insidious disease than the plague, was widespread in Spain. A few years later, when France attacked Naples, Spanish mercenaries were conscripted to defend the city. These Spaniards, newly infected with syphilis, traveled to the south of Italy where they infected local prostitutes. Prostitutes, being classic entrepreneurs, showered their favors not only on the Spanish army but also on the French. Syphilis had leaped, in less than 10 years, from Caribbean natives to Spanish soldiers to the French infantry. Ironically, typhus made its political debut in Europe during the siege of Naples, and the French army was forced to withdraw to France. During the next quarter century, however, the French armies engaged in a period of expeditionary adventures throughout Europe, successfully transmitting syphilis to larger and larger populations. During this period, syphilis was known among the English as the French disease and among the French as the Spanish disease. Each population was scapegoating someone else as the cause of the disease, and no one was prepared to accept that this was a human disease that indiscriminately attacked men and women regardless of their language or national allegiance.

Two hundred years later, as the Sandwich Islands were being settled, epidemics of measles, tuberculosis, and leprosy were widespread among the Hawaiian natives. Measles comes on suddenly and kills quickly. Tuberculosis is insidious, and patients may suffer from months to years as they lose weight and become more and more disabled. And both measles and tuberculosis are highly infectious. Leprosy, on the other hand, is a slow, insidious disease with a low rate of infectivity. The history of the Hawaiian islands records little effort to stop the epidemics of measles and tuberculosis; yet inappropriate legislation was enacted to create a permanent quarantine in the form of a leprosorium on the island of Molokai. Individuals judged to have leprosy were torn from their families and transported to this remote part of Hawaii. They were often thrown from the ship to find their own way to shore where they would remain in the company of other lepers, cut off from their families and friends for the rest of their lives. This inappropriate legislation and the creation of a leprosorium was prompted not because leprosy was a more threatening disease than measles or tuberculosis, but rather because of the widespread belief that leprosy was a loathsome disease visited by God upon sinners and transgressors.

The AIDS epidemic came like a thief in the night in 1981. Large numbers of gay men were infected before the disease was even characterized. In the late 1970s, San Francisco was truly a happy city. Twenty percent of the population of San Francisco were Asian, 12% were black, and 12% were Hispanic; 15% of adult males were gay or bisexual. There was unparalleled tolerance for racial minorities, open relationships, and experimentation with alternative lifestyles, drugs, sexual relationships, family structures, diet, dress, hairstyles, and a myriad of other social conventions. The AIDS virus escaped from Africa, and within 5 years 35,000 men, approximately half of the gay male community in San Francisco, were infected with HIV. A similar pattern was seen in other metropolitan cities in the United States, including New York, Los Angeles, and Miami.

The denial that occurred during the Black Death epidemic in 1348 occurred again in the early days of the AIDS epidemic. In a 1983 study, gay men leaving bathhouses were asked why they did not think they would catch this new, dreadful, fatal disease. The rationalization and denial were astonishing. Some men felt that they were immune from AIDS because they never had sex in the public rooms but only retired to a bedroom to have sex in private. Others suggested that they were immune because they always took a shower immediately after having sex. One man went so far as to assert that he was immune because he always changed the sheets on his bed after a sexual liaison.

In a parallel study, Hispanic men were asked why they did not have condoms available in the bar they frequented like the Caucasian gay men in the bar across the street. The interviewer was rewarded with gales of laughter and told that Hispanic men were not at risk for the same disease that was afflicting the effete Anglos in the bar across the street. This denial characterized by the notion that AIDS will always happen to someone else continues to be widespread in the United States even today. Individuals living in rural areas feel that they are protected from a disease that happens primarily in major cities. Heterosexual men feel they are immune to diseases that are happening to their homosexual brothers. Even young gay men feel they are protected from a disease that usually strikes men in their thirties and forties.

From the beginning, gay men were scapegoated as the cause of AIDS. In the first year of the epidemic, it was called the *gay cancer* and then *GRID* (gay related immune deficiency syndrome). No one seemed to ask the obvious question: Why would gay men cause a disease that was killing gay men?

Inappropriate legislation was introduced early in the epidemic. Some of it was successfully enacted; other bills were deferred or killed. The United States became one of the few countries in the world to ban visits from HIV-infected individuals. This action so outraged the international scientific community that the Sixth International AIDS Meeting at Harvard University had to be canceled and moved to Amsterdam because scientists and AIDS activists from around the world refused to come to the United States. Legislation was introduced in California to require mandatory testing and reporting of individuals at risk for AIDS. This legislation engendered tremendous support even in the face of the irrefutable knowledge that the incubation period for HIV infection was often as long as 10 years, and the individuals infected frequently had no idea where they had caught the disease or who they had infected during their period of incubation. At the same time that federal authorities were trying to limit the disease by testing individuals at risk, they refused to implement effective infection control procedures by widely promoting condom use. This prohibition was clearly politically motivated and grew out of the Catholic Church's refusal to endorse condom use to control disease transmission and fundamentalist Christian abhorrence of an open discussion of sex and the prevention of sexually transmitted diseases.

Finally, the institutions that had been created to respond to precisely this type of epidemic were ineffective. The Centers for Disease Control seemed incapable of an incisive response because of political constraints. The National Institutes of Health conducted AIDS research in an uncoordinated and haphazard fashion, spending hundreds of millions of dollars on poorly conceived projects and little or nothing on vaccine development and prevention techniques. The Food and Drug Administration proved incapable of developing a new strategy for the rapid review and approval of AIDS drugs for the first 14 years of the epidemic and finally responded only with the direct prodding of Congress.

Some families embraced their sons who were dying of AIDS and welcomed them home to die. Tragically, many other families rejected their children when they found that they were both gay and dying of AIDS. In one case, I urged a mother to travel to San Francisco and visit her dying son for the last time. She replied that she would like to come, but her husband had forbid it because he was afraid that he would contract AIDS from her. Further questioning revealed that the father was a heterosexual who had served in the Korean War. He had seen death up close and was clearly unafraid of dying. What he feared was the stigma of AIDS, the fact that if he were infected, no matter how remote the chance, his peers would discriminate against him the same way that he discriminated against his own son and he would die excluded from society. This is the same theme played out in Hawaii with leprosy. The settlers had no fear of death, shown by the fact that steps were not taken to quarantine the victims of measles and tuberculosis. Instead, the fear was of the stigma of leprosy, which was a disease visited by God, and lepers suffered the same social discrimination as the victims of AIDS.

We have learned much since 1981 about this new threat to our society. We have seen that denial and scapegoating protected no one from the epidemic and, in fact, allowed the unwitting and uninformed to become infected. Inappropriate laws have not stopped the AIDS epidemic from spreading in the United States, where almost all of the cases are acquired from other Americans living in this country rather than from tourists from other nations who are HIV infected.

Finally, the AIDS epidemic has severely undermined the faith of the affected community in the commitment and the ability of the federal government to respond in an appropriate manner to this epidemic.

The AIDS epidemic will not be the last plague to burden humanity. The author Albert Camus reminds us in *The Plague*:

> He knew what those jubilant crowds did not know but could have learned from books: that the plague bacillus never dies or disappears for good; that it can lie dormant for years and years in furniture and linen-chests; that it bides its time in bedrooms, cellars, trunks, and bookshelves; and that perhaps the day would come when, for the bane and the enlightenment of men, it would rouse up its rats again and send them forth to die in a happy city.

20
Oropharyngeal Candidiasis in HIV Infection

Deborah Greenspan
University of California School of Medicine, San Francisco, California

Oral candidiasis is the most common fungal infection of the mouth seen in association with HIV infection and has been reported to occur in more than 90% of HIV-positive people (1). Although oral candidiasis is more common as the CD4 count falls below 300 cells/mm³, it may also occur in association with acute or primary infection (2). Oral candidiasis is widely recognized as representing an important stage in the natural history of HIV infection in adults and children (3,4). Approximately 4% of HIV-infected homosexual and bisexual men followed from seroconversion develop candidiasis within 1 year, 14% within 2 years, and 26% within 5 years (5). Pseudomembranous and erythematous candidiasis were equally significant markers in the progression of HIV disease in homosexual men, independent of CD4 count (6). Oral candidiasis in women has been associated with falling CD4 counts (7) and appears after vaginal candidiasis occurs (8). Development of hairy leukoplakia or oral candidiasis was associated with the risk of progression and development of AIDS (5,9). Several studies have suggested that the same strain of *Candida* is carried throughout life, others have shown that individuals acquire different strains (10–12). These acquired strains may be more virulent. *Candida albicans* is the most common species identified with oral candidiasis, but other species such as *C. glabrata*, *C. tropicalis*, and *C. krusei* are seen. The presence of species other than *C. albicans* may have important implications for treatment, as some of these species have different susceptibilities to antifungal agents (13). *Candida albicans* is frequently recovered from the

223

oral cavity as part of the normal oral flora in 10% to 70% of individuals (14,15). Other factors may contribute to the development of oral candidiasis and may influence response to therapy. These include the use of medications such as recent or concomitant use of antibiotics, steroids including inhaled steroids, wearing dentures, dry mouth, and smoking.

CLINICAL PRESENTATION

Oral candidiasis may have distinctly different clinical appearances (16–18). These are pseudomembranous candidiasis, erythematous candidiasis, hyperplastic candidiasis, and an angular cheilitis. Pseudomembranous candidiasis, also known as thrush, appears as easily removable small white plaques, which may clump together to form large plaques, and may occur on any mucosal surface (Figure 1). Erythematous candidiasis appears as red patches, which may occur as small discrete areas or as large flat patches. These are seen most commonly on the hard and soft palate. The dorsal surface of the tongue may become

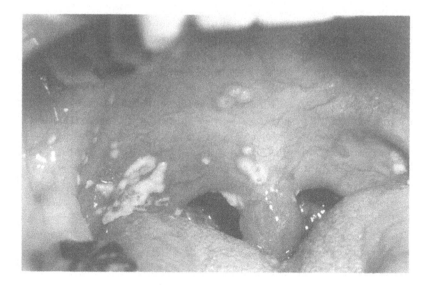

Figure 1 Pseudomembranous candidiasis.

depapillated and appear smooth and shiny. Hyperplastic candidiasis, rarely seen in association with HIV infection, usually occurs on the buccal mucosa. Angular cheilitis appears as redness or cracking at one or both corners of the mouth. More than one of these types of oral candidiasis may appear together. Candidiasis may be symptomatic causing changes in taste, a metallic taste, burning sensation, and difficulty in eating spicy food.

Candidiasis sometimes occurs in association with hairy leukoplakia (HL), and the lesions may be confused. Some cases described as candidiasis are actually HL (Figure 2). Hairy leukoplakia appears as nonremovable white patches and corrugations usually found on the lateral margin of the tongue and is caused by Epstein–Barr virus replicating within the epithelial cells (19). A trial of antifungal medication may be useful to distinguish between the two lesions. There may be some change in the clinical appearance of the lesions when *Candida* is eliminated with treatment, but HL will persist.

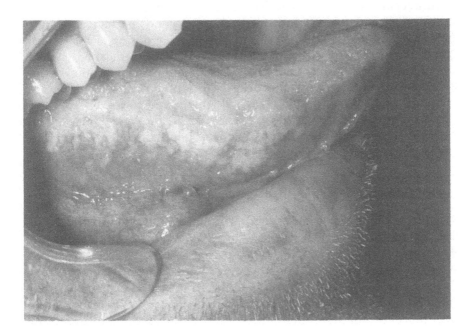

Figure 2 Hairy leukoplakia.

DIAGNOSIS

The diagnosis of oral candidiasis can be confirmed using cultures and smears. Culture is useful for the identification of *Candida* species. It may not be useful as the only confirmatory test, as 50% to 70% of individuals carry *Candida* as part of the normal oral flora. Quantitative cultures obtained from saliva, oral rinses, or imprint cultures may be useful to calculate CFU (colony forming units)/per milliliter of saliva (1). Smears taken from the lesions can be examined using Gram stain, periodic-acid–Schiff stain, or potassium hydroxide preparation. Care must be taken to obtain adequate samples from the oral lesions. Multiple hyphae are seen in smears of pseudomembranous candidiasis, but only scant hyphae are recoverable from smears of erythematous candidiasis.

TREATMENT

Many antifungal drugs are available for the treatment of oral candidiasis. Some are administered topically, others as systemic agents for either oral or intravenous use (20–23). The decision on whether to start therapy with topical medications or systemic medications depends on several factors, including compliance with the several-times-a-day dosing of the topical agents, the presence of sufficient saliva to dissolve the medication, contact time with the oral mucosa, and in the case of systemic medications, possible drug interactions with other drugs. The topical drugs can be administered as oral troches, pastilles, vaginal tablets, and rinses. Creams and ointments are used for the treatment of angular cheilitis and if there are no intraoral signs of oral candidiasis, they may be used alone, without any topical or systemic medications.

Topical Drugs

Nystatin is a topical polyene agent; it is fungicidal and is currently available as pastilles, vaginal tablets, suspension, cream, and ointment. Nystatin oral pastilles, 200,000 units, are intended for topical use, one or two pastilles to be dissolved slowly in the mouth four or five times a day. Nystatin oral suspension is used as a mouth rinse and contains 100,000 units/ml. The suspension is in contact with the oral lesion only for a short time, however, and may not be effective. The rinse and the oral pastilles both contain sucrose as a sweetening agent; consequently, there is a risk of increased susceptibility to dental caries if these medications are used frequently. Nystatin is also available as a cream or ointment. Some formulations also contain triamcinolone, which can be used for the treatment of angular cheilitis. Denture wearers have additional problems, as the surface of plastic dentures may provide a reservoir of *Candida*, and successful treatment of oral candidiasis in these individuals should include management of the denture. The denture should be left out overnight, and nystatin powder, for intraoral use, applied to the mucosal surface of the denture. Nystatin vaginal tablets 100,000 units also can be used orally, one tablet dissolved slowly in the mouth three times a day. The vaginal tablets are not flavored, and the concurrent use of a sugarless mint may improve compliance. The effectiveness of treatment depends on compliance, and lack of therapeutic response may be due to inadequate use of the medication or inadequate dissolution of the medication due to lack of saliva.

Clotrimazole is an effective topical imidazole (23), containing dextrose, and it is used as a 10 mg oral troche dissolved slowly in the mouth five times a day. Clotrimazole troches have also been shown to be effective, used as the 10 mg troche taken three times a day, in preventing oral candidiasis in individuals with leukemia undergoing chemotherapy (24). Clotrimazole is also available as a 1% cream that can be used for the treatment of angular cheilitis.

The presence of adequate saliva is essential to dissolve the medications such as troches, pastilles, and tablets. Sipping water, particularly for those who have a dry mouth, may help to dissolve the drug. Sweetening agents such as sucrose or dextrose are found in several of the topical medications, and long-term use of these preparations may lead to an increase in caries. The use of a topical fluoride rinse or gel during treatment with the antifungal medication should be encouraged. Denture wearers should leave their dentures out at night and while using topical medications.

Oral rinses that have been used for the treatment of oral candidiasis include gentian violet and chlorhexidine. Gentian violet has sometimes been used in pediatric populations, but there are reports of oral ulcers occurring with its use in neonates. In one study of oropharyngeal candidiasis and AIDS, gentian violet eliminated clinical oral candidiasis in 42% of individuals, compared with 43% in those receiving ketoconazole and 9% in those using nystatin mouth wash (25). Chlorhexidine is used as a mouth rinse and is an effective antibacterial agent. It is effective as a prophylactic agent in preventing oral candidiasis in a group of patients undergoing bone marrow transplantation (26).

Amphotericin B is available in Europe as a 10 mg lozenge and as a 100 mg/ml oral solution, 1 ml is used as a mouth rinse. Amphotericin B, 500

mg/ml, is being evaluated in an AIDS clinical trial group (ACTG) trial. A
0.1 mg/ml rinse of amphotericin B was effective in patients with clinically
proven fluconazole- resistant candidiasis (27). Mouth rinses are in contact
with the oral mucosa only for a short time, however, and may not be as
effective as troches, lozenges, or pastilles.

Systemic Drugs

Currently available systemic azoles include ketoconazole, fluconazole,
and itraconazole. They all share a similar mode of action involving inhibition of the enzyme lanosterol 14α-demethylase, which leads to changes in
the fungal membrane (28). Ketoconazole is an imidazole and was the first
azole used for the treatment of oral candidiasis and is used orally as one or
two 200 mg tablets taken once a day with food. It is an effective antifungal
agent, but its use may be limited, as individuals with hypochlorhydria
may not absorb this drug adequately. Side effects include nausea and
vomiting, pruritis, skin rash, and abnormal liver function tests (28). Ketoconazole is also available as a 2% cream that is useful for the topical
treatment of angular cheilitis. Fluconazole is a triazole and is available as
an orally administered systemic tablet 100 mg taken daily (29). Clinical
trials have demonstrated the effectiveness of fluconazole solution (30).
Changes in gastric pH do not affect the absorption of fluconazole, which is
excreted mainly through the kidney. Side effects include nausea, vomiting,
abdominal pain, and skin rash. Doses ranging from 50 to 100 mg/day and
150 mg as a single dose appear to be effective (29,31). The use of fluconazole as a prophylactic agent has been investigated in doses ranging from
50 mg/day and 50 mg every other day to 100 mg/day (32). In the last 2
years, fluconazole-resistant oropharyngeal candidiasis has emerged (33).
This has been in association with CD4 cells/mm^3 counts of less than 100
(34). The emergence of species such as C. glabrata, which is less susceptible
to fluconazole, could be partially responsible (35). The development of
true resistance as shown by in vitro susceptibility testing also seems to
occur (33). One study found that patients receiving intermittent therapy
with fluconazole carried C. albicans isolates that were less susceptible to
fluconazole than those who were on continuous therapy (36). When
fluconazole resistance occurs, treatment choices include higher doses of
fluconazole, itraconazole 200 to 400 mg/day, ketoconazole 400 mg/day,
or amphotericin oral rinse. If none of these are successful, intravenous
amphotericin B may be needed.

   Itraconazole is a recently introduced broad-spectrum, systemic, triazole antifungal agent and is available in the form of 100 mg capsule. Side

effects include nausea, headache, and altered liver function tests. Itraconazole, 200 mg/day, is as effective as clotrimazole, 10 mg troches five times daily, for the treatment of oral candidiasis (37). Those using itraconazole had a faster response to therapy and a longer period before relapse. The use of an acidic drink taken with itraconazole improves its bioavailability after administration.

Itraconazole oral solution has been evaluated in clinical trials as being an effective agent in the treatment of oral candidiasis (38), and salivary levels of itraconazole persist up to 8 hours after dosing (39).

Side effects seen with some of the azoles include drugs interactions (with antacids, H^2-receptor antagonists, sucralfate, phenytoin, rifampin, cyclosporin, terfanidine, astemizole and warfarin among others), gastrointestinal symptoms, skin rashes, and elevation of certain liver enzymes. The specific adverse effect depends on the dose and type of azole (28).

The choice of a systemic or topical agent for the treatment of oral candidiasis should be based on several factors, including cost, concomitant medications, and patient acceptability. Several studies have shown that some antifungal agents appear to be effective in the prevention of oral candidiasis. The appropriate time to start prophylactic therapy and the type and dose of the antifungal drug require further study.

REFERENCES

1. Samaranayake LP, Holmstrup P. Oral candidiasis and human immunodeficiency virus infection. J Oral Pathol Med 1989; 18: 554.
2. Dull JS, Sen P, Raffanti S, Middleton JR. Oral candidiasis as a marker of acute retroviral illness. South Med J 1991; 84: 733.
3. Royce RA, Luckmann RS, Fusaro RE, Winkelstein WJ. The natural history of HIV-1 infection: staging classifications of disease. AIDS 1991; 5: 355.
4. Katz MH, Mastrucci MT, Leggott PJ, et al. Prognostic significance of oral lesions in children with perinatally acquired human immunodeficiency virus infection. Am J Dis Child 1993; 147: 45.
5. Lifson AR, Hilton JF, Westenhouse JL, et al. Time from seroconversion to oral candidiasis or hairy leukoplakia among homosexual and bisexual men enrolled in three prospective cohorts. AIDS 1994; 8: 73.
6. Dodd CL, Greenspan D, Katz MH, et al. Oral candidiasis in HIV infection: pseudomembranous and erythematous candidiasis show similar rates of progression to AIDS. AIDS 1991; 5: 1339.
7. Shiboski CH, Hilton JF, Greenspan D, et al. HIV-related oral manifestations in two cohorts of women in San Francisco. AIDS 1994; 7: 964.

8. Imam N, Carpenter CC, Mayer KH, et al. Hierarchical pattern of mucosal candida infections in HIV-seropositive women [see comments]. Am J Med 1990; 89: 142.

9. Coates RA, Farewell VT, Raboud J, et al. Using serial observations to identify predictors of progression to AIDS in the Toronto sexual partners study. J Clin Epidemiol 1992; 45: 245.

10. Miyasaki SH, Hicks JB, Greenspan D, et al. The identification and tracking of *Candida albicans* isolates from oral lesions in HIV-seropositive individuals. J Acquir Immune Defic Syndr 1992; 5: 1039.

11. Powderly WG, Robinson K, Keath EJ. Molecular typing of *Candida albicans* isolated from oral lesions of HIV-infected individuals. AIDS 1992; 6: 81.

12. Powderly WG, Robinson K, Keath EJ. Molecular epidemiology of recurrent oral candidiasis in human immunodeficiency virus-positive patients: evidence for two patterns of recurrence. J Infect Dis 1993; 168: 463.

13. Warnock DW. Azole drug resistance in *Candida* species [editorial]. J Antimicrob Chemother 1993; 31: 463.

14. Odds FC. *Candida* and Candidosis. London: Balliere Tindall, 1988.

15. Cannon RD, Holmes AR, Mason AB, Monk BC. Oral *Candida*: clearance, colonization or candidiasis. J Dent Res 1995; 75: 1152.

16. EC-Clearinghouse on Oral Problems Related to HIV Infection and WHO Collaborating Centre on Oral Manifestations of the Immunodeficiency Virus. Classification and diagnostic criteria for oral lesions in HIV infection. J Oral Pathol Med 1993; 22: 289.

17. Greenspan D, Greenspan JS, Pindborg JJ, Schiodt M. AIDS and the Mouth. Copenhagen: Munksgaard, 1990.

18. Greenspan D. Treatment of oropharyngeal candidiasis in HIV-positive patients. J Am Acad Dermatol 1994; 31: S51.

19. Greenspan JS, Greenspan D, Lennette ET, et al. Replication of Epstein-Barr virus within the epithelial cells of "hairy" leukoplakia, an AIDS-associated lesion. N Engl J Med 1985; 313: 1564.

20. Epstein JB. Antifungal therapy in oropharyngeal mycotic infections. Oral Surg Oral Med Oral Pathol 1990; 69: 32.

21. Greenspan D, Greenspan JS. Management of the oral lesions of HIV infection. J Am Dent Assoc 1991; 122: 26.

22. Greenspan D. Treatment of oral candidiasis in HIV infections. Oral Surg Oral Med Oral Pathol 1994; 78: 211.

23. The Medical Letter. Drugs for AIDS and associated infections. 1995; 37: 87.

24. Owens NJ, Nightingale CH, Schweizer RT, et al. Prophylaxis of oral candidiasis with clotrimazole troches. Arch Intern Med 1984; 144: 290.

25. Nyst MJ, Perriens JH, Kimputu L, et al. Gentian violet, ketoconazole and nystatin in oropharyngeal and esophageal candidiasis in Zairian AIDS patients. Ann Soc Belg Med Trop 1992; 72: 45.

26. Ferretti GA, Ash RC, Brown AT, et al. Control of oral mucositis and candidiasis in marrow transplantation: a prospective, double-blind trial of chlorhexidine digluconate oral rinse. Bone Marrow Transplant 1988; 3: 483.

27. Dewsnup DH, Stevens DA. Efficacy of oral amphotericin B in AIDS patients with thrush clinically resistant to fluconazole. J Med Vet Mycol 1994; 32: 389.
28. Como JA, Dismukes WE. Oral azole drugs as systemic antifungal therapy. N Engl J Med 1994; 330: 263.
29. Hay RJ. Overview of studies of fluconazole in oropharyngeal candidiasis. Rev Infect Dis 1990; 3: s334.
30. Pons V, Greenspan D, Gallant J, et al. Comparative clinical study of oral suspension fluconazole versus topical liquid nystatin in the treatment of oropharyngeal candidiasis in AIDS, 35th ICAAC, San Francisco CA, Sep 17–20, 1995.
31. Pons V, Greenspan D, Debruin M. Therapy for oropharyngeal candidiasis in HIV-infected patients: a randomized, prospective multicenter study of oral fluconazole versus clotrimazole troches. The Multicenter Study Group [see comments]. J Acquir Immune Defic Syndr 1993; 6: 1311.
32. Just-Nubling G, Gentschew G, Meissner K, et al. Fluconazole prophylaxis of recurrent oral candidiasis in HIV-positive patients. Eur J Clin Microbiol Infect Dis 1991; 10: 917.
33. Willocks L, Leen CL, Brettle RP, et al. Fluconazole resistance in AIDS patients [letter]. J Antimicrob Chemother 1991; 28: 937.
34. Heinic GS, Stevens DA, Greenspan D, et al. Fluconazole-resistant *Candida* in AIDS patients. Report of two cases. Oral Surg Oral Med Oral Pathol 1993; 76: 711.
35. Hitchcock CA, Pye GW, Troke PF, et al. Fluconazole resistance in *Candida glabrata*. Antimicrob Agents Chemother 1993; 37: 1962.
36. Heald AE, Cox GM, Schell WA, et al. Oropharyngeal yeast flora and fluconazole resistance in HIV-infected patients receiving long-term continuous versus intermittent fluconazole therapy. AIDS 1996; 10: 263.
37. Blatchford NR. Treatment of oral candidosis with itraconazole: a review. J Am Acad Dermatol 1991; 23: 565.
38. Graybill JR, Vasquez J, Darouiche RO, Morhart R. Itraconazole oral solution versus fluconazole treatment of oropharyngeal candidiasis. Abstract 1220. 35th ICAAC, San Francisco CA 17-20 September 1995.
39. Levron JC, Reynes J, Bazin C. Bioavailability of itraconazole oral solution during treatment of oropharyngeal candidosis in HIV+ patients. Abstracts 2131. 19th International Congress of Chemotherapy, Montreal, Canada 16-20 July 1995.

21

The Clinical Impact of Antifungal Drug Resistance in Patients with AIDS

John R. Graybill
University of Texas Health Science Center at San Antonio and Audie Murphy Veterans Hospital, San Antonio, Texas

INTRODUCTION

More than 90% of patients with HIV infection develop fungal infection during the course of their disease. The most common infection is mucosal candidiasis. Although vaginosis may be increased in patients with AIDS, it does not present as much problem in severity or recurrences as does oropharyngeal candidosis. The latter first appears at modest depressions of immunity, when CD4 counts are in the range of 300 to $400/mm^3$. As immunity further wanes, both the severity and frequency of recurrence increase. Eventually, when the CD4 falls well below $100/mm^3$, mucosal infection extends to the esophagus, producing symptoms of substernal pain and dysphagia. Finally, as bone marrow reserves fail, and often under the influences of cytotoxic drugs such as ganciclovir and disruption of the integument by intravenous catheters, hematogenous disseminated disease may occur. In the end stages of AIDS, patients are also susceptible to a variety of other mycoses, including cryptococcosis, histoplasmosis, coccidioidomycosis, and aspergillosis. Together these "other" pathogens may infect between 5% and 10% of AIDS patients (1–9).

MUCOSAL CANDIDIASIS

In the setting of progressive immune deficiency and increasing fungal infections, primarily mucosal candidiasis, one of the first antifungals to be used is clotrimazole. Clotrimazole is available only topically and is successful in treatment of mild and moderately severe thrush. Clotrimazole is useful initially, but eventually tends to fail in more than half of patients (10,11). Another drug is ketoconazole, commonly used at 200 to 400 mg/day (12–14). Ketoconazole absorption is markedly increased by acid, and the achlorhydria of late AIDS patients may account for some of the ketoconazole failures (15). Thus resistance may not be due to worsening susceptibility, but to limited drug absorption. Fluconazole is better absorbed, better tolerated, renally cleared, and not as susceptible to drug interactions as ketoconazole (14,16). Fluconazole is also more effective than either clotrimazole for treatment of thrush or ketoconazole (at a low dose of 200 mg/day) for treatment of candidal esophagitis (11).

Fluconazole is benign and remarkably effective in the treatment of mucosal candidiasis, with response rate of ≥ 90% to a 2-week course of 100 mg/day (17). None of the available antifungal therapies are truly fungicidal, and *Candida* may often persist at low numbers throughout the treatment period (17). No matter what treatment is given, many patients with more severe immune depression relapse, as many as 50% within the first month after treatment is terminated (17,18). Therefore, it was a natural step to prescribe fluconazole chronically as suppression to prevent reactivation of disease (19–21). This same procedure has been used with fluconazole for suppression of cryptococcosis and itraconazole for suppression of histoplasmosis, and these have generally been successful, with fewer than 10% reported relapses (1,2).

Because of the large numbers of patients and because of the high cost of fluconazole, low doses of 50 or 100 mg/day, or 150 mg/week were used to suppress thrush and esophagitis (21). This combination of severe immune depression, low doses of antifungal drugs, and prolonged therapy prepared the stage for the development of fluconazole resistance (22).

FLUCONAZOLE-RESISTANT CANDIDA

First reports of fluconazole resistance were made in the early 1990s. Resistance occurred in a stepwise fashion. Patients who formerly responded to 50 mg/day then needed 100 mg/day, and after a while 200 mg/day, eventually failing doses as high as 800 mg/day (22–29). This process usually occurred over many months. Molecular typing studies indicated that resistance commonly emerged both by replacement of initially fluconazole-susceptible isolates with fluconazole-resistant new isolates, and also that susceptible isolates could persist and stepwise mutate to increasing resistance (30,31). Most of the fluconazole-resistant isolates associated with clinical failure were *Candida albicans*. In one study, patients with multiple *Candida* species in their mouths, with fluconazole-susceptible *C. albicans* and fluconazole-resistant *C. glabrata* or *tropicalis*, were retreated with fluconazole (32). They responded well, suggesting that fluconazole-susceptible *C. albicans* is usually the pathogen. *Candida albicans* has thus been the main focus of efforts to address antifungal resistance. Mechanisms of resistance are multiple and include decreased fungal cell penetration by fluconazole, alteration in target enzymes, overproduction of target enzymes, and production of novel sterols in the fungal cell membrane (33–36).

Initially there was no standardized in vitro testing and consequently no correlation of minimum inhibitory concentration of fluconazole in vitro with clinical failures. Eventually, the National Committee for Clinical Laboratory Standards (NCCLS) developed a standardized method for in vitro susceptibility testing (37). The first studies conducted by the NCCLS were to define a testing method that was reproducible within one laboratory and also reproducible among different laboratories (37,38). When the NCCLS method was published, it was broadly used by mycology reference laboratories. Fluconazole-susceptible organisms were identified by having minimum inhibitory concentration of ≤ 4 µg/ml, while increasing resistance was found at 8 to 32 µcg/ml and >64 µg/ml was considered highly resistant (29,39,40). There has been some uncertainty as to what minimum inhibitory concentration (MIC) to call "resistant," and some have preferred to use terms of *decreased sensitivity* to fluconazole (29). We have found that animals infected with *C. albicans* obtained before treatment of thrush respond well to treatment with fluconazole. In contrast mice infected with fluconazole-resistant isolates (obtained from the same patient with clinical failure to fluconazole, and identical in other respects to the pretreatment isolate) required higher doses of fluconazole for response (41). Also, the NCCLS method of in vitro sensitivity testing correlated increasingly well with fluconazole resistance in mice infected with *C. albicans*, *C. tropicalis*, *C. glabrata*, and with clinical failure of thrush and esophagitis (29,42–45). Therefore, at this time we believe that there is reasonably good correlation of in vitro susceptibilities with predicting clinical outcome.

The problems that persist include (a) relatively few centers with expertise in performing these tests and (b) a substantial delay in testing isolates. One way to address this may be to use an initial primary culture system that identifies *Candida* species and that screens for in vitro sensitivity. Such a system can be adapted using Chromagar impregnated with fluconazole at 8 µg/ml and cross-standardized to the NCCLS method (46). A semi-quantitative throat culture could give a suggestion of total oropharyngeal burden with which species, and whether large numbers of fluconazole-resistant *C. albicans* are present. This may be useful at the outset in predicting who will fail fluconazole therapy.

What defines failure to fluconazole? The most practical definition is failure to resolve thrush when treated with an adequate dose for an adequate time (24). What is an adequate dose? Many patients are treated with 50 mg/day. Although this dose is frequently effective, lack of response to this dose is probably too low a threshold to assess failure. In several recent or ongoing research studies there is agreement that at least 1 (or 2) weeks therapy with fluconazole at 100 (or 200) mg/day should be given without response before failure is declared (17,29) (Graybill, unpublished observations). While one might have some success in treating with doses at 200 mg/day, once resistance has begun to develop, responses at these higher doses are often only transitory (23,29).

ALTERNATIVES TO FLUCONAZOLE

After definitive fluconazole failure at higher doses, limited alternatives are available. First, there is modest cross-resistance with the other antifungal azoles, itraconazole and ketoconazole. One study evaluated ketoconazole susceptibility of isolates coming from patients treated with no fluconazole, intermittent fluconazole, or chronic fluconazole (41). Isolates from fluconazole-naive patients were exquisitely susceptible to both drugs. Conversely, patients with chronic fluconazole had a shift to much higher MIC values for the *Candida* isolates, and a similar but lesser shift of MIC to ketoconazole. This was further explored in two studies by Barchiesi et al. (39,40). Both studies identified 50 fluconazole-susceptible (MIC ≤ 4 µg/ml) wand, 50 resistant isolated with fluconazole MIC values ≥8 µg/ml, using the NCCLS method. These isolates were tested for itraconazole in one study and in the other for D0870, a new antifungal triazole with markedly heightened antifungal activity against *C. albicans*. Results of both studies were similar. While the fluconazole-susceptible isolates had extremely low MIC values to itraconazole and D0870, these values had nevertheless sifted to higher levels. What made them different was that for fluconazole they were out of the effective range, but for itraconazole and D0870 most (but not all) were still in what was thought to be an effective range. A recent publication by Martinez-Suarez and Rodriguez-Tudela (20) has confirmed these findings in a series of *C. albicans* isolates from patients in Spain.

Do these in vitro data tell us anything about drug use in vivo? For primary treatment of thrush, both itraconazole capsules and ketoconazole are about 80% effective clinically in 2 weeks. In one study, a series of patients with fluconazole-resistant thrush were treated with itraconazole and ketoconazole capsules, and here the results were not very good (47). Unfortunately, blood levels were not measured to determine whether these more variably absorbed drugs had measurable serum concentrations. A new liquid preparation of itraconazole in cyclodextrin is now under development (48,49). This preparation has also been highly effective in treatment of primary thrush, with 97% response with 200 mg/day at 2 weeks of treatment, equal or better than fluconazole at 200 mg/day for 2 weeks (17). There are few data on the use of this drug for treatment of fluconazole-resistant oral thrush, but a few preliminary studies suggest that it is effective, even though serum concentrations do not correlate well with response (50). Therefore, it is possible, if not likely, that the topical effect of the solution might have accounted for the responses. Even so, some failures were encountered, suggesting that high doses of the drug may be needed for fluconazole failures. Similar responses were seen for D0870, with excellent results in 11 of 11 patients given a 25 mg loading dose followed by 10 mg/day for 4 days as primary treatment (51). With fluconazole-resistant organisms and patients treated with 150 mg load followed by 25 mg/day for 6 days, however, only two patients were cured; 11 were suppressed, and 14 had no response (52). Thus, even these higher doses failed, and higher doses are now under investigation. I suspect that fluconazole-resistant C. albicans will in general respond to high doses of either itraconazole or D0870 (when a regimen is chosen), but it is far from clear whether these drugs will be useful for a long time under the sustained pressure of chronic therapy, as has been used for fluconazole. Other expanded spectrum triazoles are under development, but even less is known about these agents.

What other options are available? Within the next year there should be a completely new class of drugs, the pneumocandins and papulocandins in clinical trials. These drugs act by impeding β-1,3 glucan synthase and thus target the fungal cell wall (53,54). In vitro they are potent at extremely low concentrations and in our studies, mice respond at concentrations similar to those for amphotericin B (Graybill, personal observations). The only known disadvantage is that they must be given parenterally.

There is also the standby, amphotericin B, which is effective when given intravenously in most patients, at 0.3 to 0.5 mg/kg per day initially, then for suppression at once to three times a week. The new lipid-associated derivatives of amphotericin B are less noxious and likely will be effective in mucosal candidiasis, although they have both been clinically studied in this setting. Amphotericin B Lipid Complex (ABCLCET The Lipisome Company, Princeton, NJ) has been licenzed for treatment of Aspersillosis.

RESISTANCE TO OTHER MYCOSES

What about resistance to other mycoses? There is some concern about *Cryptococcus neoformans* developing a rising MIC to fluconazole. Isolates with high MIC values have been more resistant to fluconazole mouse models, but whether this is a major problem clinically is unclear (55,56). Casadevall et al. (57) have suggested that isolates from patients with relapsing or persisting disease are as susceptible as patients before treatment and have argued indirectly that patients must be noncompliant; however, their observations are based on only a few patients. There is no evidence of in vitro resistance of *Histoplasma capsulatum* or *Coccidioides immitis* to amphotericin B or to azole antifungals. However, histoplasmosis is far more readily and predictably treated than coccidioidomycosis and has fewer than 10% relapses (1,2,5,6). *Coccidioides immitis*, while remaining susceptible in vitro, has traditionally been poorly responsive to antifungals in vivo, both in HIV and non-HIV-infected patients (3,6). Responses of 50% to 60% are as much as we hope to achieve with current antifungals in non-HIV patients (3). In AIDS patients, responses correlate more with the level of immune depression than with a specific drug. Patients with very low CD4 counts have severe disseminated disease and usually die within a month or two, while those less compromised respond better (4). This response is also reminiscent of aspergillosis, a disease that in leukemic patients responds better to neutrophil recovery than to any specific antifungal regimen. In HIV patients, aspergillosis occurs late, when there is terminal depression of bone marrow. Neutropenia and steroid use are frequent but not universal, and other risk factors are incompletely defined. The disease tends to progress inexorably, sometimes with remissions or slowdowns induced by amphotericin B or itraconazole, but usually the result is death with or caused by aspergillosis (58,59). There is no clear correlation with drug resistance, but there is an excellent correlation of response with poor host resistance.

SUMMARY

Mucosal candidiasis is the most common mycotic infection seen in patients with AIDS. The frequent recurrences as immunity wanes have led to increasing use of fluconazole, with recalcitrance to this drug increasingly shown. We have some new developments in triazole for treatment of these patients, but we have no experience with these drugs being used under long, hard pressure. My fear is that ultimately they will fail as well, and we may be left with amphotericin B, highly toxic and still not completely effective.

REFERENCES

1. Wheat LJ, Hafner R, Wulfsohn M, et al. Prevention of relapse of histoplasmosis with itraconazole in patients with the acquired immunodeficiency syndrome. Ann Intern Med 1993;118: 610–616.
2. Norris S, Wheat J, McKinsey D, et al. Prevention of relapse of histoplasmosis with fluconazole in patients with the acquired immunodeficiency syndrome. Am J Med 1994; 96: 504–508.
3. Stevens DA. Coccidioidomycosis. N Engl J Med 1995; 332: 1077–1082.
4. Fish DG, Ampel NM, Galgiani JN, et al. Coccidioidomycosis during human immunodeficiency virus infection: a review of 77 patients. Medicine 1990; 69: 384–391.
5. McKinsey DS, Gupta R, Riddler SA, Driks MR, Smith DL, Kurtin PJ. Long term amphotericin B therapy for disseminated histoplasmosis in patients with the acquired immunodeficiency syndrome (AIDS). Ann Intern Med 1989; 111: 655–659.
6. Denning DW, Stevens DA. Antifungal and surgical treatment of invasive aspergillosis: review of 2,121 published cases. Rev Infect Dis 1990; 12: 1147–1201.
7. Saag MS Powderly WG, Cloud GA, et al. Comparison of amphotericin B with fluconazole in the treatment of AIDS-associated cryptococcal meningitis. N Engl J Med 1992; 26: 83–89.
8. Supparatpinyo K, Khamwan C, Baosoung V, et al. Disseminated *Penicillium marneffi* infection in Southeast Asia. Lancet 1994; 344: 110–113.
9. Denning DW, Lee JY, Hostetler JS, et al. NIAID Mycoses Study Group multicenter trial of oral itraconazole therapy for invasive aspergillosis. Am J Med 1994; 97: 135–144.
10. Powderly WG, Finkelstein DM, Feinberg J, et al. A randomized trial comparing fluconazole with clotrimazole troches for the prevention of fungal infections in patients with advanced human immunodeficiency virus infection. N Engl J Med 1995; 332: 700–705.
11. Koletar SL, Russel JA, Fass RJ, Plouffe JF. Comparison of oral fluconazole and clotrimazole troches as treatment for oral candidiasis in patients infected with human immunodeficiency virus. Antimicrob Agents Chemother 1990; 34: 2267–2268.

12. Como J, Dismukes WE. Oral azole drugs as systemic antifungal therapy. N Engl J Med 1994; 330: 263–272.
13. Horsburgh CR, Kirkpatrick CH. Long-term therapy of chronic mucocutaneous candidiasis with ketoconazole: experience with twenty-one patients. Am J Med 1983; 74: 23–29.
14. Meunier F, Aoun M, Gerard M. Therapy for oropharyngeal candidiasis in the immunocompromised host: a randomized double-blind study of fluconazole versus ketoconazole. Rev Infect Dis 1990; 12(suppl 3): S364–S368.
15. Chin TWF, Loeb M, Fong IW. Effects of an acidic beverage (Coca-Cola) on absorption of ketoconazole. Antimicrob Agents Chemother 1995; 39: 1671–1675.
16. Bailey EM, Krakovsky DJ, Rybak MJ. The triazole antifungal agents: a review of itraconazole and fluconazole. Pharmacotherapy 1990; 10: 146–153.
17. Graybill JR, Vazques J, Darouiche RO, et al. Itraconazole solution (IS) versus fluconazole (F) treatment of oropharyngeal candidiasis (OC). Thirty Fifth Interscience Conference on Antimicrobial Agents and Chemotherapy, San Francisco, California, September 17–20, 1995.
18. Stevens DA, Green SI, Lang OS. Thrush can be prevented in patients with acquired immunodeficiency syndrome-related complex. Randomized, double-blind, placebo-controlled study of 100 mg oral fluconazole daily. Arch Intern Med 1991; 151: 2458–2464.
19. Parente F, Ardizzone S, Cernuschi M, et al. Prevention of symptomatic recurrences of esophageal candidiasis in AIDS patients after the first episode: a prospective open study. Am J Gastroenterol 1994; 89: 416–420.
20. Martinez-Suarez JV, Rodriguez-Tudela JL. Patterns of in vitro activity of itraconazole and imidazole antifungal agents against *Candida albicans* with decreased susceptibility to fluconazole from Spain. Antimicrob Agents Chemother 1995; 39: 1512–1516.
21. Sangeorzan JA, Bradley SF, He X, et al. Epidemiology of oral candidiasis in HIV infected patients: colonization, infection, treatment, and emergence of fluconazole resistance. Am J Med 1994; 97: 339–346.
22. DuPont B, Improvisi L, Eliaszewicz M, et al. Resistance of *Candida albicans* to fluconazole in AIDS patients. Thirty Second Interscience Conference on Antimicrobial Agents and Chemotherapy, Anaheim, California, 1992.
23. Redding S, Smith J, Farinacci G, et al. Resistance of *Candida albicans* to fluconazole during treatment of oropharyngeal candidiasis in a patient with AIDS: documentation by in vitro susceptibility testing and DNA subtype analysis. Clin Infect Dis 1994; 18: 240–242.
24. Ng TTC, Denning DW. Fluconazole resistance in *Candida* in patients with AIDS—a therapeutic approach. J Antimicrob Chemother 1993; 26: 117–125.
25. Moreno F, Allendoerfer R, Pfaller MA, et al. In vivo significance of mutation to fluconazole resistance in *C. albicans*. 94th General Meeting of the American Society for Microbiology, Adelaide, Australia, 1994.
26. Pfaller MA, Rhine-Chalberg J, Redding SW, et al. Variations in fluconazole susceptibility and electrophoretic karyotype among oral isolates of *Candida*

albicans from patients with AIDS and oral candidiasis. J Clin Microbiol 1994; 32: 59–64.

27. Sanguineti A, Carmichael JK, Campbell K. Fluconazole-resistant *Candida albicans* after long-term suppressive therapy. Arch Intern Med 1993; 153: 1122–1124.

28. Bailey GG, Perry FM, Denning DW, Mandal BK. Fluconazole resistant candidiasis in an HIV cohort. IXth International Conference on AIDS. Berlin, Germany, 1993.

29. Rex JH, Rinaldi MG, Pfaller MA. Resistance of *Candida* species to fluconazole. Antimicrob Agents Chemother 1995; 39: 1–8.

30. Millon L, Manteaux A, Reboux G, et al. Fluconazole-resistant recurrent oral candidiasis in human immunodeficiency virus-positive patients: persistence of *Candida albicans* strains with the same genotype. J Clin Microbiol 1994; 32: 1115–1118.

31. Powderly WG, Robinson K, Keath EJ. Molecular epidemiology of recurrent oral candidiasis in human immunodeficiency virus-positive patients; evidence for two patterns of recurrence. J Infect Dis 1993; 168: 463–466.

32. Dronda F, Chaves F, Alonso-Sanz M, et al. Clinical significance of mixed oropharyngeal candidiasis due to *Candida albicans* and non-*albicans* strains in HIV-infected patients. Thirty-Fourth Interscience Conference on Antimicrobial Agents and Chemotherapy, Orlando, Florida, October 4–7, 1994.

33. Parkinson T, Falconer DJ, Hitchcock CA. Fluconazole resistance due to energy-dependent drug efflux in *Candida glabrata*. Antimicrob Agents Chemother 1995; 39: 1696–1699.

34. Hitchcock CA. Resistance of *Candida albicans* to azole antifungal agents. Biochem Soc Trans 1993; 21: 1039–1047.

35. Hitchcock CA, Pye GW, Troke PF, et al. Fluconazole resistance in *Candida glabrata*. Antimicrob Agents Chemother 1993; 37: 1962–1965.

36. Barchiesi F, Restrepo M, McGough DA, Rinaldi MG. In vitro activity of a new antifungal triazole: UK109,496. Thirty Fifth Interscience Conference on Antimicrobial Agents and Chemotherapy, San Francisco, California, September 17–20, 1995.

37. Galgiani JN. Susceptibility testing of fungi: current status of the standardization process. Antimicrob Agents Chemother 1993; 37: 2517–2521.

38. National Committee for Clinical Laboratory Standards. Reference method for broth dilution antifungal susceptibility testing of yeasts. National Committee for Clinical Laboratory Standards, Villanova, Pennsylvania, 1992.

39. Barchiesi F, Colombo AL, McGough DA, et al. In vitro activity of a new antifungal triazole, D0870, against *Candida albicans* isolates from oral cavities of patients infected with human immunodeficiency virus. Antimicrob Agents Chemother 1994; 38: 1530–1533.

40. Barchiesi F, Colombo AL, McGough DA, et al. In vitro activity of itraconazole against fluconazole-susceptible and resistant *Candida albicans* isolates from oral cavities of patients infected with human immunodeficiency virus. Antimicrob Agents Chemother 1994; 38: 2553.

41. Barchiesi F, Najvar LK, Luther MF, Scalise G, Rinaldi MG, Graybill JR. Variation in fluconazole efficacy for *Candida albicans* sequentially isolated from the oral cavities of patients with AIDS in an experimental murine candidiasis. Antimicrob Agents Chemother 1996; 40: 1317–1320.

42. Graybill JR, Najvar LK, Holmberg JD, Luther MF. Fluconazole, D0870, and flucytosine treatment of disseminated *Candida tropicalis* infections in mice. Antimicrob Agents Chemother 1995; 39: 924–929.

43. Najvar LK, Holmberg J, Luther M, Graybill JR. Fluconazole (F) and D0870 (D) treatment of murine candidiasis with *C. albicans* (CA) resistant in vitro to fluconazole. Thirty Fifth Interscience Conference on Antimicrobial Agents and Chemotherapy, San Francisco, California, September 17–20, 1995.

44. Atkinson BA, Bouthet C, Bocanegra R, et al. Comparison of fluconazole, amphotericin B and flucytosine in treatment of a murine model of disseminated infection with *Candida glabrata* in immunocompromised mice. J Antimicrob Chemother 1995; 35: 631–640.

45. Cameron ML, Schell WA, Bruch S, et al. Correlation of in vitro fluconazole resistance of *Candida* isolates in relation to therapy and symptoms of individuals seropositive for Human Immunodeficiency Virus Type 1. Antimicrob Agents Chemother 1993; 37: 2449–2453.

46. Patterson TF, Revankar SG, Kirkpatrick WR, et al. Simple method for detecting fluconazole–resistant yeasts with chromogenic agar. J Clin Microbiol 1996; 34: 1794–1797.

47. Bailey GC, Perry FM, Denning DW, Mandal BK. Fluconazole resistant candidiasis in an HIV cohort. Ninth International Conference on AIDS, Berlin, Germany, June 6–11, 1993.

48. Hostettler JS, Hanson LH, Stevens DA. Effect of cyclodextrin on the pharmacology of antifungal azoles. Antimicrob Agents Chemother 1992; 36: 477–480.

49. Prentice AG, Warnock DW, Johnson SAN, et al. Multiple dose pharmacokinetics of an oral solution of itraconazole in autologous bone marrow transplant recipients. J Antimicrob Chemother 1994; 34: 247–252.

50. Ganger G, Just-Nubing G, Eichel M, et al. Itraconazole solution in patients with non-response to fluconazole. Ninth International Conference on AIDS. Berlin, Germany, June 6–11, 1993.

51. deWit S, Dupont B, Cartledge JD, et al. Pilot study of a new triazole derivative (D0870) in HIV patients with oral candidiasis (OC). Thirty Fourth Interscience Conference on Antimicrobial Agents and Chemotherapy, Orlando, Florida, 1994.

52. Cartledge JD, Dupont B, et al. Treatment of fluconazole (FCZ) resistant (res) oral candidosis (OC) with D0870 in patients with AIDS (PWA). Thirty Fourth Interscience Conference on Antimicrobial Agents and Chemotherapy, Orlando, Florida, 1994.

53. Abruzzo GK, Flattery AM, Gill CJ, et al. Evaluation of water-soluble pneumocandin analogs L-733450, L-705589, and L-731373 with mouse models of disseminated aspergillosis, candidiasis, and cryptococcosis. Antimicrob Agents Chemother 1994; 38: 2750–2757.

54. Bartizal K, Scott T, Abruzzo GK, et al. In vitro evaluation of the pneumocandin antifungal agent L-733560, a new water soluble hybrid of L-705589 and L-731373. Antimicrob Agents Chemother 1994; 39: 1070–1076.
55. Nguyen MH, Barchiesi F, McGough DA, et al. In vitro evaluation of combination of fluconazole and flucytosine against *Cryptococcus neoformans* var *neoformans*. Antimicrob Agents Chemother 1995; 39: 1691–1695.
56. Velez JD, Allendoerfer R, Luther MF, et al. Correlation of an in vitro azole susceptibility with in vivo response in a murine model of cryptococcal meningitis. J Infect Dis 1993; 168: 508–510.
57. Casadevall A, Spitzer ED, Webb D, Rinaldi MG. Susceptibilities of serial *Cryptococcus neoformans* isolates from patients with recurrent cryptococcal meningitis to amphotericin B and fluconazole. Antimicrob Agents Chemother 1993; 1383–1386.
58. Pursell KJ, Telzak EE, Armstrong D. *Aspergillus* species colonization and invasive disease in patients with AIDS. Clin Infect Dis 1992; 14: 141–148.
59. Lortholary O, Meyohas MC, Dupont B, et al. Invasive aspergillosis in patients with acquired immunodeficiency syndrome: report of 33 cases. Am J Med 1993; 95: 177–187.

22

Current Approaches to Diagnosis and Treatment of Candidiasis in Children

Thomas J. Walsh
National Cancer Institute, Bethesda, Maryland

Invasive fungal infections are emerging as important causes of morbidity and mortality in immunocompromised children. *Candida* spp. now constitute one of the most common causes of nosocomial infections, particularly in the setting of prolonged antibacterial therapy, chronic indwelling central venous catheters, granulocytopenia, complicated surgical procedures, and very low birth weight. Mucosal candidiasis is the most common opportunistic infection in HIV-infected patients. Therapeutic advances have improved understanding of existing antifungal drugs, particularly amphotericin B, and development of new compounds, especially antifungal triazoles. This chapter reviews the patterns of candidiasis in children and current approaches to antifungal therapy.

Candidiasis is the most common mucosal and deeply invasive mycosis affecting children. *Candida albicans* is the most common species of the genus *Candida* causing infections. Other species such as *C. tropicalis*, *C. parapsilosis*, *C. krusei*, *Torulopsis glabrata* (considered by some authorities to belong to the genus *Candida*), are increasing in incidence and may cause serious infection. The term *candidiasis* is a general one, which refers to a spectrum of infection, including cutaneous candidiasis, mucosal candidiasis, candidemia, disseminated candidiasis, and single organ infection.

Candida infections are classified as cutaneous candidiasis, mucosal candidiasis, and deeply invasive candidiasis. Mucosal candidiasis may be further classified as cutaneous, oropharyngeal, and esophageal infection.

Deeply invasive candidiasis may be further classified as fungemia, acute disseminated candidiasis, chronic disseminated candidiasis, and single-organ candidiasis.

OROPHARYNGEAL CANDIDIASIS

The clinical manifestations of oral candidiasis are variable, including a punctate mucosal erythema, a diffuse mucosal erythema, and white-beige pseudomembranous plaques on the buccal mucosa, hard palate, oropharyngeal mucosa, and gingivae (1). These lesions may be become confluent plaques, involving extensive regions of the mucosa of the oral cavity. These plaques can be removed with difficulty to reveal a granular base that bleeds easily. A more chronic form of oropharyngeal candidiasis, known as atrophic *Candida* glossitis, may develop on the dorsum of the tongue, appearing as an erythematous lesion associated with the loss of papillae. The lesions may become sufficiently severe as to impair alimentation. Oral candidiasis in immunocompromised patients may also be complicated by extension to esophageal candidiasis (2–4), laryngeal candidiasis, or *Candida* epiglottitis, which may cause hoarseness or threaten patency of the airway (2,5–9).

As white mucosal plaques are not necessarily pathognomonic for oropharyngeal candidiasis, direct microscopic examination of scrapings of lesions and culture confirmation is the most reliable means of establishing this diagnosis. Many cases of apparent thrush, particularly in granulocytopenic patients, may have other causes including herpes simplex or mixed oral bacterial flora.

Topical antifungal treatment is usually effective in controlling most cases of oropharyngeal candidiasis and is recommended as the initial therapeutic intervention. Nystatin has limited activity in moderate to advanced forms of oropharyngeal candidiasis in severely immunocompromised hosts. It is also limited by its somewhat bitter taste, which may be a major impediment to compliance. In this regard, clotrimazole, administered four to five times a day, appears to be more active than nystatin in the treatment of oropharyngeal candidiasis, possibly because of improved compliance. The more prolonged exposure of the oral cavity to clotrimazole also may substantially contribute to its antifungal activity. Nevertheless, administration of clotrimazole troches requiring retention of the troche in the oral cavity until it is completely dissolved may be difficult in younger children. In cases where the child is not able to maintain a clotrimazole troche under the tongue or under buccal mucosal for a sustained time, the clotrimazole troches may be pulverized and formulated into a suspension given by syringe.

Children with oropharyngeal candidiasis refractory to topical therapy are candidates for systemic therapy using ketoconazole or, when approved, fluconazole. Ketoconazole and fluconazole for oropharyngeal candidiasis may be administered at 3.0 mg/kg in two divided doses (10,11). Recent reports of itraconazole also suggest a potential role for this agent in treatment of oropharyngeal candidiasis in children, including those with chronic mucocutaneous candidiasis (12,13). For smaller children, a tablet may be divided and pulverized into a suspension and administered as a fraction of that suspension twice a day. The optimal use of the antifungal azoles, however, in HIV-associated oropharyngeal candidiasis has at this point not been clearly elucidated. Children with particularly depressed cell-mediated immunity may have oropharyngeal and esophageal candidiasis that becomes completely refractory to topical and oral therapy (14). Such patients may respond well to intermittent courses of amphotericin B at 0.5 mg/kg a day for approximately 7 to 14 days, depending on therapeutic response. Lower doses of amphotericin B for refractory mucosal candidiasis may not be successful in eradicating the infection. In addition to treating the oropharyngeal candidiasis, one should treat any concomitant infections such as those caused by herpes simplex virus, which may occur concomitantly with invasive candidiasis. Advanced stages of oropharyngeal candidiasis in HIV-infected children and granulocytopenic children may often be accompanied by esophageal candidiasis. Recent findings indicate that azole resistant C. *albicans* may emerge in HIV-infected children as a cause of esophageal candidiasis (15).

ESOPHAGEAL CANDIDIASIS

Esophageal candidiasis is associated with risk factors that are similar to those of oropharyngeal candidiasis, but may occur in the absence of conspicuous oropharyngeal *Candida* infection (2–4,16). Radiation to the mediastinum and gastroesophageal reflux are additional risk factors for esophageal candidiasis (17). Concomitant infections caused by herpes simplex, cytomegalovirus, and bacteria may coincide with or precede esophageal candidiasis.

Esophagoscopy with mucosal biopsy is the most definitive method for establishing a diagnosis of esophageal candidiasis. Although biopsy of the esophageal mucosa is the gold standard for diagnosis of esophageal candidiasis, this may not be feasible in many children. Accordingly, an empirical approach is often warranted in children with suspected esophageal candidiasis. Such an empirical approach in children with granulocytopenia may consist of initial clotrimazole and/or systemic azole. Because the esophagus may be the portal of entry for candidiasis, however, failure to respond symptomatically and promptly is an indication for empirical amphotericin B. One must also be aware that the resolution of symptoms does not necessarily signify the eradication of esophageal candidiasis in granulocytopenic patients. Thus, a persistently febrile patient with proven esophageal candidiasis may still require empirical amphotericin B therapy, despite resolution of esophageal symptoms. Children with HIV infection, who are also highly susceptible to development of esophageal candidiasis, may initially receive therapy, depending on the severity of symptoms and level of immunosuppression, with ketoconazole, fluconazole, or amphotericin B. Nystatin appears to have little or no effect in the management of esophageal candidiasis. Initial studies in children indicate that fluconazole is effective in the treatment of esophageal candidiasis. Appropriate doses of fluconazole for treatment of esophageal candidiasis have yet to be defined, but 3 mg/kg in non-neutropenic patients is active.

GENITOURINARY CANDIDIASIS

The management and diagnostic significance of candiduria depend on the host and location of infection. Removal of urinary catheters and other foreign bodies (e.g., urinary stents), when possible, is a basic principle for the management of urinary catheter infections. Candiduria proven through a reliable clean-catch specimen or a straight catheterized specimen in a low-birth-weight infant or child with granulocytopenia should be considered significant and treated as evidence of disseminated candidiasis until proven otherwise. By comparison, the nonimmuno-compromised child with candiduria and temporary placement of a urinary catheter or congenital anatomical ureteral and bladder abnormalities most likely does not have disseminated candidiasis. Such patients are more likely to have infection restricted to the mucosa. Thus, treatment of *Candida* cystitis with systemic antifungal therapy depends on the probability of concomitant deeply invasive candidiasis.

Medical management of uncomplicated *Candida* cystitis may include fluconazole (3 mg/kg a day), intravenous amphotericin B (0.3–0.5 mg/kg per day), or oral flucytosine (5-FC; 150 mg/kg per day in three to four divided doses). With the advent of fluconazole, amphotericin B bladder washouts may be avoided in most instances. Single doses or short courses of intravenous amphotericin B achieve sufficiently high fungicidal concentrations in the urine to eradicate *Candida*. Nevertheless, candiduria may recur as long as the patient remains catheterized. Given its high urinary concentrations, fluconazole may be highly effective in the treatment of urinary tract infections due to *C. albicans, C. tropicalis*, and possibly *C. parapsilosis* (17). Other yeastlike fungi, such as *C. parapsilosis, T. glabrata, Candida krusei*, and *Hansenula anomala*, however, may emerge as resistant superinfecting pathogens when fluconazole is used as therapy (18–20).

The management of vaginal candidiasis, another manifestation of genitourinary candidiasis, includes establishing a direct microscopic and microbiological diagnosis, ruling out other causes of vaginal discharge, and administration of appropriate antifungal chemotherapy. Recurrent vulvovaginal candidiasis in a sexually active or intravenous drug–using adolescent may be the first manifestation of HIV infection. Most cases of vaginal candidiasis may be treated by topical therapy such as clotrimazole or miconazole cream or clotrimazole troches. Ketoconazole or fluconazole may be used for treatment of recurrent vaginal candidiasis.

Tracheobronchial candidiasis, particularly in HIV-infected patients, is yet another manifestation of impaired mucosal immunity. This process is generally an asymptomatic infection that does not require antifungal treatment. Notably, pulmonary candidiasis reflecting deep tissue parenchymal invasion, although well described as a complication of neutropenia and very-low-birth-weight infancy (21–24), is seldom a complication of tracheobronchial candidiasis in HIV-infected patients.

CANDIDEMIA

The risk factors for hospital-acquired candidemia include the simultaneous use of more than two antibiotics, use of chronic Silastic indwelling catheters (e.g., Hickman–Broviac catheters), granulocytopenia, and abdominal surgery (25). These risk factors for candidemia are frequently encountered in very-low-birth-weight infants and children with neutropenia, as well as HIV infection. Diagnosis of suspected fungemia depends on the blood culture detection system (26,27). The lysis centrifugation system is as sensitive or more sensitive than other systems and is especially valuable in conveying a semiquantitative determination of the number of yeast cells per quantity of blood. A recent study comparing the frequency of detection by fungmeia by lysis centrifugation and the frequency of autopsy-proven invasive candidiasis, however, demonstrated that lysis centrifugation blood cultures may not detect as much as 50% of patients with deep tissue candidiasis (27).

Detection of *Candida* in blood cultures in virtually all cases should be considered evidence of invasive candidiasis, thereby warranting a course of antifungal therapy. Untreated candidemia may be followed in non-granulocytopenic patients by approximately 10% to 20% frequency of late complications, including *Candida* endophthalmitis, meningitis, osteo-myelitis, arthritis, endocarditis, and renal candidiasis (28–33). Dissemi-nated candidiasis in neonates and granulocytopenic patients is often reflected by fungemia and carries a high mortality rate if treatment is delayed (34–46). Fungemia may be followed in granulocytopenic patients by the complication of hepatosplenic candidiasis (47–50). Candidemia may be a reflection of clinical occult deep tissue seeding. Indeed, candidemia should be considered with the same therapeutic sig-nificance as that of a positive blood culture for *Staphylococcus aureus*, whose complications following bacteremia are as dangerous as those of candidemia.

Management of candidemia depends on the host and isolated organism. Although the optimal dosage and duration for treatment of fungemia amphotericin B have not been well defined, sufficient experi-ence exists to suggest some general principles. Uncomplicated candidemia can be treated by a 2-week course of amphotericin B at 0.5 mg/kg per day, particularly if the fungemia is due to *C. albicans* in a nongranulocytopenic patient, and removal of the intravascular catheter. Given the higher level of resistance of *C. tropicalis* and *C. parapsilosis*, fungemia caused by these organisms may require higher doses of amphotericin B (e.g., 0.75 to 1.0 mg/kg per day) and more protracted courses (e.g., 3 to 4 weeks). Fluconazole was equivalent to amphotericin B in the treatment of uncom-plicated catheter-associated fungemia in non-neutropenic, nonimmuno-suppressed adults (51). Whether these findings can be extended to children, particularly immunosuppressed children and low-birth-weight infants, warrants further study. Persistent fungemia, despite treatment with amphotericin B, is treated by increasing the dosage of amphotericin B, the addition of 5-FC, and removal of any intravascular foreign bodies. Fungemia caused by *C. parapsilosis* is highly associated with intravascular catheters (32,41,52,53).

The gastrointestinal tract is an important portal of entry for *Candida* spp. in immunocompromised hosts (54,55). Intravascular catheters, how-ever, also may be a source of fungemia, as well as a target for attachment of circulating *Candida* spp. from a different portal of entry (e.g., the gastrointestinal tract). Intravascular catheters in either circumstance serve as a source for continued seeding of the bloodstream. Thus, intravascular catheters should be removed, whenever feasible, in patients with fungemia. Several studies have demonstrated the importance of removal of central venous catheters in patients with fungemia (30,31,40). Peripheral intravenous catheters clearly can be a portal of entry and a focus for *Candida* suppurative thrombophlebitis (55,56). In addition to intravenous amphotericin B, removal of the peripheral vascular catheter and segmental resection of the infected vein are important for complete therapeutic response. Delay in resecting the infected venous segment can result in persistent fungemia, progressive thrombophlebitis, or relapse of infection after discontinuation of antifungal chemotherapy.

Fungemia seldom occurs as a direct complication of mucosal candidiasis in HIV-infected patients. Instead, fungemia in HIV-infected hosts classically has been considered as developing as a nosocomial infection following the typical previously described risk factors (57). These children have a high mortality rate because of invasive candidiasis. A recent study from the National Cancer Institute, however, found that fungemia among our HIV-infected children most frequently presented in the ambulatory clinic as a vascular catheter-associated community-acquired infection (58). Fungemia was detected in the outpatient clinic by blood cultures in the process of evaluating patients for new onset of fever. There was a strong association between the presence of chronic indwelling central venous catheters and the development of fungemia. Vascular catheters appeared to be the portal of entry for fungemia in these patients. All patients with fungemia had vascular catheters, but no patient without catheters had fungemia. The organisms causing fungemia in more than half of all cases consisted of non-*albicans Candida* species of other species of fungi. These patients were managed consistently with an approach using (a) early detection of fungemia by blood cultures at the new onset of fever presenting in the outpatient clinic, (b) prompt initiation of amphotericin B at 0.5 to 1 mg/kg per day upon recovery of fungus from blood, and (c) removal of the central venous catheter within 2 days of initiating antifungal therapy. This strategy resulted in a 95% survival rate and no posttherapeutic infectious sequelae. These findings contrast with the high mortality rate of nosocomial invasive candidiasis in HIV-infected children observed by Leibovitz et al. (57). Such differences may be related to concomitant underlying diseases and timing of detection of *Candida* as the cause of fever in these seriously ill children.

Central venous catheters associated with candidemia in neonates may cause severe complications of superior or inferior vena caval thrombosis (33,59). Early recognition, catheter removal, administration of amphotericin B in high dosages and extended duration (≥4 weeks), as well as administration of heparin are important elements of management. Long durations of high-dose amphotericin B (1.0 mg/kg per day) appear to be a critical element in ensuring clearance of this endovascular infection.

Yeastlike organisms resistant to conventional antifungal compounds may also cause fungemia. These organisms include *C. lusitaniae* (60–62), *C. guilliermondii* (63,64), *C. krusei* (19,65), *T. (Candida) glabrata* (18,66–68), *C. lipolytica* (69), and *Trichosporon beigelii* (70). *Candida lusitaniae, C. guilliermondii,* and *C. lipolytica* may have high minimum inhibitory concentrations (MICs) in vitro and may be the cause of fungemia-refractory amphotericin B. *Candida krusei* and *T. glabrata* may emerge as superinfecting causes of fungemia in neutropenic patients receiving prophylactic antifungal azole therapy (19,65–68). Most isolates of *C. krusei* are intrinsically resistant to antifungal azoles, whereas some isolates of *T. glabrata* may be initially susceptible but become resistant during the course of antifungal azole therapy.

DISSEMINATED CANDIDIASIS IN CHILDREN WITH NEOPLASTIC DISEASES

Tissue-proven disseminated candidiasis may be classified as acute disseminated or chronic disseminated candidiasis. The syndromes of acute and chronic disseminated candidiasis occupy two ends of a spectrum that is particularly well demonstrated in granulocytopenic patients. Acute disseminated candidiasis is manifested typically in granulocytopenic children by persistent fungemia, hemodynamic instability, multiple cutaneous and visceral lesions, and high mortality rates despite antifungal therapy. By comparison, chronic disseminated candidiasis, otherwise known as hepatosplenic candidiasis, is characterized by an indolent process of disseminated candidiasis, often without detectable fungemia in a hemodynamically stable patient with a relatively high survival rate from disseminated candidiasis when antifungal therapy is administered. Of course, there is a continuum of patterns of infection between these two distinctive syndromes of disseminated candidiasis. A similar syndrome of acute disseminated candidiasis may develop in low-birth-rate infants and may be manifested by apnea, hypotension, and fever or hypothermia (70). We treat acute disseminated candidiasis with high-dose amphotericin B at doses ≥1.0 mg/kg per day plus 5-FC. Prompt initiation of aggressive antifungal therapy is necessary in such patients.

Candida tropicalis has been increasingly implicated as an important cause of disseminated candidiasis in neutropenic children. Flynn et al. (39) reported from St. Jude Children's Research Hospital on 19 children treated for leukemia in whom *C. tropicalis* infections developed. Fungemia without meningitis in 11 children was treated successfully, whereas *C. tropicalis* meningitis in 7 children was uniformly fatal. A high index of suspicion and the early use of aggressive amphotericin B therapy are critical to the successful management of *C. tropicalis* infections in neutropenic children with leukemia.

Chronic disseminated candidiasis is a more indolent condition that develops during the course of granulocytopenia, but usually only becomes apparent on recovery from granulocytopenia. A computed tomography (CT) scan or a magnetic resonance imaging (MRI) scan performed at this time often demonstrates multiple lesions in liver, spleen, and at times other organs such as kidney and lungs. A biopsy of hepatic lesions is important in the management of these patients. For several reasons—other infections (including other mycoses), neoplastic processes, and inflammatory lesions that may simulate the conditions of hepatosplenic candidiasis—the administration of long-term amphotericin B is justified only with definitive evidence of the candidiasis. Biopsy confirmation of candidiasis is necessary for the delivery of investigational agents (e.g., lipid preparations of amphotericin B), which are often required in refractory cases. Our initial approach in managing hepatosplenic candidiasis is administration of amphotericin B usually with 5-FC, followed by long-term fluconazole (6 to 60 mg/kg per day) until resolution or calcification of lesions. Such a course of therapy may require 6 months to 1 year. Hepatosplenic candidiasis caused by *C. tropicalis* may be particularly refractory to fluconazole therapy and may be amenable only to long-term amphotericin B for 6 to 12 months. Fluconazole also has been used in patients with hepatosplenic candidiasis refractory to amphotericin B or amphotericin B-associated nephrotoxicity (71,72). During this interim of therapy for chronic disseminated candidiasis, children requiring continued cycles of chemotherapy may receive such cycles without progression of hepatosplenic candidiasis or with breakthrough fungemia, provided that the disseminated candidiasis has stabilized or is resolving (73). Clearly, an infection that is not responding to antifungal therapy precludes concomitant administration of cytotoxic chemotherapy.

DISSEMINATED CANDIDIASIS IN CHILDREN WITH
LOW-BIRTH-WEIGHT INFANTS

Candida spp. have become increasingly common pathogens among infants requiring neonatal intensive care. Disseminated candidiasis occurs predominantly in premature infants with birth weights <1500 g. Previous studies have estimated an incidence of disseminated *Candida* infections of 2% to 4% in these very-low-birth-weight premature infants, a rate two to four times higher than the incidence of candidemia in the overall neonatal population (23,35,70,74–80). Very-low-birth-weight infants have a high predilection for development of disseminated candidiasis because of tenuous cutaneous anatomical barriers and immunological deficits. These deficits include low serum immunoglobulins and complement levels (81), impaired opsonic ability, and defective neutrophil and monocytic functions, specifically chemotaxis, intracellular killing, and oxidative burst (82).

Among the many risks factors reported, all are related to prolonged hospitalizations of usually more than 7 days under intensive care support. Antimicrobial therapy was the strongest risk factor associated with the development of fungemia in a case control study performed in this population of patients (36). The protracted use of antibiotics increases the risk of gastrointestinal and cutaneous colonization by *Candida* spp. (53). Recently, an outbreak of *C. tropicalis* fungemia in a neonatal intensive care unit as a result of cross-infection between medical staff and patient was described, underscoring *Candida* spp. as contact-transmissible nosocomial pathogens (34).

Most neonates with systemic candidiasis are symptomatic at the onset of their disease. Signs and symptoms are virtually identical to those of the sepsis caused by other etiological agents. The affected infants may develop respiratory deterioration, bradycardia, abdominal distention, temperature instability, hypotension, and erythematous rash or skin pustules. The most frequent laboratory abnormalities associated with fungemia in preterm infants are elevated band count, thrombocytopenia, hyperglycemia, and glycosuria. Acute disseminated candidiasis in newborns may ensue as a postpartum nosocomially acquired infection or may be acquired as a congenital infection (74). These authors also emphasized that histopathological examination of the umbilical cord vessels may be an effective means of early detection of congenital candidemia. Umbilical cords typically demonstrated pseudohyphae amid an acute necrotizing inflammation.

Candida has a well-documented predilection for the invasion of specific tissue sites in neonates. Analysis of 89 cases of systemic candidiasis reported in the literature revealed that central nervous system (32%), eye (4%), kidneys (67%), and lungs (32%) are the most common sites involved in disseminated diseases in infants (41,70,75).

Skin rash or pustules positive for *Candida* spp are also associated findings in these patients (15%), as is osteoarthritis (1%). Catheter-related septic thrombosis and endocarditis associated with refractory candidemia is an uncommon but serious complication in these infants that may be further complicated by the development of intracardiac fungal masses (33,77,83). *Candida* peritonitis in newborns is uncommon and generally occurs as a consequence of gastrointestinal disease such as necrotizing enterocolitis or gastrointestinal perforations (84,85). Morbidity resulting from the consequences of disseminated candidiasis is serious and includes poor vision or blindness attributable to macular or perimacular lesions, osteoarthritis, venous septic thrombosis, multiple cerebral abscesses, and chronic neurological deficits.

Antifungal therapy is recommended for all infants with at least one positive blood culture or those highly suspected of having an invasive fungal infection (86,87). Butler et al. (87) reviewed 38 neonates with invasive candidiasis, including 28 (74%) with disseminated candidiasis and 10 with catheter-associated candidemia. These investigators concluded that catheter-associated candidiasis could be treated effectively with removal of the vascular catheter and administration of amphotericin B alone for a total dosage of 10 to 15 mg/kg per day. By comparison, higher total dosages of 25 to 30 mg/kg per day were encouraged for treatment of disseminated candidiasis. For acute disseminated candidiasis, particularly when caused by non-*albicans Candida* spp., we recommend amphotericin B (0.5 to 1 mg/kg) combined with 5-FC (50 to 100 mg/kg per day) as the treatment of choice. Most side effects of 5-FC can be prevented or managed by monitoring and adjusting dosage, as described later. The relatively high frequency of central nervous system infection during proven disseminated candidiasis suggests that initial therapy of systemic candidiasis should include fluorocytosine, which readily penetrates the blood–brain barrier. Data concerning treatment with the antifungal triazole compounds, itraconazole, and fluconazole in very-low-birth-weight infants are sparse; however, current findings warrant further investigation of these agents in this high-risk population (88–92).

Fluconazole was evaluated prospectively by Fasano et al. (93) in 40 neonates and infants with invasive candidiasis between the ages of 2 days and 3 months in whom conventional antifungal therapy was ineffective or contraindicated. The patients received therapy on an individual compassionate request basis for microbiologically documented or presumed fungal infection. The mean fluconazole dosage was 5.3 mg/kg per day (range 1 to 16 mg/kg per day), and the mean duration of therapy was 26 days (range, 2 to 80 days). Efficacy was evaluated in neonates with proven fungal infection as documented by the presence of a pathogen at baseline. A positive clinical response was achieved in 97% (31 of 32) of the clinically evaluable patients; eradication of the fungal organism was achieved in 97% (30 of 31) of evaluable patients. Adverse events occurred in two patients (5%); therapy was not discontinued in either patient. These favorable safety and efficacy data are similar to results obtained with fluconazole in older children and adults. These findings warrant further investigation comparing fluconazole and amphotericin B for treatment of invasive candidiasis in a thoughtfully designed and carefully conducted randomized clinical trial in neonates and infants. Recently, two cases of systemic candidiasis treated with liposomal amphotericin B (AmBisome) were reported showing good therapeutic response and lower toxicity than with conventional therapy (94).

Candida albicans and other Candida spp. may be transferred by contact transmission from patient to patient on the hands of medical staff. Various outbreaks in pediatric intensive care units by strains of Candida spp. have been identified (34,63). As discussed by Betremieux et al. (95), molecular epidemiological studies demonstrate that a given strain of Candida spp. is transmissible to patients from medical personnel. Thus, hand washing becomes paramount in preventing this mode of nosocomial acquisition of pathogenic fungi.

DEEP CANDIDIASIS INVOLVING SINGLE NONMUCOSAL ORGAN SITES

Candida Peritonitis

Candida peritonitis in children is well described in three different clinical settings: gastrointestinal surgery, necrotizing colitis, and peritoneal dialysis (78,84,85,96–99). The first setting of gastrointestinal surgery usually follows leakage of lumenal contents into the peritoneum from an anastomotic site, particularly in children receiving broad-spectrum antibacterial antibiotics. Management of this condition requires reexploration of the abdominal cavity, drainage of the infection, and administration of intravenous amphotericin B. Perforation of necrotic bowel in infants who are receiving broad-spectrum antibiotics may result in Candida peritonitis. Surgical drainage, resection of necrotic bowel, and amphotericin B are the foundations of management in these critically ill patients. Peritoneal dialysis, catheter-associated *Candida* peritonitis requires removal of the catheter and administration of intravenous amphotericin B therapy for optimal therapy. Failure to remove the peritoneal dialysis catheter often results in relapses after discontinuation of antifungal therapy. Direct intraperitoneal administration of amphotericin B is not recommended. Intraperitoneal instillation of amphotericin B administered intraperitoneally may cause abdominal pain and peritoneal adhesions, which may compromise subsequent courses of peritoneal dialysis. Intravenously administered amphotericin B obtains levels within peritoneal fluid that are fungicidal against most susceptible strains of *Candida* spp. Oral antifungal azoles, specifically ketoconazole and fluconazole, have been useful in selected children with *Candida* peritonitis related to chronic ambulatory peritoneal dialysis (100,101).

Candida Meningitis

Candida meningitis in children is most frequently encountered in low-birth-weight infants and older immunosuppressed patients (28,39,102–104). *Candida* meningitis also is increasingly recognized as a complication of ventricular shunts and drains (105). Chiou et al. (105) recently reported that fungi accounted for 8 (17%) of 48 shunt infections. All babies were born prematurely and required a ventriculoperitoneal shunt for hydrocephalus. Diagnosis of *Candida* meningitis may be elusive because of subtle clinical findings and the inherent difficulty in culturing the organism from cerebrospinal fluid (CSF). Elevated protein, hypoglycorrhachia, and pleocytosis may be present, but are not characteristic.

Amphotericin B plus 5-FC in combination is the most appropriate regimen for treatment of *Candida* meningitis. Despite this aggressive therapy, *Candida* meningitis is notorious for relapses of infection, particularly in patients in whom immunosuppression persists. Cultures of CSF may be initially negative despite symptomatic relapse. As a general guideline, antifungal therapy must be continued as long as pharmacological or intrinsic immunosuppression persists. Among patients with *Candida* meningitis emerging as a complication of ventricular shunts and drains, removal of any ventricular prosthetic device is especially important for successful eradication of *Candida* from the CSF (105). As intraventricular administration of amphotericin B can cause chemical ventriculitis, arachnoiditis, severe headache, and seizures, all of the aforementioned interventions should be exhausted before pursuing this approach. Although fluconazole penetrates CSF well and has reported activity in *Candida* meningitis (106), cases of pediatric *Candida* meningitis not responding to this agent warrant caution in the use of antifungal triazoles for this infection (92,107).

Candida Osteomyelitis

Candida osteomyelitis may develop as a complication of fungemia in low-birth-weight infants, older immunosuppressed children, and immunocompetent patients. Multiple bony lesions may evolve in immunocompromised hosts (108,109). *Candida* osteomyelitis requires surgical debridement of the bone for both diagnostic and therapeutic effects and subsequently will require amphotericin B. Monitoring of bone scan (scans) or MRI, as well as erythrocyte sedimentation rate, permits therapeutic end points to be evaluated.

Candida Endocarditis

Candida endocarditis requires a timely diagnosis of fungemia with valvular involvement. Diagnosis may be difficult to establish and may be heralded by the abrupt onset of an embolic event to a major artery. The recent introduction of transesophageal echocardiography may substantially improve detection of valvular vegetations in suspected cases with negative transthoracic echocardiograms (110). Definitive treatment requires resection of the valve and administration of amphotericin B ± 5-FC. Rare cases of *Candida* endocarditis treated with medical therapy alone (52,111) do not justify this approach as a standard of care. Given the risk and unpredictability of lethal or neurologically catastrophic embolization, surgical resection should be promptly pursued in fungal endocarditis.

Candida Endophthalmitis

The presence of characteristic white vitreal opacities in a patient with candidemia signifies the development of *Candida* endophthalmitis (112). Management is conducted in concert with pediatric ophthalmological consultation (113). Amphotericin B plus 5-FC is recommended for this infection. Timely use of vitrectomy, however, may be critical to saving vision. The role of intravitreal amphotericin B in children is not well defined.

Pulmonary Candidiasis

Pulmonary candidiasis may be a primary bronchopneumonia or secondary process arising from hematogenous dissemination (114). Primary *Candida* bronchopneumonia may be found in neutropenic patients with extensive chemotherapy-induced oral mucositis, very-low-birth-weight infants, and low-birth-weight deliveries associated with *Candida* chorio-amnionitis (21–24). Aspiration of infected oral secretions into the tracheo-bronchial tree with extension into pulmonary parenchyma is the primary route of infection for *Candida* bronchopneumonia. True pulmonary candidiasis develops most frequently as hematogenous infection of the lungs in granulocytopenic children or *Candida* bronchopneumonia in low-birth-weight-infants.

Fever and pulmonary infiltrates in an immunocompromised patient should not be ascribed solely to *Candida* unless proven by biopsy. Biopsy of lung tissue is the only reliable means of establishing a diagnosis in patients with pulmonary candidiasis. Lung biopsy also may demonstrate other unsuspected causes of infiltrates in such patients. The presence of *Candida* spp. in bronchoalveolar lavage fluid from a patient with pulmonary infiltrates is sufficiently nonspecific as to preclude a definitive diagnosis. Treatment of *Candida* bronchopneumonia or hematogenous disseminated candidiasis is initiated with amphotericin B with or without flucytosine. Among patients unable to tolerate amphotericin B, fluconazole may be considered for treatment of infection because of *C. albincans*.

Candida Epiglottitis and Laryngeal Candidiasis

Candida epiglottitis and laryngeal candidiasis may emerge as a life-threatening cause of airway obstruction in neutropenic children, very-low-birth-weight infants, and patients with chronic mucocutaneous candidiasis (2,5–9).

Candida epiglottitis presents initially as refractory odynophagia in the hypopharyngeal and epiglottic regions. The patient may point directly to these areas as the most intense locations of pain. Laryngeal stridor may develop in more advanced cases. Diagnosis is corroborated by an otolaryngologist using appropriate methods for laryngoscopy-guided visualization and swabbing of the epiglottis. The swab material is cultured, smeared, strained, and examined microscopically. Treatment consists of intravenous amphotericin B and airway protection (5).

SUMMARY

Refractory mucosal candidiasis and deeply invasive candidiasis are formidable problems in immunocompromised children. Identification of high-risk children through improved epidemiological understanding, early recognition of invasive candidiasis, aggressive therapeutic intervention, and reversal of immunosuppression are essential principles in management of invasive candidiasis.

REFERENCES

1. Leggott P, Robertson P, Greenspan D, et al. Oral manifestations of primary and acquired immunodeficiency diseases in children. Pediatr Dent 1987; 9: 98–104.
2. Leggott PJ. Oral manifestations of HIV infection in children. Oral Surg Oral Med Oral Pathol 1992; 73: 187–192.
3. Buckley RH. Immunodeficiency diseases. JAMA 1992; 268: 2797–2806.
4. Selik R, Starcher E, Curran J. Opportunistic diseases reported in AIDS patients: frequencies, associations, and trends. AIDS 1987; 1: 175–182.
5. Walsh TJ, Gray W. *Candida* epiglottitis in immunocompromised patients. Chest 1987; 91: 482–485.
6. Balsam D, Sorrano D, Barax C. Candida epiglottitis presenting as stridor in a child with HIV infection. Pediatr Radiol 1992; 22: 235–236.
7. Hass A, Hyatt AC, Kattan M, et al. Hoarseness in immunocompromised children: association with invasive fungal infection. J Pediatr 1987; 111: 731–733.
8. Tashjian LS, Peacock JE Jr. Laryngeal candidiasis. Arch Otolaryngol 1984; 10: 806–809.
9. Jacods RF, Yasuda K, Smith AL, Benjamin DR. Laryngeal candidiasis presenting as inspiratory stridor. Pediatrics 1982; 69: 234–236.
10. Hay RJ, Clayton YM. Fluconazole in the management of patients with chronic mucocutaneous candidosis (letter). Br J Dermatol 1988; 119: 683–684.
11. Hernandez-Sampelayo T. Fluconazole versus ketoconazole in the treatment of oropharyngeal candidiasis in HIV-infected children. Eur J Clin Microbiol Infect Dis 1994; 13: 340–344.
12. Burke WA. Use of itraconazole in a patient with chronic mucocutaneous candidiasis. J Am Acad Dermatol 1989; 21: 1309–1310.
13. DePadova-Elder SM, Ditre CM, Kantor GR, Koblenzer PJ. Candidiasis endocrinopathy syndrome. Treatment with itraconazole. Arch Dermatol 1994; 130: 19–22.
14. Kobayashi RH, Rosenblatt HM, Carney JM, et al. *Candida* esophagitis and laryngitis in chronic mucocutaneous candidiasis. Pediatrics 1980; 66: 380–384.
15. Walsh T, Peter J, Damron S, et al. Emergence of resistance to fluconazole in HIV-infected children. Abstracts of the Annual Meeting of the Infectious Diseases Society of America, 1994.

16. Kodsi BE, Wickremesinghe PC, Kozinn PJ, et al. *Candida* esophagitis: a prospective study of 27 cases. Gastroenterology 1976; 71: 715–719.
17. Walsh T, Belitsos N, Hamilton S. Bacterial esophagitis in immunocompromised patients. Arch Intern Med 1986; 146: 1345–1348.
18. Hoppe JE, Klingebiel T, Niethammer D. Selection of *Candida glabrata* in pediatric bone marrow transplant recipients receiving fluconazole. Pediatr Hematol Oncol 1994; 11: 207–210.
19. Wingard JR, Merz, Rinaldi MG, et al. Increase in *Candida krusei* infection among patients with bone marrow transplantation and neutropenia treated prophylactically with fluconazole. N Engl J Med 1991; 325: 1274–1277.
20. Alter SJ, Farley J. Development of *Hansenula anomala* infection in a child receiving fluconazole therapy. Pediatr Infect Dis J 1994; 13: 158–159.
21. Haron E, Vartivarian S, Anaissie E, et al. Primary *Candida* pneumonia. Experience at a large cancer center and review of the literature. Medicine (Baltimore) 1993; 72: 137–142.
22. Hughes WT. Pneumonia in the immunocompromised child. Semin Respir Infect 1987; 2: 177–183.
23. Loke HL, Szymonowicz W, Yu VYH. Systemic candidiasis and pneumonia in preterm infants. Aust Paediatr J 1988; 24: 138–142.
24. Mamelok RJ, Richardson CJ, Mamlok V, et al. A case of intrauterine pulmonary candidiasis. Pediatr Infect Dis 1985; 4: 692–693.
25. Wey SB, Mori M, Pfaller MA, et al. Risk factors for hospital-acquired candidemia. A matched case-control study. Arch Intern Med 1989; 149: 2349–2353.
26. Walsh TW, Lyman CA, Pizzo PA. Laboratory diagnosis of invasive fungal infections in patients with neoplastic diseases. Balliére's Clinical Infectious Diseases International Practice and Research 1994; 1: 469–498.
27. Berenguer J, Buck M, Witebsky F, et al. Lysis–centrifugation blood cultures in the detection of tissue-proven invasive candidiasis: disseminated versus single organ infection. Diagn Microbiol Infect Dis 1993; 17: 103–109.
28. Faix RG. *Candida parapsilosis* meningitis in premature infants. Pediatr Infect Dis 1983; 2: 462–464.
29. Brooks R. Prospective study of *Candida* endophthalmitis in hospitalized patients with candidemia. Arch Intern Med 1989; 149: 2226–2228.
30. Dato V, Dajani A. Candidemia in children with central venous catheters: role of catheter removal and amphotericin B therapy. Pediatr Infect Dis J 1990; 9: 309–314.
31. Eppes SC, Troutman JL, Gutman LT. Outcome of treatment of candidemia in children whose central catheters were removed or retained. Pediatr Infect Dis J 1989; 8: 99–104.
32. Weems JJ, Chamberland ME, Ward J, et al. Candida parapsilosis fungemia associated with parenteral nutrition and contaminated blood pressure transducers. J Clin Microbiol 1987; 25: 1029–1032.
33. Walsh TJ, Hutchins GM. Postoperative *Candida* infections of the heart in children: clinicopathologic study of a continuing problem of diagnosis and therapy. J Pediatr Surg 1980; 15: 325–331.

34. Finkelstein R, Reinhertz G, Hashman N, Merzbach D. Outbreak of *Candida tropicalis* fungemia in a neonatal intensive care unit. Infect Control Hosp Epidemiol 1993; 14: 587–590.
35. Shian W, Chi C, Wang C, Chen C. Candidemia in the neonatal intensive care unit. Acta Paediatr Sin 1993; 34: 349–355.
36. Weese-Mayer D, Fondriest DW, Brouillette R, Shulman ST. Risks factors associated with candidemia in the neonatal intensive care unit: a case control study. Pediatr Infect Dis J 1987; 6: 190–197.
37. Wiley JM, Smith N, Lenethal B, et al. Invasive fungal disease in pediatric leukemia patients with fever and neutropenia during induction chemotherapy. A multivariate analysis of risk factors. J Clin Oncol 1990; 8: 280–286.
38. Hughes WT. Systemic candidiasis: a study of 109 fatal cases. Pediatr Infect Dis J 1982; 1: 11–18.
39. Flynn PM, Marina NM, Rivera GI, Hughes WT. *Candida tropicalis* infections in children with leukemia. Leuk Lymphoma 1993; 10: 369–376.
40. Lecciones JA, Lee JW, Navarro E, et al. Vascular catheter-associated fungemia in cancer patients: analysis of 155 episodes. Rev Infect Dis 1992; 14: 875–883.
41. Faix R. Invasive neonatal candidiasis: comparison of *albicans* and *parapsilosis* infection. Pediatr Infect Dis J 1992; 11: 88–93.
42. Bodey GP, Luna M. Skin lesions associated with disseminated candidiasis. JAMA 1974; 229: 1466–1468.
43. Jarowski CI, Fialk MA, Murray HW, et al. Fever, rash and muscle tenderness. A distinctive clinical presentation of disseminated candidiasis. Arch Intern Med 1978; 138: 544–546.
44. Dick JD, Rosenguard Br, Merz WG, et al. Fatal disseminated candidiasis due to amphotericin B-resistant *Candida guilliermondii*. Ann Intern Med 1985; 102: 67–68.
45. Faix R. Systemic *Candida* infections in infants in intensive care nurseries: high incidence of central nervous system involvement. J Pediatr 1984; 105: 616–622.
46. Johnson DE, Thompson TR, Green TP, Ferrieri P. Systemic candidiasis in very low-birth-weight infants (<1500 grams). Pediatrics 1984; 73: 138–143.
47. Maaksymiuk AW, Thongprasert S, Hopfer R, et al. Systemic candidiasis in cancer patients. Am J Med 1984; 77 (suppl): 20–27.
48. Tashjian LS, Abramson JS, Peacock JE Jr. Focal hepatic candidiasis: a distinct clinical variant of candidiasis in immunocompromised patients. Rev Infect Dis 1984; 6: 689–703.
49. Miller JH, Greenfield LD, Wald BR. Candidiasis of the liver and spleen in childhood. Radiology 1982; 142: 375–380.
50. Thaler M, Pastakia B, Shwaker TH, et al. Hepatic candidiasis in cancer patients: the evolving picture of the syndrome. Ann Intern Med 1988; 108: 88–100.
51. Rex JH, Bennett JE, Sugar AM, et al. A randomized trial comparing fluconazole with amphotericin B for the treatment of candidemia in patients without neutropenia. N Engl J Med 1994; 17: 331: 1325–1330.

52. Faix R, Feick H, Frommelt, P, Snider AR. Successful medical treatment of *Candida parapsilosis* endocarditis in a premature infant. Am J Perinatol 1990; 7: 272–275.
53. El-Mohandes AE, Johnson-Robbins L, Keiser JF, et al. Incidence of *Candida parapsilosis* colonization in an intensive care nursery population and its association with invasive fungal disease. Pediatr Infect Dis J 1994; 13D: 520–524.
54. Walsh TJ, Merz W. Pathologic features in the human alimentary tract associated with invasiveness of *Candida tropicalis*. Am J Clin Pathol 1986; 85: 498–502.
55. Malfroot A, Verboven M, Levy J, et al. Suppurative thrombophlebitis with sepsis due to *Candida albicans*: an unusual complication of intravenous therapy in cystic fibrosis. Pediatr Infect Dis 1986; 5: 376–377.
56. Walsh TJ, Bustamente C, Vlahov D, Standiford HC. *Candida* suppurative peripheral thrombophlebitis: prevention, recognition and management. Infect Control 1986; 7: 16–22.
57. Leibovitz E, Rigaud M, Chandwan S, et al. Disseminated fungal infections in children infected with human immunodeficiency virus. Pediatr Infect Dis J 1991; 10: 888–894.
58. Walsh TJ, Gonzalez C, Roilides E, et al. Fungemia in HIV-infected children: new epidemiologic patterns, emerging pathogens, and improved antifungal outcome. Clin Infect Dis 1995; 20: 900–906.
59. Ashkenazi S, Pickering LK, Robinson LH. Diagnosis and management of septic thrombosis of the inferior vena cava caused by *Candida tropicalis*. Pediatr Infect Dis J 1990; 9: 446–447.
60. Christenson JC, Guruswamy A, Mukwaya G, Rettig PJ. *Candida lusitaniae*: an emerging human pathogen. Pediatr Infect Dis J 1987; 6: 755–757.
61. Merz WG. *Candida lusitaniae*: frequency of recovery, colonization, infection, and amphotericin B resistance. J Clin Microbiol 1984; 20: 1194–1195.
62. Yinnon AM, Woodin KA, Powell KR. *Candida lusitaniae* infection in the newborn: case report and review of the literature. Pediatr Infect Dis J 1992; 11: 878–880.
63. Yagupsky P, Dagan R, Chipman M, et al. Pseudooutbreak of *Candida guilliermondii* fungemia in a neonatal intensive care unit. Pediatr Infect Dis J 1991; 10: 928–932.
64. Dick JD Rosenguard BR, Merz WG, et al. Fatal disseminated candidiasis due to amphotericin B resistant *Candida guilliermondii*. Ann Intern Med 1985; 102: 67–68.
65. Tam JY, Blume KG, Prober CG. Prophylactic fluconazole and *Candida krusei* infections (letter). N Engl J Med 1992; 325: 891.
66. Glick C, Graves G, Feldman S. Torulopsis glabrata in the neonate: an emerging fungal pathogen. South Med J 1993; 86: 969–970.
67. Quirke P, Hwang WS, Validen CC. Congenital *Torulopsis glabrata* infection. Am J Clin Pathol 1980; 73: 137–140.
68. Walter EB, Gingras JL, McKinney RE. Systemic *Torulopsis glabrata* infection in a neonate. South Med J 1990; 86: 837–838.

69. Walsh TJ, Salkin I, Dixon DM, Hurd M. *Candida lipolytica*. Clinical, microbiological, and animal studies. J Clin Microbiol 1989; 27: 927–931.
70. Butler K, Baker C. *Candida*: an increasingly important pathogen in the nursery. Pediatr Clin North Am 1988; 35: 543–563.
71. Kauffman CA, Bradley SF, Ross SC, Weber DR. Hepatosplenic candidiasis: successful treatment with fluconazole. Am J Med 1991; 91: 137–141.
72. Anaissie E, Bodey GP, Kantarjian H, et al. Fluconazole therapy for chronic disseminated candidiasis in patients with leukemia and prior amphotericin B therapy. Am J Med 1991; 91: 142–150.
73. Walsh TJ, Whitcomb P, Ravankar S, et al. Successful treatment of hepatosplenic candidiasis during repeated episodes of neutropenia. Program & Abstracts of the 33rd Intersci Conf Antimicrob Agents Chemother. 1993, #809.
74. Schwartz DA, Reef S. *Candida albicans* placentitis and funisitis: early diagnosis of congenital candidemia by histopathologic examination of umbilical cord vessels. Pediatr Infect Dis J 1990; 9: 661–665.
75. Baley JE, Kliegeman RJ, Fanaroff A. Disseminated fungal infections in very low-birth-weight infants: clinical manifestations and epidemiology. Pediatrics 1984; 73: 144–152.
76. Baley JE, Kliegman RM, Fanaroff AA. Disseminated fungal infections in very low-weight infants: therapeutic toxicity. Pediatrics 1984; 73: 153–157.
77. Johnson DE, Bass JL, Thompson TR, et al. Candida septicemia and right atrial mass secondary to umbilical vein catheterization. Am J Dis Child 1981; 135: 275–277.
78. Johnson DE, Conroy MM, ThompsonTR, et al. *Candida* peritonitis in the newborn infant. Pediatrics 1980; 97: 298–300.
79. Johnson DE, Thompson TR, Ferrieri P. Congenital candidiasis. Am J Dis Child 1981; 135: 273–275.
80. Smith H, Congdon P. Neonatal systemic candidiasis. Arch Dis Child 1985; 60: 365–369.
81. Conway SP, Dear PRF, Smith I. Immunoglobulin profile of the preterm baby. Arch Dis Child 1985; 60: 208–212.
82. Xanthou M, Valassi-Adam E, Kintzonidou E, Matsaniotis N. Phagocytosis and killing ability of *Candida albicans* by blood leukocytes of healthy term and preterm babies. Arch Dis Child 1975; 50: 72–75.
83. Ho NK. Systemic candidiasis in premature infants. Aust Pediatr J 1984; 20: 127–130.
84. Karlowicz MG. Risk factors associated with fungal peritonitis in very low birth weight neonates with severe necrotizing enterocolitis: a case-control study. Pediatr Infect Dis J 1993; 12: 574–577.
85. Kaplan M, Eidelman A, Dollberg L, Abu-dalu K. Necrotizing bowel disease with *Candida* peritonitis following severe neonatal hypothermia. Acta Pediatr Scand 1990; 79: 876–879.
86. Glick C, Graves G, Feldman S. Neonatal fungemia and amphotericin B. South Med J 1993; 86: 1368–1371.

87. Butler KM, Rench MA, Baker CJ. Amphotericin B as a single agent in the treatment of systemic candidiasis in neonates. Pediatr Infect Dis J 1990; 9: 51–56.
88. Bhandari V, Narang A. Oral itraconazole therapy for disseminated candidiasis in low birth weight infants (letter). J Pediatr 1992; 120: 330.
89. Viscoli C, Castagnola E, Corsini M, et al. Fluconazole therapy in an underweight infant. Eur J Microbiol Infect Dis 1993; 8: 925–926.
90. Saxen H, Hoppu K, Pohjavuori M. Pharmacokinetics of fluconazole in very low birth weight infants during the first two weeks of life. Clin Pharmacol Ther 1993; 54: 269–277.
91. Hitchcock RJ, Pallett A, Hall MA, Malone PS. Urinary tract candidiasis in neonates and infants. Br J Urol 1995; 76: 252–256.
92. Epelbaum S, Laurent C, Morin G, et al. Failure of fluconazole treatment in *Candida* meningitis (Letter). J Pediatr 1993; 123: 168–169.
93. Fasano C, O'Keeffe J, Gibbs D. Fluconazole treatment of neonates and infants with severe fungal infections not treatable with conventional agents. Eur J Clin Microbiol Infect Dis 1994; 13: 351–354.
94. Lackner H, Schwinger W, Urban C, et al. Liposomal amphotericin B (AmBisome) for treatment of disseminated fungal infections in two infants of very low weight. Pediatrics 1992; 89: 1259–1261.
95. Betremieux P, Chevrier S, Quindos G, et al. Use of DNA fingerprinting and biotyping methods to study a *Candida albicans* outbreak in a neonatal intensive care unit. Pediatr Infect Dis J 1994; 13: 899–905.
96. Eisenberg ES, Leviton I, Soeiro R. Fungal peritonitis in patients receiving peritoneal dialysis: experience with 11 patients and review of the literature. Rev Infect Dis 1986; 8: 309–321.
97. McClung MR. Peritonitis in children receiving continuous ambulatory peritoneal dialysis. Pediatr Infect Dis J 1983; 2: 328–332.
98. Oh SH, Conley SB, Rose GM, et al. Fungal peritonitis in children undergoing peritoneal dialysis. Pediatr Infect Dis 1985; 4: 62–66.
99. Tapson JS, Mansy H, Freeman R, Wilkinson R. The high morbidity of CAPD fungal peritonitis—description of 10 cases and review of treatment strategies. Q J Med 1986; 61: 1047–1053.
100. Johnson RJ, Blair AD, Ahmad S. Ketoconazole kinetics in chronic peritoneal dialysis. Clin Pharmacol Ther 1985; 37: 325–329.
101. Reuman PD, Neiberger R, Kondor DA. Intraperitoneal and intravenous fluconazole pharmacokinetics in a pediatric patients with end state renal disease. Pediatr Infect Dis J 1992; 11: 132–133.
102. Buchs S. *Candida* meningitis: a growing threat to premature and full-term infants. Pediatr Infect Dis 1985; 4: 122–291.
103. Walsh TJ, Hier DB, Caplan LR. Fungal infections of the central nervous system: analysis of risk factors and clinical manifestations. Neurology 1985; 35: 1654–1657.
104. Leggiadro RJ, Collins T. Postneurosurgical *Candida lusitaniae* meningitis. Pediatr Infect Dis J 1988; 7: 368–369.

105. Chiou C, Wong T, Lin H, et al. Fungal infection of ventriculoperitoneal shunts in children. Clin Infect Dis 1994; 19: 1049–1053.
106. Byers M, Chapman S, Feldman S, Parent A. Fluconazole pharmacokinetics in the cerebrospinal fluid of a child with *Candida tropicalis* meningitis. Pediatr Infect Dis 1992; 11: 895–896.
107. Walsh TJ, Lee JW, Seibel N, Pizzo PA. Failure of fluconazole treatment in *Candida* meningitis. J Pediatr 1993; 123: 168–169.
108. Oleinik E, Della-Latta P, Rinaldi M, Saiman L. *Candida lusitaniae* osteomyelitis in a premature infant. Am J Perinatol 1993; 10: 313–315.
109. Poplack DG, Jacobs SA. *Candida* arthritis treated with amphotericin B. J Pediatr 1975; 87: 989–900.
110. Johnston P, Lee J, Demanski M, et al. Late recurrent *Candida* endocarditis. Chest 1991; 99: 1531–1533.
111. Sanchez PJ, Siegel JD, Fishbein J. *Candida* endocarditis: successful medical management in three preterm infants and review of the literature. Pediatr Infect Dis J 1991; 10: 239–243.
112. Edwards JE Jr. *Candida* endophthalmitis. In: Bodey GP, Fainstein V, eds. Candidiasis, New York: Raven Press, 1985; 211–225.
113. Annable WL, Kachmer ML, De Santis D. Long term follow-up of *Candida* endophthalmitis in the premature infants. J Pediatr Ophthalmol Strabismus 1990; 27: 103–106.
114. Panos R, Barr L, Walsh TJ, et al. Factors associated with fatal hemoptysis in cancer patients. Chest 1988; 94: 1008–1013.

23

Antiviral Drug Development for Herpesvirus Infections: History, Status, and Future of Antiviral Drugs

Richard J. Whitley
The University of Alabama at Birmingham, Birmingham, Alabama

Compared with the remarkable progress made in the treatment of bacterial infections during the last five decades, only a few antiviral drugs have had clinical value, and such drugs are available only for a limited number of indications. It is possible to divide the development of antiviral therapeutics into three chronological periods: (a) the past, including the early antiviral agents (idoxuridine, vidarabine, and trifluorothymidine); (b) the present, including acyclovir, prodrugs (famciclovir and valaciclovir) and the numerous drugs for the management of human immunodeficiency virus (HIV) infection and its viral complications; and (c) the future, namely hopes for improving antiviral drugs. The characteristics of a good antiviral agent are listed in Table 1. These characteristics should be sought in most new therapeutics. Each of the first two periods have provided important lessons for the development of antiviral drugs in the future.

THE PAST

Early development of antiviral therapies paralleled the discovery of drugs used to treat malignancy. The unique problems associated with the development of antiviral agents as opposed to anticancer therapies became apparent at the outset. Three fundamental principles are summarized.

267

Table 1 Characteristics of a
Good Antiviral Agent

Safe
Selective
Orally bioavailable
Crosses blood–brain barrier
Cost effective

First, viruses are obligate intracellular parasites that use many biochemical pathways of the infected cell. It has been difficult to achieve clinically useful antiviral activity without also adversely effecting normal host cell metabolism, which resulted in unwanted toxicity. The route of drug administration was limited to topical application. The hurdles encountered in the development of idoxuridine illustrate this point. Idoxuridine was the first compound identified as active in the inhibition of herpes simplex virus (HSV) replication in cell culture in the late 1950s (1). Subsequently, in the early 1960s, the efficacy studies of idoxuridine *topical* therapy of HSV keratoconjunctivitis in the rabbit model and, ultimately, humans, established the value of this compound as the first licensed therapeutic agent for HSV infections (2). Despite the efficacy of topically applied idoxuridine for the treatment of HSV infections of the eye, the lack of a selective mechanism of action, namely its inability to differentiate host cell from viral functions, precluded its use as a *systemic* antiviral therapy. This latter point was well illustrated by the toxicity induced with idoxuridine treatment of HSV encephalitis in the early 1970s (3). Thus, the key principle learned in the early development of idoxuridine and, subsequently, vidarabine was the requirement of a selective mechanism of action that distinguished host cell from viral functions. Such a selective mechanism of action should preclude significant host toxicity.

Another unique problem is the requirement for early diagnosis of viral infection. Diagnosis must be early for successful antiviral therapy because by the time symptoms appear several cycles of viral multiplication have usually occurred and replication is waning. Precise diagnosis is exceedingly difficult for many viral infections because the associated clinical syndromes lack specificity. For example, coryza and cough arising from rhinovirus infection, pneumonitis attributable to cytomegalovirus (CMV), or encephalopathy associated with HSV encephalitis all can be attributed to a variety of viral agents in addition to those listed. Effective antiviral therapy, therefore, depends on rapid, sensitive, specific, and practical means of diagnosing specific viral diseases. Nevertheless, there are some viral infections such as herpes zoster or genital herpes for which clinical diagnosis is straightforward.

A third unique problem is that many of the disease syndromes caused by viruses are common, relatively benign, and self-limited. The therapeutic index (efficacy/toxicity ratio) must be extremely high, as was illustrated in the case of the development of idoxuridine, in order for therapy to be acceptable. Life- or sight-threatening diseases such as HSV or progressive CMV retinitis in immunocompromised patients are, of course, exceptions. The therapeutic index can be assessed only in the context of the severity of the disease targeted for therapy.

During this past chronological period of antiviral drug development, other medications came to the forefront that provided important practical lessons in the deployment of antiviral therapeutics. In parallel with development of idoxuridine for the treatment of HSV keratoconjunctivitis, amantadine was evaluated for prophylaxis of influenza infections in high-risk (i.e., elderly) populations. Amantadine successfully prevented influenza A infections with an efficacy rate of approximately 70% when administered daily for 2 to 3 months during influenza outbreaks (4). The licensure of an orally administered drug for the prevention of influenza disease was a landmark in antiviral drug development. Unfortunately, amantadine receives less than optimal use because of adverse clinical effects in elderly individuals and the general lack of interest in prophylaxis for routine disease. This later point warrants emphasis, particularly stressing that for such diseases prevention by vaccination is more desirable than prevention by daily dosing with medication.

The first successful intravenously administered antiviral agent was vidarabine, a compound evaluated during the 1970s and early 1980s. Intravenous therapy was proved efficacious for the treatment of HSV encephalitis, neonatal HSV disease, and varicella zoster virus (VZV) infections in immunocompromised patients. Several important lessons were learned from these early studies of vidarabine. First, parenteral vidarabine had a major impact on disease manifestations. For example, a disease such as HSV encephalitis, mortality was reduced and morbidity improved (5). Second, vidarabine is deaminated in the blood by adenosine deaminase to arabinosyl hypoxanthine, a compound with antiviral activity, albeit less than the parent compound. Vidarabine is not orally bioavailable and is poorly soluble; therefore, continuous intravenous administration was required over a period of 12 hours. The requirement for continuous infusion with the attendant fluid load, as well as evidence of limited, but documented toxicity, precluded its routine and continued use for the treatment of herpes virus infections. The lack of oral bioavailability is a significant deterrent for the use of any antiviral drug, including vidarabine for the treatment of routine mucocutaneous HSV and VZV infections. Thus, the profile of antiviral drugs for routine mucocutaneous herpes virus infections must reflect oral bioavailability and water solubility, although there are exceptions to this rule. Parenthetically, the final clinical studies of vidarabine brought an end to the first-generation antiviral drugs, namely, those compounds that did not have selective mechanisms of action.

THE PRESENT

Although the present era is characterized by the availability of a number of antiviral agents (Table 2), agents active against herpes viruses, especially the first second-generation antiviral agent, acyclovir, and anti-HIV nucleoside analogs, predominate.

Therapy for HSV Infections

The era of present antiviral therapy began in the 1980s, the period of contemporary antiviral therapy. The introduction of acyclovir into clinical

Table 2 Antiviral Drugs Licensed
for Systemic Administration in the
United States Nucleoside Analogs

Acyclovir
Didanosine
Famciclovir
Ganciclovir
Ribavirin
Stavudine
Vidarabine
Zalcitabine
Zidovudine
Tricyclic amine
Amantadine
Rimantadine
Pyrophosphate analogs
Foscarnet
Cytokine
Interferon alpha

trials provided a landmark, identifying a second-generation antiviral drug by which standards for the future must be set. The value of acyclovir has been established since the early 1980s in detailed clinical evaluations, and its development is a model for the development of future antiviral therapies. The development of this compound indicates safety, efficacy, and oral bioavailability (6). To date, more than 35 million acyclovir prescriptions have been written worldwide with uniform acceptance of clinical utility. Acyclovir is selectively activated by thymidine kinase of HSV and, therefore, has a selective mechanism of action not found with other antiviral drugs defined during the 1980s. Acyclovir is a synthetic acyclic nucleoside analog, which selectively inhibits HSV types 1 and 2 and VZV (6). It is converted to its monophosphate derivative by virally coded thymidine kinase, an event that does not occur to any significant extent in uninfected cells. Subsequent diphosphorylation and triphosphorylation are catalyzed by cellular enzymes, resulting in acyclovir triphosphate concentrations 40- to 100-fold higher in HSV-infected cells than in uninfected cells.

Acyclovir triphosphate inhibits viral DNA synthesis by competing with deoxyguanine triphosphate as a substrate for viral DNA polymerase. Viral DNA synthesis is then terminated because acyclovir triphosphate lacks a 3'-hydroxyl group for DNA chain elongation. Viral DNA polymerase is tightly associated with a terminated DNA chain and is functionally inactivated. In addition, the viral polymerase has greater affinity for acyclovir triphosphate than cellular DNA polymerase, resulting in little incorporation of acyclovir into cellular DNA. In vitro, acyclovir is most active against HSV-1 (average EC_{50} 0.04 μg/ml), HSV-2 (0.10 μg/ml) and VZV (0.50 μg/ml). The Epstein–Barr virus and CMV, which both lack a virus-specific thymidine kinase, require higher concentrations of acyclovir for inhibition. Because of its selective mechanism of action, acyclovir has been studied against a variety of clinical conditions associated with herpes virus diseases.

Clinical development of acyclovir had to incorporate increasing knowledge about the changing natural history of routine viral infections. For example, the use of immunosuppressive drugs dramatically increased with the advent of organ transplantation. The ultimate effectiveness of any antimicrobial therapy often depends on host defenses, and this principle is clearly of paramount importance when considering the value of antiviral agents such as acyclovir. The susceptibility of the immunocompromised patients to the development of symptomatic herpes virus infections deserves special consideration. The ability of all herpes viruses to become latent results in an extremely high incidence of reactivated infection in this patient group. In renal transplantation recipients, for example, reactivation rates of 40% to 70% for HSV infections, 80% to 100% for CMV infection, and 5% to 35% for VZV infections are seen within 1 year of transplantation. Not only is the incidence of reactivation high, but these infections are often more severe in the immunocompromised population; examples of this include varicella in children with leukemia, mucocutaneous HSV infections in organ transplantation recipients, and CMV infections, especially retinitis and colitis, in bone marrow transplantation recipients and patients with the acquired immunodeficiency syndrome (AIDS).

Ironically, the first clinical trial that proved the value of acyclovir was published in 1981 where anticipatory drug administration to HSV-seropositive bone marrow transplantation recipients suppressed reactivation of latent HSV infection (7). This clinical trial introduced the concept that suppressive therapy could be achieved in high-risk patient populations. Since 1981, acyclovir has proved valuable under a variety of clinical circumstances. Diseases that proved amenable to therapy included mucocutaneous HSV infections in the immunocompromised host, HSV encephalitis and neonatal HSV infections, chickenpox and herpes zoster in both normal and immunocompromised hosts, and, most important, primary and recurrent genital HSV infections. Long-term suppression of recurrent disease is achievable with oral acyclovir administration for frequently recurrent genital herpes and HSV infections of the immunocompromised host (6). In each of these conditions, a toxicity profile that supports the safety of this compound has evolved.

Despite the established value of acyclovir as a therapeutic agent, outcome remains poor, indicating a need for further improvement in approaches to the therapy of HSV infections of the central nervous system, whether in the newborn or older individuals. Furthermore, available therapies, even the most effective (i.e., acyclovir), have no impact on the establishment of latency and the frequency of recurrences. Thus, future therapeutic efforts should attempt to alter the interaction between HSV and the nervous system in order to have an impact on such relatively benign issues as recurrences to the more severe complications of morbidity and mortality. The relatively low oral bioavailability of acyclovir has prompted the development of two prodrugs, valaciclovir and famciclovir, designed specifically for the treatment of HSV and VZV infections.

Resistance of both HSV and VZV to acyclovir has been documented. Resistance has been associated with progressive disease, particularly in the immunosuppressed host. However, a putatively normal host has been documented to have progressive disease with an acyclovir-resistant virus isolated from his lesions despite appropriate therapy (8). The development of acyclovir resistance in a normal host is of concern and must be monitored over time.

Therapy of CMV Infections

The licensure of foscarnet and ganciclovir provided therapies that slowed the rate of progressive CMV disease, especially CMV retinitis, in patients with advanced HIV disease. Neither agent, however, cures CMV infection; both drugs merely provide temporary relief in the overall course of the infection. The limitations of foscarnet and ganciclovir illustrate the need for improvement in therapy in these areas, as both drugs must be administered intravenously for optimal therapeutic benefit and are associated with varying degrees of toxicity.

Recently, advances in the management of CMV infections in individuals with HIV infection have been realized. Oral administration of ganciclovir as maintenance therapy following induction has been useful in the management of CMV retinitis. Oral ganciclovir therapy is associated with very poor bioavailability. Nevertheless, as shown by retinal photographs, this modality of therapy was similar to intravenous ganciclovir therapy. The role of oral ganciclovir therapy in the management of CMV retinitis has yet to be established. Likely, it will be used early after the diagnosis of CMV retinitis and when patients wish to vacation without the need for daily infusions.

Cidofovir, a nucleotide analog, delays reactivation of CMV retinitis in HIV-infected patients with relapsing disease. This medication has the advantage of being administered every other week. However, administration requires careful attention to renal function and its monitoring during therapy. Treatment regimens must include the concomitant administration of probenecid and intravenous hydration. Nevertheless, of all the medications tested to date, is will probably be the most active for CMV infections of the eye.

Therapy of Herpes Zoster

The recent introduction of new therapies for herpes zoster marks an additional landmark in the development of antiviral therapy. Famciclovir, recently licensed for the treatment of herpes zoster in the normal host, is the first prodrug for antiviral therapy. Famciclovir is cleaved on absorption and passage through the liver to penciclovir, which is then phosphorylated to its triphosphate derivative intracellularly. In two well-controlled trials, famciclovir was proven superior to placebo and equivalent to acyclovir for the management of herpes zoster. A significant advantage of famciclovir over acyclovir is its ease of administration. The carcinogenicity profile of penciclovir appears increased compared to acyclovir.

The development of valaciclovir, a prodrug of acyclovir, should provide similar advances in decreased dosing frequency and enhanced plasma levels when compared to the parent compound acyclovir. It was recently licensed in the United States for the treatment of herpes zoster. Valaciclovir recipients had statistically significantly less persistence of pain when compared to those patients who received acyclovir. This finding would suggest a dose-dependent effect on the resolution of this key end point.

Finally, bromovinyl arabinosyl uracil (sorivudine) is the most active of all drugs against VZV in vitro. This drug can be administered once a day with resulting plasma levels of drug well in excess of inhibitory concentrations. Preliminary analyses of three clinical trials indicate that this drug will accelerate the cessation of lesion formation in immunocompromised patients with AIDS.

THE FUTURE

The future era of antiviral drug development will reflect the convergence of many ongoing biomedical research efforts. The rapid explosion of research in molecular biology will help solve two of the problems that have been previously identified. First, it has been possible to determine enzymes unique to viral replication and, therefore, to distinguish clearly between virus and host cell functions. The unique events of viral replication serve as ideal targets for antiviral agents; examples include thymidine kinases, proteases, or protein kinases of specific herpes viruses. Second, several early, sensitive, and specific diagnostic methods for viral illnesses have resulted from advances in biotechnology. For example, the use of monoclonal antibodies, DNA hybridization techniques, and polymerase chain reaction assays should all accelerate the ability to diagnose viral infections early in the course of illness and, therefore, allow for timely intervention with specific antiviral therapies.

Future therapeutic efforts must be directed toward the development of safe, selective, and relatively inexpensive antiviral agents. A favorable safety profile is essential if antiviral agents are to find a role for patients whose viral disease is not life- or sight-threatening. These agents should be orally bioavailable and have the capability of crossing the blood–brain barrier.

Among the herpes viruses, the greatest need can be recognized in such areas as the treatment of CMV disease, whereby existing antiviral agents, for the most part, have to be administered intravenously. It should be noted, however, that oral formulations of both ganciclovir and foscarnet are under evaluation for both treatment and prophylaxis of CMV retinitis in high-risk populations.

The application of molecular biology to the development of novel therapeutic strategies is well underway. Drugs directed against HSV protease and the Ul_{97} gene of CMV (a protein kinase) are currently in development in a variety of laboratories. Clinical studies of such compounds may lead to the development of drugs that have mechanisms other than those identified by compounds such as acyclovir for treatment of HSV and VZV. This issue becomes extremely important in attempts to identify drugs that can be used for resistant viruses encountered in the community at large.

The future of antiviral drug development is one of great hope for the practicing physician. With the development of drugs that have alternative mechanisms of action compared to acyclovir, safety must not be compromised. It is hoped that the introduction of new antiviral agents will improve outcome for patients with life-threatening HSV infections of the central nervous system and diseases caused by CMV. Further advances are also anticipated in the management of patients with HIV infection, particularly with the introduction of inhibitors of unique viral functions, which have not been previously targeted (e.g., HIV protease), as well as a variety of other clinical diseases.

A fundamental issue that confronts the development of such drugs will be the availability of targeted patient populations in which adequate data can be accumulated to define therapeutic response. Future approaches include not only new antiviral drugs, but also gene therapy and vectors that express antiviral agents.

ACKNOWLEDGMENT

Financial support from NIAID N01-AI-15113, NCI CA RO-1-13148, DRR RR-032, an unrestricted infectious diseases grant from Bristol Myers Squibb and a grant from the state of Alabama.

REFERENCES

1. Alford CA, Whitley RJ. Treatment of infections due to herpesviruses in humans: a critical review of the state of the art. J Infect Dis 1976; 133: A101–A108.
2. Kaufman HE, Martola EL, Dohlman CH. The use of 5-iodo-2'-deoxyuridine in the treatment of herpes simplex keratitis. Arch Ophthalmol 1962; 68: 235–239.
3. Boston Interhospital Virus and the NIAID Cooperative Antiviral Study Groups. Failure of high dose 5-iodo-2'-deoxyuridine therapy of herpes simplex encephalitis: evidence of unacceptable toxicity. N Engl J Med 1975; 292: 600–603.
4. Couch RB. Respiratory Diseases. In: Galasso GJ, Whitley RJ, Merigan TC, eds. Antiviral Agents and Viral Diseases of Man. New York, Raven Press, 1990: 327–362.
5. Whitley RJ, Soong SJ, Dolin R, et al. Adenine arabinoside therapy of biopsy-proved herpes simplex encephalitis. N Engl J Med 1977; 297: 289–294.
6. Whitley RJ, Gnann JW. Acyclovir: a decade later. N Engl J Med 1992; 327: 782–789.
7. Saral R, Burns WH, Laskin O, et al. Acyclovir prophylaxis of herpes simple virus infections: a randomized double-blind controlled trial in bone marrow transplant recipients. N Engl J Med 1981; 305: 63–66.
8. Kost RG, Hill EL, Tigges M, Straus S. Brief report: recurrent acyclovir resistant genital herpes in an immunocompetent host. N Engl J Med 1993; 329: 1777–1781.

24

Neonatal Herpes Simplex:
Management of Mother and Infant

Charles G. Prober
Stanford University Medical Center, Stanford, California

INTRODUCTION

Neonates who contract infection caused by herpes simplex virus (HSV) are at substantial risk of death, and survivors often have substantial long-term sequelae. More than 90% of neonatal HSV infections are contracted from infected mothers at delivery (1). In addition to neonatal infection, potential morbidity attributable to maternal gestational genital herpes infection include premature delivery, intrauterine growth retardation (IUGR), and congenital infection (1). Understanding the epidemiology and manifestations of gestational and neonatal HSV infections is critical to the development of effective management strategies.

This chapter outlines current understanding of the epidemiology of genital HSV infections, with emphasis on observations specific to pregnant women. Data with regard to the likelihood of adverse consequences of gestational HSV infections are summarized; and neonatal manifestations of infection, currently recommended treatment options, and prognosis are discussed. A series of recommendations relevant to the management of infected women during pregnancy and at delivery and infected neonates are presented. Concluding comments focus on potential ways of ultimately reducing the frequency and consequences of neonatal HSV infections.

EPIDEMIOLOGY OF GENITAL HSV INFECTIONS

The frequency of clinically apparent genital herpes infections has been steadily increasing; currently about half a million new cases occur each year (1). Approximately 10% of sexually active adults have a history consistent with genital herpes infection. More than 90% of recurrent and 70% of primary genital herpes infections are caused by HSV type 2 (HSV-2). The true frequency of infection caused by HSV-2 is not accurately estimated on the basis of clinically evident infections because infections are more likely to be silent than symptomatic (2). The true prevalence of HSV-2 infection can be determined only by serological surveillance studies that use sensitive and specific serological assays.

Historically, reliable conclusions from serologically based studies have been hampered by extensive antigenic homology between HSV-1 and HSV-2. However, we and others have developed assays that accurately distinguish HSV-1 from HSV-2 antibodies. These assays are based on the detection of antibodies directed against unique HSV-2 epitopes located within glycoprotein G (3–5). Several studies conducted in different populations in the United States consistently have shown HSV-2 seroprevalence rates of 20% to 30%. Incidence increases with increasing age and is higher among blacks than whites and among those of lower socioeconomic status (2).

Serological studies conducted specifically among pregnant women also have demonstrated seroprevalence rates of 20% to 30% (6,7). To define how often pregnant women are at risk of contracting primary HSV-2 infection from their spouses, we evaluated 249 pregnant women and their spouses for serological evidence of HSV-2 infection. Seventy-one percent of the couples studied were serologically concordant for HSV-2 antibodies; 53% were seronegative and 18% seropositive. Twenty-nine percent of the couples were discordant for antibodies to HSV-2, despite having been sexually intimate for more than 6 years. A total of 33 women among the cohort of couples (13%) were seronegative for HSV-2 antibodies with HSV-2 seropositive partners. Half of the partners of these women at risk of contracting a primary infection with HSV-2 had no history of genital herpes. Therefore, it appears that a substantial number of women are at risk of contracting a primary HSV-2 infection from their partners, at least half of whom could not be aware of this risk in the absence of serological screening (8).

POTENTIAL CONSEQUENCES OF GESTATIONAL HSV INFECTIONS

Gestational genital herpes infections may result in spontaneous abortion, premature delivery, IUGR, congenital infection, and neonatal infection. The risk of adverse consequence appears to be greater after maternal primary compared with recurrent infection. The association between gestational HSV infection and spontaneous abortion has not been established. Although a study published more than 20 years ago suggested that the frequency of spontaneous abortion was increased in women who contracted genital infection during pregnancy, diagnosis of genital HSV infection was based on cervical cell morphology (9). More recent studies, which have based the diagnosis of HSV infection on viral culture, fail to confirm any relationship between genital herpes infections and spontaneous abortion (10,11).

Limited data support an association between symptomatic, first episode, late gestational, genital herpes infections and prematurity and IUGR. Five of 15 (33%) women with presumed primary gestational infections described by Brown et al. (12) delivered prematurely, and three of five infants had IUGR. Neither premature delivery nor IUGR were associated with presumed primary infections occurring earlier in gestation or with nonprimary infections.

Intrauterine infection as a result of HSV-2 infection in pregnant women is uncommon. Of 192 infected infants enrolled in the National Institutes of Allergy and Infectious Diseases Collaborative study evaluating antiviral treatment, 9 (5%) were identified with congenital infection (13). Manifestations of intrauterine infection in these infants included skin lesions and scars, chorioretinitis, microcephaly, hydranencephaly, and microphthalmia. The type of maternal infection (primary vs recurrent) that resulted in the congenital manifestations could not be determined.

The most serious consequence of maternal genital herpes is neonatal infection. The majority of neonates contract HSV infection from exposure to maternal virus shed in the genital tract at delivery. Risk of infection is influenced most by the type of maternal infection. Neonates exposed to mothers with primary infections at delivery have a much higher risk of infection than those exposed to mothers with recurrent episodes. Infection occurs in approximately 50% of neonates exposed to primary infections compared to less than 5% exposed to reactivated infections (1). Infants born to women with primary infections are exposed to a higher titer of virus than those born to women with reactivated infections. In addition, neonates born to mothers with primary infections do not receive HSV antibodies transplacentally, whereas those exposed to recurrent infection do receive these possibly protective antibodies.

Neonates infected with HSV may have disease limited to the skin, eye, and mouth (SEM) or to the central nervous system (CNS) or they may have widely disseminated infection. The SEM form of disease represents about 40% of cases, CNS disease about 35%, and disseminated about 25% (14).

Neonates with SEM disease usually present between the first and second weeks of life, although some have skin lesions evident immediately after birth. Skin lesions evolve from macules to vesicles on an erythematous base over 1 to 2 days. Typical locations for initial skin lesions include sites of trauma such as the place of attachment of fetal electrodes, conjunctival margins, or over the presenting body part. Material obtained from skin lesions suspected to be caused by HSV should be submitted to the diagnostic laboratory for direct examination and viral culture. Sensitive and specific direct tests, such as direct immunofluorescence examination, use immunologic reagents for antigen detection. Compared to tissue culture isolation, this test has a sensitivity of >90%, and there are few false-positive reactions (1). Direct examination by Papanicolaou stain or Tzanck test for typical cytological changes should not be relied on because they have an unacceptably low sensitivity rate (1).

Babies with localized SEM disease usually do well if diagnosis is made promptly and antiviral therapy is administered. If infants with SEM disease are not treated, however, about 75% will progress to disseminated or CNS disease (15).

Neonates with HSV infection localized to the CNS typically develop signs and symptoms of infection at 2 to 3 weeks of age. Fever and lethargy are followed by the sudden onset of focal seizures which are difficult to control. Cerebrospinal fluid (CSF) examination usually reveals 50 to 100 white blood cells/mm^3, a reduced glucose and a high protein concentration. The electroencephalogram tends to be diffusely abnormal, but the computer tomography (CT) scan of the head early in the course usually is normal. More than half of all neonates with untreated CNS disease will die and <10% of survivors develop normally. In the absence of skin lesions, the definitive diagnosis of CNS infection requires the performance of a brain biopsy for virological evaluation. The presence of HSV DNA, detected in CSF by polymerase chain reaction, is promising as a diagnostic aid.

Disseminated infection is the most serious form of neonatal herpes (15). Symptoms often are suggestive of severe bacterial sepsis. Onset commonly is during the first several days of life, with common signs including hepatosplenomegaly, jaundice, abnormal liver functions tests, coagulopathy, and radiographical evidence of pneumonia. About two-thirds of patients develop skin lesions sometime during their illness, but these lesions often are absent at the onset of symptoms. Progression of infection is rapid and untreated mortality rate exceeds 70%. Death results from progressive shock, liver failure, or respiratory failure (15). Evaluation of infants with suspected disseminated HSV infection should include viral cultures of specimens obtained from the nasopharynx, rectum, blood buffy coat, and skin or mucosal lesions.

MANAGEMENT OF INFECTED WOMEN DURING PREGNANCY

Most infants born to women with recurrent HSV-2 infections have no problems attributable to the maternal infection. Therefore, the most important element of managing these women is to provide education and reassurance. They should be assured that gestational recurrent HSV infections rarely are associated with fetal compromise, and most infants can be safely delivered vaginally. Furthermore, because prenatal cultures from women with recurrent herpes fail to predict shedding of virus at delivery, the practice of obtaining these cultures late in pregnancy has been abandoned (16).

Primary infections are associated with a higher risk of fetal and neonatal morbidity than are recurrent infections (12). Many first episode infections do not represent *true* primary infections but rather are the first clinical manifestations of a distant infection. The only way to distinguish primary from recurrent infections is by serological evaluation of the subject with reliable type-specific assays for HSV antibodies. These assays currently are available only in research laboratories.

Women with suspected primary infections should be advised of the possible adverse consequences of their infection. Primary infections are associated with prolonged viral shedding and an increased risk of asymptomatic reactivations proximal to the initial episode. Therefore, it is reasonable to perform weekly cultures on these women if they contract infection during the last trimester. If these cultures are positive close to the onset of labor, a cesarean delivery should be performed.

MANAGEMENT OF INFECTED WOMEN AT DELIVERY

Management of infected women at delivery depends on whether the infection is clinically active or inactive. All women with recurrent genital herpes should be closely examined at delivery. To facilitate prompt examination, they should enter the hospital soon after labor begins. If genital lesions are present, cesarean delivery should be performed, before rupture of amniotic membranes or as soon as possible thereafter.

Women without evidence of active genital HSV infection at delivery should be allowed to deliver vaginally unless they have had a recent primary infection with continued viral shedding.

MANAGEMENT OF NEONATES WITH HSV INFECTION

Treatment with antiviral agents has improved the outcome of neonates infected with HSV. Nonetheless, substantial morbidity and mortality remain. Vidarabine (Ara-A) was the first agent shown to be of benefit in the treatment of neonatal HSV infections (17). The efficacy of acyclovir, a more selective and specific inhibitor of HSV, also has been demonstrated (18). The best therapeutic results with either agent are observed in infants with localized SEM disease. With treatment before progression of their infection, virtually all of these infants survive and more than 90% are developmentally normal (18). In stark contrast, about 15% of those with localized CNS disease will die, but only about one-third of survivors will be normal at follow-up examination (18). Disseminated disease has the highest mortality rate; whether treated with vidarabine or acyclovir mortality rates are about 50% (18). Despite the similar efficacies of vidarabine and acyclovir, the ease of administration and safety profile of acyclovir generally favor its use. It is administered intravenously at a daily dosage of 30 mg/kg, given in three equally divided doses for 10 to 14 days. The use of higher doses of acyclovir given for longer periods is under investigation.

Parents of neonates known to have been exposed to HSV at delivery should be advised about the symptoms and signs of infection and the necessity for prompt evaluation if any occur. If exposure has resulted from a recurrent maternal infection, the parents should be reassured that the risk of neonatal HSV infection is low, approximately 2% to 3%. More concern is warranted if exposure was to a primary maternal infection. These exposed neonates should have viral cultures performed on specimens obtained from their eyes, throat, urine, stool, and CSF, and acyclovir therapy should be initiated if any of these cultures are positive.

METHODS OF REDUCING THE RISK OF NEONATAL HSV

Reducing the risk of neonatal HSV infections could be accomplished by either reducing the chance of maternal infection or the likelihood that a mother shedding virus at delivery will transmit it to her neonate. The only means of preventing reactivation of infection is antiviral therapy. Acyclovir consistently reduces the frequency of clinically evident recurrent genital herpes infections in nonpregnant individuals by 70% to 90%. Although asymptomatic shedding of virus has been demonstrated in individuals receiving suppressive therapy, the frequency of shedding is reduced. It is impractical, however, to consider prescribing acyclovir to all pregnant women at risk of reactivating HSV. Unless all pregnant women were to be tested serologically for evidence of prior HSV-2 infection, the majority of women at risk of viral reactivation would not be identified. In the future, it might be possible to reduce reactivation of HSV infection by modulating host immunity. For the foreseeable future, however, women with latent genital HSV infections will continue to pose a risk to their offspring. Fortunately, this risk is low even in the absence of any intervention. The chance of viral reactivation on any given day, including the day of delivery, is about 1%, and the chance of a neonate contracting infection as a result of exposure to virus shed by a woman with prior infection is 2% to 3% (1).

Preventing acquisition of new genital HSV infections during pregnancy is more feasible than preventing reactivated infections. If a woman susceptible to HSV-2 infection has a sexual partner infected with the virus, primary infection could be prevented by abstinence or reduced by the use of condoms. Successful application of this strategy requires serological testing of partners to detect asymptomatically infected individuals. The current limitation of this strategy is the lack of availability of reliable type-specific serological assays for HSV-2.

Ultimately, preventing primary genital herpes infections depends on the availability of a safe and effective vaccine. Vaccine could be administered to women at risk of contracting infection from their sexual partner. Efficacy studies of vaccines against HSV are in progress, including clinical trials focused on couples discordant for HSV infection.

The second approach to lowering the incidence of neonatal herpes, reducing the likelihood that a mother shedding virus at delivery will transmit virus to her neonate, requires the rapid identification of infected women. Promptly identifying women with lesions at delivery is plausible, whereas identifying women asymptomatically shedding HSV is problematic, requiring a highly sensitive and specific rapid diagnostic test.

Although tests capable of rapidly identifying virus in clinical lesions are available, they are not sufficiently reliable to be used in the identification of asymptomatic viral shedding. It is unlikely that any test will be developed that will be useful in determining the optimal mode of delivery. Even if a test were 99% specific, 40,000 women in the United States each year (1% of the 4 million mothers delivering each year in the United States) would be falsely identified as shedding virus. These women would suffer the potential consequences of unnecessary abdominal deliveries.

Currently, the prevention of adverse consequences attendant to perinatal HSV infections depends on reducing new acquisitions of genital HSV infections during gestation and careful evaluation of women at delivery for the presence of active HSV infection. If a neonate contracts infection, adverse outcome can be reduced by prompt recognition of infection and initiation of antiviral therapy. Ultimate control of this infection depends on the availability of an effective vaccine program.

REFERENCES

1. Prober CG, Arvin AM. Genital herpes and the pregnant woman. In: Swartz M, Remington JS, eds. Current Clinical Topics in Infectious Diseases 10. Boston: Blackwell Scientific Publications, 1989: 1–26.
2. Koutsky LA, Stevens CE, Holmes KK, et al. Underdiagnosis of genital herpes by current clinical and viral-isolation procedures. N Engl J Med 1992; 326: 1533–1539.
3. Sullender WM, Yasukawa L, Schwartz M, et al. Type specific antibodies to herpes simplex virus-2 glycoprotein G in pregnant women, infants exposed to maternal HSV-2 infection at delivery, and infants with neonatal herpes. J Infect Dis 1988; 157: 164–171.
4. Coleman RM, Pereira L, Bailey PD, et al. Determination of herpes simplex virus type-specific antibodies by enzyme-linked immunosorbent assay. J Clin Microbiol 1983; 18: 287–291.
5. Johnson RE, Nahmias AJ, Magder LS, et al. A seroepidemiologic survey of the prevalence of herpes simplex virus type 2 infection in the United States. N Engl J Med 1989; 321: 7–12.
6. Boucher FD, Yasukawa LL, Bronzan RN, et al. A prospective evaluation of primary genital herpes simple virus type 2 infections acquired during pregnancy. Pediatr Infect Dis J 1990; 9: 499–504.
7. Prober CG, Corey L, Brown ZA, et al. The management of pregnancies complicated by genital infections with herpes simplex virus. Clinical Infect Dis 1992; 15: 1031–1038.

8. Kulhanjian JA, Soroush V, Au DS, et al. Identification of women at unsuspected risk of contracting primary herpes simplex virus type 2 infections during pregnancy. N Engl J Med 1992; 326: 916–920.

9. Nahmias AJ, Josey WE, Naib ZM et al. Perinatal risk associated with maternal genital herpes simplex virus infection. Am J Obstet Gynecol 1971; 110: 825–837.

10. Vontver LA, Hickok DE, Brown Z, et al. Recurrent herpes simplex virus infection in pregnancy: infant outcome and frequency of asymptomatic recurrences. Am J Obstet Gynecol 1982; 143: 75–84.

11. Grossman JH, Waller WC, Sever JL. Management of genital herpes simplex virus infection during pregnancy. Obstet Gynecol 1981; 58: 1–4.

12. Brown ZA, Vontver LA, Benedetti J, et al. Effects of infants of a first episode of genital herpes during pregnancy. N Engl J Med 1987; 317: 1246–1251.

13. Hutto C, Arvin AM, Jacobs R, et al. Intrauterine herpes simplex virus infections. J Pediatr 1987; 110: 97–101.

14. Whitley RJ, Corey L, Arvin A, et al. Changing presentation of herpes simplex virus infection in neonates. J Infect Dis 1988; 158: 109–116.

15. Whitley RJ. Herpes simplex virus infections. In: Remington JS, Klein JO, eds. Infectious Diseases of the Fetus and Newborn Infant. 3rd ed. Philadelphia: Saunders, 1990.

16. Arvin AM, Hensleigh PA, Prober CG, et al. Failure of antepartum maternal cultures to predict the infant's risk of exposure to herpes simplex virus at delivery. N Engl J Med 1986; 315: 796–800.

17. Whitley RJ, Nahmias AJ, Soongt S-J, et al. Vidarabine therapy of neonatal herpes simplex virus infection. Pediatrics 1980; 66: 495–501.

18. Whitley RJ, Arvin A, Prober C, et al. A controlled trial comparing vidarabine with acyclovir in neonatal herpes simplex virus infection. N Engl J Med 1991; 324: 444–449.

25

Current Treatment of Genital Warts

Geo von Krogh
Karolinska Hospital, Stockholm, Sweden

INTRODUCTION

Epidemiology—The Iceberg Dilemma

Risk of acquiring genital papillomavirus infection (GPVI) covariates with early sexual debut, frequent partner changes, concurrent and previous other sexually transmitted diseases (STDs), and heavy smoking habits. An inverse relationship exists with consistent use of condoms (1). In Western countries, the incidence of patients self-attending for genital and anal warts is about 0.5% to 1% of sexually active 15- to 25-year olds (2,3). In sexually active males in their upper teens, the rate of warts detectable by magnification equipment ("penoscopy") is as high as 6% to 7% (1). The true prevalence, however, of virologically detectable GPVI among adolescents is in the upper range of 30% to 50% (4–6), and estimated lifetime risk is 80% (7). The fact that most lesions induced by oncogenic ("high-risk") human papilloma virus (HPV) types remain asymptomatic and undetectable by naked eye examination appears as a sociomedical paradox and an intriguing clinical dilemma.

As a rule, multifocal epithelial alterations are induced, and the infection is generally regional rather than local (8). Overt warts frequently coexist with subclinical lesions (9,10). Benign warts often coexist with dysplastic lesions ("intraepithelial neoplasia"), often being parts of a morphological spectrum of continuity. Fluctuations often occur from a state of subclinical or latent infection to overt wart disease, or vice versa (4,7,10).

Depending on severity HPV-associated epithelial dysplasia is classified as grade I (mild), II (moderate), or III (severe). The denominations

CIN, VAIN, VIN, PIN, PEIN, and AIN are commonly used when intra-epithelial neoplasia engages, respectively, the cervix, vagina, vulva, penis, perineum, or anus. The cervix uteri represents a locus minoris for subsequent cancer development (11,12), where the relation to HPV infection satisfies most classic criteria for causal interference. The relative risk of malignant transformation is very low in remaining genital and anal areas. Even on the cervix, however, cancer seems to arise only in a fraction of cases, when dysplasia persists for at least 5 to 10 years and is associated with cofactors such as chronic infections, chemical cocarcinogens, and local or systemic immunological dysfunctions (13). The relative risk of persistent moderate-severe CIN ("high-grade squamous lesions") increases significantly by age >30 years and among women infected with, above all, the oncogenic HPV types 16, 18, 31, 33 and 45. About two-thirds of mild CIN ("low-grade squamous lesions") regress spontaneously within 5 to 7 years. Such lesions are caused by both low- and high-risk HPV types.

Regulatory Mechanisms for Biological Expression

A state of subclinical/latent infection may be sustained by down-regulatory control mechanisms exerted by tumor suppressor gene products of the keratinocytes and/or cell-mediated immunological surveillance. HPV, as "non-self" antigens, may potentially lead to immunogenic responses, causing an ultimate rejection of biological tumor activity. In many cases, however, an alternative route of tolerance ("not seen") may rather develop. A detrimental effect by some yet unidentified product(s) from HPV has been postulated as a contributing cause of faint immune reactions that may lead to persistent viral infection in immunologically otherwise healthy individuals. Such mechanisms include partial depletion and morphological alteration of Langerhans' cells, suboptimal cytokine release, and depletion of natural killer (NK) cell responses. Also, impaired human leucocyte antigen-DR (HLA-DR) and intercellular adhesion molecule-1 (ICAM-1) associated antigen presenting capacity of infected keratinocytes have been demonstrated in persistent HPV lesions (14). Significant increase of biological expression, with a high degree of recalcitrance, recurrence, and malignant transformation, also occurs during immunosuppression associated with malignancies and with HIV (15–17), or induced iatrogenically in allograft recipients (18). The hereditary condition epidermodysplasia verruciformis is associated with genetically deranged immunological homeostatic mechanisms (19). Up-regulatory influences also include life-style related factors, such as tobacco smoking and high alcohol consumption (20), factors that often covariate with the presence or history of other STDs. Influence of hormonal factors, exerted by stimulation of a common receptor for progesterone and glucocorticoid on keratinocytes (21), is also demonstrated during pregnancy when warts tend to become florid and coalescent (22). Similar growth potential is also associated with diabetes mellitus.

There is a strong inclination for HPV types 6 and 11 to induce acuminate warts, and for HPV types 16 and 18 to be present in subclinical lesions. This propensity, however, is not sufficient for a differentiation on a clinical basis among individuals infected with the various HPV types. Thus, "high-risk" HPV types may be harbored in all clinical wart types, and concurrent infection with several HPV types is common (22–25).

When to Investigate and Treat

Genitoanal warts are of *cosmetic* and *psychosexual significance*. Patients experience them as distasteful and disfiguring, and consider them as a major hindrance to sexual performance. Psychosexual and psychosocial effects, possibly more frequent in females than in males, include profound influence on sexuality, mood, social life, emotional relationship with partner, and fear of cancer (26–28). Naturally, overt warts must be properly managed and cured, whenever possible.

Concerns have been raised about the medicolegal dilemma of missing or underdiagnosing genital HPV disease. This aspect is significant for the diagnosis of CIN and cervical cancer, but less valid for the outer genitalia. It has been suggested that women with CIN may benefit from examination and treatment of clinical and/or subclinical lesions of their male partners, aiming at optimizing the cure rates of CIN. This might seem rational, as these men appear to have a high frequency of severe penile intraepithelial neoplasia (PIN) when their acetowhite lesions are biopsied. Nevertheless, treatment failure rates of women with CIN whose partners are carefully examined and treated for subclinical penile lesions do not, so far, differ from that of women whose partners remain untreated (29,30).

As it is not the HPV itself that is harmful to the patient, the primary task at the time must be to focus on *lesions* that are either of psychosexual importance, giving rise to symptoms, or represent significant risk of cancer sequelae. Management of patients with overt disease already puts a notable strain on medical resources; a much larger challenge is ahead if subclinical cases are diagnosed and treated. Even if sufficient resources are created, no antiviral therapy is available and we will hardly be able to remove all these multifocal lesions. Accordingly, routine screening for subclinical lesions on the outer genitals of asymptomatic individuals seems pointless and may cause unnecessary fear and anguish in otherwise healthy people.

Management—A Multidisciplinary Challenge

Decentralized primary management by primary health care providers is often most feasible in many clinical settings. Many patients, estimated in the range of 20% to 40% of cases, require subsequent transfer to specialist care, including dermatovenereologists and/or gynecologists. Occurrence of urinary meatus and anal warts may require a specialist team including urologists and proctologists. Children with condylomas should be referred for pediatric and sociomedical evaluation (31–33). Routine vaginocervical cytology examination (Pap smear) of females older than 25 years of age must be performed liberally, aiming at detection of persistent CIN II–III.

Condylomas are often difficult to treat. Regardless of available therapeutic modalities (Table 1), removal of overt warts may be incomplete because of occult subclinical HPV infection occurring concurrently with and adjacent to lesions being treated, contributing to recurrence rates in the range of 38% to 81% (34). In a retrospective evaluation of therapy demands in 230 male patients attending an STD clinic in Stockholm (35), a long-term complete cure of penile and/or anal warts was accomplished in only 33% of the patients following either a single course of home treatment with 0.5% podophyllotoxin–ethanol applied twice a day for 3 days or one course of surgical intervention using scissor excision and/or electrodesiccation (Table 2). Although 55% were cured after one to four courses,

Table 1 Current Treatment Modalities of Genital Warts

Cytotoxic agents
  Podophyllin
  Podophyllotoxin
  Trichloroacetic acid
  5-Fluorouracil
Surgery
  Scissor excision/curretage
  Electrosurgery/loop excision
  Cryotherapy (liquid nitrogen, nitrous oxide)
  Laser (CO_2 laser, Neodynium: YAG laser)
Adjuvant interferons

Table 2 Retrospective Evaluation of Therapy
Demands in Men

Management level	Patients
• STD clinic therapy—number of courses[a] required for cure	
1	77 (33%)
2–4	51 (22%)
5–12 first year	28 (12%)
Recurrences > 1 year	46 (20%)
• Proctology referral	19 (8%)
• Urology referral	9 (4%)
Total	230 men

[a]A therapy course refers to home treatment with 0.5%
podophyllotoxin (applied twice a day for 3 days) or
outpatient surgery using excision and/or electrodessication.
From Ref. 35.

recurrences were observed after the first year of therapy in as many as 20% of the men. Another 8% of the men primarily required referral to the proctology department because of extensive anal growths, and 4% were referred to the urology department for the management of intrameatel warts; thus, the study also emphasizes the importance of multidisciplinary management of some condylomata cases.

As for other STDs, principles recommended by the World Health Organization (WHO) should be applied (36), including the encouragement of condom use for primary and secondary prevention, as well as the promotion of examining and counseling sexual partners. The presence of other STDs should be sought. Patients suffering from visible warts and/or lesions that otherwise give rise to symptoms should always be offered therapy. This is not unequivocally the case for subclinical lesions where the decision about management is more difficult.

TOPICAL TREATMENT USING CYTOTOXIC AGENTS

Podophyllin

Podophyllin has so far been a popular front-line treatment for genital warts because it is relatively inexpensive to produce. Podophyllin is a crude plant resin extracted from the roots of either the North American *Podophyllum peltatum* or the Indian *Podophyllum emodi* species. Its efficacy, as based on short-term "cure" of penile warts afflicting American military troops, was first described in 1942 (37). Subsequent reports, however, have focused on major shortcomings including lack of satisfactory long-term efficacy (38–45), frequent occurrence of painful tissue reactions, significant risks of systemic toxicity (46–49), and the potential for mutagenic influences of the epithelium (50,51). The latter aspect is distressing; many condyloma patients are concurrently coinfected with oncogenic HPV types, when the influence from mutagenic cofactors may be of potential pathogenetic significance for malignant transformation of the keratinocytes.

Podophyllin is an impure, semiquantitatively produced, nonstandardized substance composed of numerous chemical substances and a varying amounts of cytotoxic compounds known as lignans. Lignans act predominantly as antimitotics, arresting the cellular spindle formation in metaphase (38,52,53). The ingredients may vary significantly among various batches. Furthermore, stability is unreliable and degradation of biologically active lignans into inactive isomers may occur rapidly (38). Quercetin and kaempherol are components lacking therapeutic properties but that potentially may act as strong mutagenic compounds (50,51). In the light of current insight that multicentric genital intraepithelial neoplasia induced by oncogenic HPV types often coexists with benign condylomas, it seems rather doubtful whether podophyllin has any further place in condylomata therapy, as both quercetin and kaempherol potentially could act as oncogenic cofactors in the progress of intraepithelial neoplasia.

Podophyllin is applied as a 20% to 25% solution in ethanol or tincture of benzoin. Podophyllin can cause severe and aggressive burning, swelling, and ulcerations on application sites. For this reason, it must be applied under careful medical supervision and washed off within 4 to 6 hours. Applications repeated once or maximally twice a week because of a high risk of skin irritation must be made by a physician or a specially trained nurse.

It is somewhat surprising that podophyllin treatment remains a popular method for treating condylomata acuminata despite the fact that recurrences are likely to occur. Although an average primary cure rate of 50% (range 22% to 78%) has been reported, recurrence rates appear to be as high as 65% to 74% (34,40,54) and appear to be considerably higher than from surgical excision (40). In prospective trials by von Krogh (38), examining efficacy at 3 months follow-up from freshly prepared podophyllum preparations against penile warts, it was evident that efficacy is far below that originally claimed; only 22% of the men were cured after a single application, and a second course of treatment for residual warts showed a cumulative effect of 38%.

Thus, podophyllin treatment suffers disadvantages of low efficacy, heavy demands on the medical and nursing staff, and inconvenience to the patient. The cost/benefit aspects of such therapy deserves questioning (54,55). Furthermore, potential systemic toxicity of podophyllin is another major problem and drawback of the remedy. When applied in large volumes on florid warts, severe systemic toxicity symptoms have been observed. In a few instances, toxicity has caused fatal outcome because of central nervous system (CNS) influence and cardiovascular crisis (46–49).

Safety and Precaution

Podophyllin should not be stored for more than a month. Office applications more frequently than once a week is not recommended. Patients must be instructed to wash away the remedy within 4 to 6 hours (34,38). Self-treatment should never be prescribed. Maximum volume for topical use with 20% preparations should not exceed 0.9 ml for *P. peltatum*- and 0.4 ml for *P. emodi*-based remedies (48). Podophyllin should not be given during pregnancy (48). Females must use a reliable contraceptive method or abstain from sexual intercourse during the days of active therapy.

Podophyllotoxin

Podophyllotoxin is a purified podophyllin ingredient, which appears to be the most biologically active lignan (56–58). The drug binds to tubulins, which are essential for mitotic cell division, preventing tubulin polymerization into microtubules (38,48,52,55). Biological effects include mitotic arrest of keratinocyte division in metaphase, nucleoside transport inhibition and a detrimental influence on epidermal capillaries (57). Therapeutic effect is associated with necrotic involution of condylomas that is maximal 3 to 5 days after initial administration. Histopathologically, drug influence is demonstrable for up to 1 to 2 weeks, presenting as a degenerative keratinocyte damage and/or the occurrence of abnormal bizarre mitotic figures that may occasionally be confused with epithelial dysplasia (59). Thus, any biopsy evaluation from podophyllin/podophyllotoxin treated areas should be avoided until 2 drug-free weeks have passed. No long-term risk of dysplasia is associated with the regimen.

In studies on penile warts in uncircumcised men, using low concentrations (0.5% to 1%) podophyllotoxin, self-applied as an ethanolic solution twice a day for 3 days, was highly effective (53). After a single 3-day course, preputial cavity warts (the glans penis, the coronal sulcus, the fraenulum, and the inner aspect of the foreskin) were cured in 70% of cases. Altogether, 49% of the patients were completely wart-free after one 3-day course, and the cumulative cure rate was 82% when self-treatment was repeated once more. Efficacy at 3 months' follow-up was significantly superior ($P < 0.001$) to that after use of freshly prepared 20% podophyllin (Table 3). Several subsequent single-blind prospective trials comparing patient-applied podophyllotoxin (Wartec, Warticon, Perstorp Pharma, Lund, Sweden; Condyline, Nycomed Pharma, Oslo, Norway) with clinic-applied podophyllin resin confirm a superior efficacy from podophyllotoxin compared to that of podophyllin (41–44). In these reports, varying rates of local irritation of the treated areas have been documented. A complete absence of subjective and/or objective local toxicity has been reported in 31% to 83% of cases. Mild to moderate local side effects associated with wart involution has occurred in 17% to 63% of patients. More notable phenomena such as burning, pain, and/or balanoposthitis are rare, but may occur in 5% to 14% of cases afflicted with relatively large or numerous warts (42–45). These studies, however, all confirm that local reactions tend to be considerably lower than those reported after podophyllin. A highly satisfactory degree of efficacy and tolerance from multiple self-treatment courses of podophyllotoxin against genitoanal warts has also been documented in a large British multicenter study based on 303 uncircumcised males (60).

In the urinary meatus and on the penile shaft, efficacy tends to be less impressive than under the foreskin (Table 4), where an occlusive influence

Table 3 Self-Treatment with Podophyllotoxin Versus Office Application of Podophyllin Against Penile Warts (About 3 Months Follow-Up)

	No. cycles	Podophyllo-toxin	Podo-phyllin	P value
von Krogh (1981) (53)	1–2	82% (142/173)	38% (40/105)	<0.001
Lassus (1987) (41)	1–4	77% (37/48)	44% (23/52)	<0.01
Edwards et al. (1988) (43)	1–6	88% (28/32)	63% (12/19)	<0.05
Mazurkiewicz and Jablonska (1990) (44)	1–6	79% (11/14)	38% (5/13)	<0.05

Table 4 Self-Treatment with 0.5% Podophyl-
lotoxin as a Single Cycle (Bid for 3 Days):
Efficacy on Penile Warts in Uncircumcised
Males

Wart distribution	Efficacy
Preputial cavity	70%
Transitional area of the foreskin	48%
Urinary meatus	33%
Penile shaft	10%

From Ref. 53.

apparently contributes to the success rates (53). In subsequent studies
(61,62), it has been demonstrated that in about half of such cases, warts
may resolve completely, and about 80% of the original wart bulk disappears, when three to four repeated 3-day courses of 0.5% podophyllotoxin
(Condylox, Oclassen Pharmaceuticals, Inc., San Rafael, California) are
given at 4 to 7 days of drug-free intervals. In the trials accounted for by
Beutner et al. (61), 109 circumcised males with warts predominantly
located to the penile shaft (88%) were randomly allocated to 0.5% podophyllotoxin or placebo. Therapy was self-administered in treatment courses
of twice daily applications for 3 consecutive days followed by a 4-days
drug-free period. Patients administered a minimum of two and a maximum of four such treatment courses. None of the 53 placebo patients, but
45% (25/56) podophyllotoxin-treated patients were completely wart-free
at some time during the study. At the end of the treatment period, 74% and
8% of treated warts in the active or placebo groups, respectively, were no
longer present. Analogous results have been accounted for by Kirby et al. (62).

Von Krogh (38) reported absence of any local irritation in 49% of
patients. Painful tissue reactions similar to those associated with
podophyllin did not occur. Altogether, 46% of patients experienced a
slight burning and/or tenderness in association with the occurrence of
superficial erosions and some erythema on days 3 to 5 after initiated
treatment. Only 5% experienced some pain in association with necrosis
of extensive warts. It was concluded that, analogous to surgery, some
"adverse effects" are inevitable when warts are destroyed and should be
considered as part of the therapeutic effect. Most important, however,
podophyllotoxin-associated erosions heal considerably faster than those
after surgical procedures (45,63).

Self-treatment with 0.5% podophyllotoxin–ethanol has also been tested as repeated 3-day courses against vulvar warts. Results are analogous to those reported for circumcised males (64). Approximately half of the podophyllotoxin-treated women experienced mild and tolerable local erosions causing some burning and/or pain.

The optimal concentration of podophyllotoxin formulation for self-treatment of genital warts is yet to be determined. Von Krogh et al. (65) compared ethanolic solutions of 0.5% and 0.25% podophyllotoxin against penile warts. While the placebo solution exerted a marginal influence, primary cure was documented in 72% (13/18) and 81% (13/16) of 34 men self-treating their warts with 0.25% or 0.50% podophyllotoxin, respectively. Follow-up investigations (range 5 to 23 weeks) revealed some degree of relapse in nine men (38%), when warts occurred on previously untreated sites in 33% and in another 44% on podophyllotoxin-treated sites, as well as on adjacent sites. Analysis of the debulking potential of podophyllotoxin on the original warts showed that 0.25% podophyllotoxin cured 85% (184/217) and the 0.5% preparation eradicated 96% (130/135) of the original warts, a difference not being statistically significant. Side effects, generally being mild to moderate, did not differ between the two drug concentrations.

While some therapies come into use through "breakthroughs," other useful therapies evolve (63). By its nature evolution continues. Podophyllotoxin–ethanol self-applications seem convenient against penile warts. Less accessible vulvar, perineal, and anal warts, however, might potentially be reached more feasibly by cream preparations, allowing the assistance of tactile acid from the patient's own fingers during applications. This has been successfully demonstrated in subsequent studies (66–69), signaling that further refinements may be expected for self-therapy with podophyllotoxin in a near future. In a double-blind, placebo-controlled study (67), self-treatment with 0.5% podophyllotoxin cream, administered twice a day in 3-day courses once a week for up to 3 weeks, was evaluated among women afflicted with outer vulvoanal warts. Placebo lacked therapeutic influence. Cure at 3-months' follow-up occurred in 77% of the 44 women receiving the 0.5% podophyllotoxin cream formulation. A slight-to-moderate tenderness, burning, and/or pain was noted by 60% of them. Similar encouraging results from a 0.5% cream formulation has been documented also in more recent studies (67) when one to four 3-day cycles of home treatment cleared vulva warts more often (71%) than one to four office applications of podophyllin (48%; $P < 0.05$). Therapy was generally well tolerated. In recent trials of 0.15% to 0.3% of podophyllotoxin cream preparations (68), a trend has been documented that is in favor of a somewhat higher efficacy when using 0.3% of the drug, while the 0.15% formulations (Table 5) tend to induce somewhat less local irritancy. Use of 0.3% cream might possible be most favorable with regard to efficacy, although the 0.15% cream potentially may be of value in highly sensitive areas, such as the anal verge and other intertriginous areas, where a minimizing of side effects may be of major importance. Efficacy of 0.30% to 0.15% creams for self-application against penile warts was recently demonstrated by Strand et al. (69), who reported few and mild local side effects even in uncircumcised males.

Patient-applied podophyllotoxin is becoming widely available and has become increasingly recognized as a valuable first-line therapy for external genital warts, with several advantages compared to podophyllin (Tables 6 and 7). Currently available podophyllotoxin preparations have highly satisfactory shelf-life stability, which is not the case for podophyllin preparations. The low toxic potential for podophyllotoxin has initiated a change in the generic name to "podofilox" (61–63) in the United States.

Safety and Precaution

An optimal regimen for use of podophyllotoxin preparations entails application twice a day for 3 days (63). No washing off is required between applications. When large warts occur, ethanol solutions of podophyllotoxin may induce a temporary unpleasant stinging when warts necrotize on day 2 or 3 of therapy (53). If problems occur because of unpleasant erosions of the foreskin in retracting the foreskin in an uncircumcised male, the patient requires medical supervision and assistance until the condition resolves, which usually happens within a few days. Any local discomfort is otherwise easily suppressed by topical antiinflammatory remedies. Podophyllotoxin should not be given during pregnancy.

Table 5 Podophyllotoxin Solution Versus Cream Formulations Applied (Bid for 3 Days as 1 to 4 Weekly Courses)

Formulation	Cure rates ≥ 3 months
0.5% solution	85% (127/148)
0.3% cream	83% (126/151)
0.15% cream	75% (112/149)

(Rosén, personal communication, Conpharm AB, Sweden)

Table 6 Composition of 25% Podophyllum Resin and 0.5% Podophyllotoxin

	25% Podophyllum resin[a]	0.5% Podophyllotoxin purified
Podophyllotoxin mg/ml	25–100	5
Other lignans mg/ml[b]	2–25	0
Quercetin	Yes	No
Kaempherol	Yes	No
Systemic absorption	Yes	Minimal
Known stability	No	Yes
Patient applied	No	Yes

[a]Content varies with species and source.
[b]Alpha-peltatin, beta-peltatin, and 4-demethylpodophyllotoxin.

Females must use a contraceptive or abstain from penetrative sexual activity.

Trichloroacetic Acid

This caustic acid is applied as an ethanolic solution at weekly intervals at concentrations of 50% to 85%. Although the efficacy has been poorly documented, it is clear that, similar to podophyllin, numerous treatments are usually required. Overall efficacy has been purely documented; especially efficacy against cervical and vaginal HPV-associated lesions is not

Table 7 Some Major Aspects of Podophyllin Versus Podophyllotoxin[a] (Podofilox[b])

20% Podophyllin preparations—disadvantages	≤0.5% Podophyllotoxin preparations—advantages
Nonstandardized, unstable remedy	Standardized, stable remedy
Local toxicity high and unpredictable	Local toxicity low and predictable
Systemic toxicity risk considerable	Systemic toxicity risk negligible
Mutagenic properties	No mutagenic properties
Low efficacy	High efficacy
Office treatment required	Home treatment feasible

[a]Original chemical term
[b]Change of generic name in the United States because of a lack of significant toxicity of the drug in current low-concentration formulations derived for home treatment.

yet fully clarified, although there are reports on an 80% cure rate in benign HPV infections of the cervix when using 85% trichloracetic acid (34,70).

Safety and Precaution

In contrast to podophyllotoxin, however, trichloracetic acid is painful at the moment of applications and, thus, must be applied by a specialist. Because there is no report on systemic toxicity, trichloroacetic acid may be used during pregnancy.

5-Fluorouracil

The pyrimidine antagonist 5-fluorouracil (5-FU), acting by inhibition of nucleic acid synthesis, is a powerful cytotoxic drug and has been tried with varying success as a 5% cream (Fluoro-uracil cream, Hoffman-La Roche AG, Basel, Switzerland) for the treatment of resistant genital warts of the vulva and the penis, and especially of urethral warts in men (71,72). Side effects are common and include painful epithelial erosions, sometimes accompanied also by intolerable posttreatment pain. For this reason, and because efficacy has been highly variable, with a cure rate of 33% to 100% after daily applications for up to 8 weeks (34), use of 5-FU on the outer anogenital area must be performed with great caution (70–77).

Localized areas of large wart plaques, as well as bowenoid papulosis, have been successfully treated with 5-FU cream used twice a day for 1 to 3 weeks (71–77). Also, a 5-FU cream may be tried for self-treatment against otherwise recalcitrant lesions of the urinary meatus (71). Urinary meatus warts disappear in up to 70% to 90% of cases when the cream is applied after each voiding for 2 to 3 weeks. On this site, medication can be confined to a limited area, and in general ulcerations emanating from therapy cause merely a tolerable dysuria. Applications are often best performed using a Q-tip; the meatus is first dried from excess urine with one end of the cotton swab, and the other end is used for cream application. The procedure is followed by squeezing the distal urethra with the patient's fingers, and excess of 5-FU cream is subsequently wiped away with paper tissue to avoid unnecessary spread to the glans and to other penile sites, which could otherwise cause unnecessary local epithelial irritation. Some dysuria and purulent discharge frequently occur during the second or third week of therapy (71). When patients are informed of this, most can be motivated to continue therapy for a 3-week period. Furthermore, intra-urethral instillations of the cream may be performed in an inpatient setting, using a syringe when extensive intraurethral growths have been encountered (77,78). In such cases, the patient must be monitored carefully, particularly with regard to the potential development of urinary retention.

Some investigators have found 5-FU valuable for treating vulvovaginal warts. Ferenczy (72) applied 2.5 g of the cream intravaginally for five consecutive evenings and found that the failure rate against condylomata was as low as 3.5% after two separate treatment courses. When the drug is used in the vagina, the vulvar area should be protected by zinc oxide cream to avoid erosive vulvitis.

Various schedules have been suggested for treatment of vulvar warts. Krebs (73) reported a 41% cure rate when 5-FU cream was applied twice a week at two subsequent nights for 10 weeks, while Pride (74) found a cure rate of 68% after one to three treatment cycles when 5-FU was applied with fingers or by using a vaginal applicator (10 ml) twice a day for 1 week per cycle, followed by a rest period for another 7 to 10 days. A mild vulvovaginitis was reported in only 16% of females following the proposed application schedule.

5-FU cream has also been tried as prophylactic treatment after surgery on vulvovaginal warts. Krebs (74) inserted the cream intravaginally once every 2 weeks for 6 months subsequent to surgical treatment of vaginal warts. Of the 5-FU-treated women, only 13% developed recurrences as compared with 38% of women who were not 5-FU treated. Similarly, a significant reduction of the recurrence rate for vulvar warts has been reported by Reid et al. (76), who used 5-FU applications twice a week for up to 6 months after laser ablation.

Safety and Precaution

5-FU should not be used during pregnancy. Local side effects are common and often pronounced and may require regular and repetitive monitoring.

SURGERY

As with chemical therapy, surgical methods are based on the destruction of tissue and comprise scalpel surgery, the scissor-snip method, sharp curettage, electrosurgery, cryotherapy and laser therapy (34,79–81). Which of the different types of surgical approaches is used depends on the clinical picture and location of disease. Often, however, local traditions and the practice of individual physicians are more important.

Anesthesia

With the exception of the cervix, all surgical methods more or less require analgesia, which is mostly provided by local infiltration anesthesia or, when larger areas are afflicted, by general anesthesia. Recently, some progress has been achieved by a new local anesthetic cream containing lidocaine and prilocaine (EMLA, Astra Pharmaceuticals, AB, Södertälje, Sweden), which is valuable for reduction of pain produced by electrosurgery or CO_2 laser treatment of circumscribed vulvar or penile lesions. Its use is especially favorable in children suffering from genitoanal warts (82). Many physicians use EMLA cream as a premedication before using local infiltration anesthesia as a means of reducing the needle stick pain, in particular in anxious patients. Postoperative regimens comprise proper hygiene, coital rest, analgesics, baths, and creams.

Scissor Excision/Curettage

Simple excision is especially appropriate for limited disease and solitary or few small-sized genital, perianal, and intraanal warts and can usually be performed as outpatient treatment. Inpatient care and general anesthesia, however, may be more suitable when wart growth is massive and when patients are psychologically sensitive. For anal warts, referral to specialized proctoscopy units may be advantageous (80,81,83,84). Extensive wart proliferation on the foreskin sometimes may be managed best by circumcision rather than by topical application of cytotoxic drugs, which may be associated with risks of transient phimosis. Surgery is also suitable for removal of well-circumscribed papular lesions such as bowenoid papulosis. Infiltration of anesthesia into the affected skin area leads to separation and elevation of the lesions, which then can be easily removed individually using scissors, leaving islands of epithelium between treated areas. Bleeding is easily controlled by diathermy. Initially described by Thomson (80,81) to minimize posttreatment scarring (Figure 1), the method has subsequently been widely used (76,83–86). Warts are excised across the base, using fine-toothed dessecting forceps and pointed curved scissors, creating small elliptical skin deficits. Healing is usually excellent within 10 to 14 days, with minimal scar tissue formation, provided that destruction does not extend beyond the upper part of the reticular dermis.

The use of a sharp spoon curette, combined with electrocautery, leads to acceptable results against pedunculated or filiform warts of the perianal and inguinal areas, but is less suitable for warts of the prepuce, glans penis, introitus vaginae, vagina, cervix, or anus.

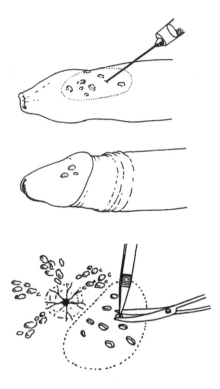

Figure 1 In circumscribed lesions, surgery is performed using infiltration anesthesia applied subepidermally. Separation of warts is achieved, and individual lesions can be removed by scissor-snip excision, curettage, electrocautery, or CO_2 laser. Infiltration anesthesia may be performed on the penile shaft, foreskin, and glans penis. Infiltration anesthesia of the perianal and the vulvar area is best performed with adrenalin as an adjuvant to promote hemostasis. Separation of individual warts will facilitate an accurate removal of the warts and sparing of uninvolved skin bridges. Application of EMLA cream before infiltration anesthesia helps minimize pain from the needle stick.

Electrosurgery/Loop Excision

Electrosurgery uses a generator, converting household current into high-frequency alternating current (500 Hz to 3.3 MHz), which is passed through a monopolar electrode to cut or coagulate tissue. The active electrode is either a fine wire loop for cutting ("electroresection") or needles and balls of different sizes for coagulation. Physical principles and various techniques are accounted for in further detail by Scoular (85). Electrosurgery can be used for both limited and extensive disease, widespread lesions, and recalcitrant anogenital warts, as well as exuberant growing giant condylomata acuminata. When required, loop resection can be combined with subsequent curettage or CO_2 laser therapy (84–86). Electrocautery also appears to be the surgical method of choice for intrameatal warts (87).

Loop excision is considered the treatment of choice for CIN (88), eliminating most problems raised by scalpel ("cold knife") and laser conization, such as postoperative bleeding for cold knife cone and high equipment costs for laser cone. Similarly to the CO_2 laser, the diathermy loop can cut and coagulate simultaneously, and the procedure is usually performed under local anesthesia, rendering the loop technique usable for outpatient treatment. The technique is associated with low recurrence rates (89) and a minimization of complications such as bleeding and stenosis (90). Furthermore, loop excision allows a thorough histological control of the entire transformation zone. Microscopic analysis of specimens removed by loop excision has shown that target biopsies taken before therapy usually tend to underestimate the true nature and extent of dysplastic cervical lesions by one or two degrees in about 10% of cases investigated (91). In lesions with an exocervical squamocolumnar junction, excision to a depth of 7 mm is sufficient, as this is the maximal depth of CIN within glandular tubes. CIN lesions extending onto the cervix or even to the vagina should be treated by laser. The same is true for CIN without detectable junctions in postmenopausal women. Because a loop excision deeper than 15 mm is rather difficult, in these patients laser or cold knife conization should preferentially be used.

Safety and Precautions

The disadvantage of both electrocoagulation and loop excision is the difficulty in knowing the extent of the warty tissue to be destroyed. Excessive coagulation may lead to fibrosis and scarring. A hazard is that of fire or explosion if electrosurgery is conducted in the presence of alcohol, oxygen, or bowel gases (methane). These problems also occur with CO_2 laser. Safety features in modern electrosurgery equipment prevent the delivery of dangerous amounts of electricity by the active electrode in cases of malfunction.

The use of disposable or sterilized electrodes is recommended to prevent transmission of virus by the electrode. As for CO_2 laser surgery, electrocoagulation generates smoke plume. As HPV DNA has been recovered from the smoke, a smoke evacuator is currently considered mandatory for both methods. Members of the treatment team should wear a surgical mask (34).

Cryotherapy

Cryotherapy, turning cellular water into intracellular ice crystals that leads to destruction of the cells (92), has a number of advantages. It is simple, inexpensive, well tolerated, and does not create any smoke. Liquid nitrogen, producing cold at $-196°C$, is applied as a spray directly to the lesion, or is applied by dipping cotton-tipped applicators into liquid nitrogen kept in a small thermos. Nitrous oxide gas, leading to cold at $-88°C$, is often used in closed systems where the gas is delivered through specially designed cryoprobe tips of varying sizes. Some probes are especially designed for therapy of portiocervical lesions. In general, most warts must be retreated at intervals of 1 to 3 weeks, and sometimes up to 10 or more sittings may be required. Nevertheless, according to Bashi (39) properly applied cryotherapy is certainly superior to podophyllin therapy against external warts.

A cure rate of about 70% and a recurrence rate of 21% to 40% has been reported (34,92). No significant differences exist between cryosurgery, laser surgery and electrocautery with regard to recurrence rates, which may be as high as 75% (86).

Giving treatment in the second half of pregnancy carries the risks of bleeding and secondary infections. Cryotherapy has its special niche as a safe and efficacious method to be used in pregnant women even during the last two trimesters (93,94). Cryotherapy is also useful for the treatment of CIN; complication rates are low and therapeutic success rates after refreezing persistent CIN lesions have been as high as 97% (95,96). Large lesions and CIN extending into the endocervical canal, however, respond less favorably. Also, as a slight risk of vasomotor symptoms and uterine cramps exist during long-lasting cryotherapy sessions, lesions >3 cm in diameter should not be treated by cryosurgery.

Safety and Precautions

Local anesthesia is necessary. Most patients experience varying degrees of pain after cryotherapy. The time required to final cure is rather long. After intensive cryosurgery, urtication, edema, and frequent blister formation can be expected. A profuse watery discharge, sometimes lasting up to 3 weeks, occurs in a high proportion of patients. The principle criticism to cryosurgery, however, is the lack of control of depth by destruction because removal of treated tissue is not visualized during treatment (95,96).

Laser Surgery

As an instrument for both cutting and vaporization, the CO_2 laser has a wide spectrum of applications. CO_2 lasers emit light energy at a wavelength of 10.600 nm, which superheats intracellular and extracellular water to 100°C, resulting in cellular evaporation. CO_2 lasers have become the method of choice against intraepithelial neoplasia (97) because of advantages such as precision, clean incisions, minimal tissue damage (especially to the surrounding tissue), minimal postoperative swelling, good hemostasis, fine scar formation, and rare occurrence of subsequent pain and wound secretions.

Equipment costs and mandatory safety requirements are disadvantages of CO_2 lasers. The main limitation of cryotherapy is lack of histological control, implying a potential incomplete destruction of and/or a missed diagnosis of early invasive cancer despite multiple pretherapy biopsies (34,97).

Coagulation depth can be controlled by power, spot size, and exposure time. A focused beam of 0.1 mm diameter penetrates into the tissue, enabling the laser to be used as a cutting instrument, whereas a defocused beam of up to 2 mm spot size only causes vaporization of superficial cell layers, with a coagulation zone of about 0.3 mm. Within this zone, vessels up to a diameter of 0.5 mm are sealed. A recently developed CO_2 laser operating principle, which enables ablation of surface ultrathin char-free epithelial layers, has been applied mainly against vulvar lesions (98). Neodymium (Nd:YAG) lasers, emitting a beam of 1060 mm that is less absorbed than visible light and penetrates more deeply (96) does not induce bleeding. Accordingly, Nd:YAG lasers are recommended for treatment of HIV-positive patients. Also, as the beam can be transmitted by specially designed flexible light-guidance systems, it can be used successfully in hollow spaces such as the urethra.

Intraepithelial neoplasia of the cervix extending into the stroma ≤5 mm is best treated with the CO_2 laser by evaporization, excisional biopsy, or a combination of both approaches (98,99) performed through colposcope or an operating microscope-guided instrument without anesthesia. Vaporization should be achieved down to a 5 to 7 mm depth to treat CIN in cervical glands. The advantages of excisional conization compared with electrocauterization are a rare occurrence of hemorrhage and postoperative stenosis (98,99). The cutting technique is especially favorable for removal of CIN lesions expanding into the endocervical canal and for early invasive carcinoma, when the procedure normally is performed in general anesthesia. Failure rates for destructive and excisional laser therapy ranges from 2% to 10% after one to three sittings. A follow-up period of at least 12 months is recommended. Laser surgery is superior to cryotherapy in treating cervical lesions >3 cm in diameter (34). CO_2 laser is also a good tool for the treatment of VIN, VAIN, and PIN, including bowenoid papulosis. Extensive disease, however, often requires multiple treatment courses and disagreeable discomfort for patients (34,97,98). Because of the risk of missing early invasive carcinoma in hair-bearing areas, surgical excision followed by suturing should be performed for severe dysplasia and for cases of Morbus Bowen and Queyrat's erythroplasia (34,100–105).

Safety and Precautions

Potential hazards associated with laser therapy in general refer primarily to injuries of the eye. Whereas CO_2 is more apt to damage the cornea, sclera or surrounding skin, the Nd:YAG laser can injure the retina. Eye protection using special protective lenses, therefore, is mandatory for patients, physicians, and personnel. As for electrosurgery, CO_2 laser surgery must be flanked by a smoke evacuator (106–108).

ADJUVANT INTERFERON ADMINISTRATION

Successful immune response to viral infections involves a complex cascade of events that include presentation of viral antigens to the immune system, proliferation of antigen-specific lymphocytes, and activation of a diverse array of cytokines. Viral infection of target cells normally causes the release of cytokines such as interferons (IFNs), tumor necrosis factor (TNF), interleukin I (IL-1), and others. IFN exerts potential antiviral, antiproliferative, and/or immunomodulatory effects. Recombinant IFN products contain single interferon subtypes. Natural products comprise interferon from pooled units of human leukocytes that have been induced by incomplete infection with avian Sendai virus (109).

Despite a number of optimistic open studies using IFN beta gels (34, 110,111), no beneficial effects have consistently been demonstrated from topical application as compared to placebo. Available preparations probably do not deliver adequate quantities of IFN to infected epidermal basal cell layers. Intralesional administration of IFNs was long favored as a promising approach; however, several studies demonstrate that limited beneficial effect occurs on noninjected lesions (112–117). Such treatment requires frequent visits and causes repetitive local pain, as multiple injections are required. Advantages over traditional ablative methods include lack of ulcerations and scarring. Intralesionally administered recombinant IFN alpha 2b[1] has recently been licensed in the United States by the Food and Drug Administration for treatment of genital warts. More newly developed leukocyte-derived interferon alpha-n3 may possibly be more efficacious than recombinant alpha-2b (109).

Placebo-controlled studies on parenteral IFN administration have also yielded controversial results (34,117). The most favorable approach comprises IFN administered as an adjuvant to surgical procedures (Table 8). In contrast to the disappointing effects of topical IFN used as single therapy, application of IFN beta hydrogel after destruction of the epithelial barrier by either CO_2 laser, electrocautery, or cryotherapy leads to lower recurrence rates as compared with patients receiving adjuvant IFN beta gel (40% versus 78%) (118). Although still somewhat controversial (119), adjuvant systemic IFN therapy seems to decrease recurrence rates (120–124). Subcutaneous injections of 1 MU IFN alpha 2a, given cyclically in three cycles consisting of 5 days of therapy with a 4-week interval between the cycles, seems favorable and well tolerated. The potential value of the noncontinuous cyclic therapy regimen is demonstrated in a study by Hohenleutner et al. (119) showing reduced recurrence rates by comparison of laser (81% cure) with two courses of 1MU IFN alpha 2b given subcutaneously daily for 6 days with a 2-week interval between the courses (42% cure without IFN). The combination of laser surgery and IFN appears to be superior (121) to that of laser followed by 5-FU administration (Table 9). Accordingly, in problem cases surgery should be followed by adjuvant IFN administration to break a vicious cycle or recalcitrance. Naturally, use of this approach requires a high degree of motivation and compliance by the patient.

Safety and Precautions

Side effects of IFNs are dose-dependent, the most common being flulike symptoms a few hours after administration. Mild leukopenia, thrombocytopenia, and temporary elevation of liver function tests may also occur.

---

[1] Intron A recombinant, and Alferon N Injection leucocyte derived 14 interferon-α subtypes = alpha-n3 (Schering Corp, Kenilworth, New Jersey).

Table 8 Influence of Adjuvant IFN on the Recurrence Rates of Condylomas

Ablative therapy	Recurrence rate no IFN	IFN	IFN type	Adminis-trative form	Study
Electrocautery	78%	40%	beta	topical	Gross (1990) (117)
CO_2 laser	81%	42%	alpha 2b	sc	Hohenleutner et al. (1990) (119)
CO_2 laser	38%	19%	alpha 2b	il	Vance and Davis (1990) (120)
CO_2 laser	77%	48%	alpha 2b	sc	Petersen et al. (1991) (121)
CO_2 laser	45%	21%	alpha 2b	il	Davis and Noble (1992) (122)
CO_2 laser	29%	35%	alpha 2a	sc	Cond. Internat Collabor. Study Group (1993) (123)

Table 9 Combination of Laser, 5-FU, and IFN

	Cure
• Laser alone	40%
• Laser + 5-FU	50%
• Laser + alpha 2b IFN sc × 3/week for 10 weeks	82%

From Ref. 124.

These side effects are well tolerated and last only for the first two to three treatments.

REFERENCES

1. Hippeläinen M, Syrjänen S, Koskela H, et al. Prevalence and risk factors of genital human papillomavirus (HPV) infections in healthy males: a study on Finnish conscripts. Sex Transm Dis 1993; 20: 321–328.
2. Koutsky LA, Wölner-Hanssen P. Genital papillomavirus infections: current knowledge and future prospects. Obstet Gynecol Clin North Am 1989; 16: 541–564.

3. Krogh von G. Genitoanal papillomavirus infection: diagnosis and therapeutic objectives in the light of current epidemiological observations. Int J STD AIDS 1991; 2: 391–404.
4. Schneider A, Kirchhoff T, Meinhardt G, Gissman L. Repeated evaluation of human papillomavirus 16 status in cervical swabs of young women with a history of normal Papanicolaou smears. Obstet Gynecol 1992; 79: 683–688.
5. Villiers de E-M, Wagner D, Schneider A, et al. Human papillomavirus DNA in women without and with cytological abnormalities: results of a 5-year follow-up study. Gynecol Oncol 1992; 44: 33–39.
6. Wheeler CM, Parmenter CA, Hunt WC, et al. Determinants of genital human papillomavirus infection among cytologically normal women attending the University of New Mexico student health care center. Sex Transm Dis 1993; 20: 286–289.
7. Syrjänen K, Syrjänen S. Epidemiology of human papillomavirus infections and genital neoplasia. Scand J Infect Dis 1990; 60: 7–17.
8. Rymark P, Forslund O, Hansson BG, Lindholm K. Genital HPV infection not a local but a regional infection. Genitourin Med 1993, 69: 18–22.
9. Wikström A, Hedblad M-A, Johansson B, et al. The acetic test in evaluation of subclinical genital papillomavirus infection: a comparative study on penoscopy, histopathology, viology and scanning electron microscopy findings. Genitourin Med 1992; 68: 90–99.
10. Wikström A, von Krogh G, Hedblad M-A, Syrjänen S. Papillomavirus-associated balanoposthitis. Genitourin Med 1994; 70: 175–181.
11. Crum CP, Nuovo GJ, eds. Genital Papillomaviruses and Related Neoplasms. New York: Raven Press, 1991.
12. Syrjänen KJ. Long-term consequences of genital HPV infections in women. Ann Med 1993; 24: 233–235.
13. Singer A, Ho L, Terry G, Sun Kwie T. Association of human papillomavirus with cervical cancer and precancer. In: Mindel A, ed. Genital Warts. Human Papillomavirus Infection. London, Boston, Melbourne, Auckland: Edward Arnold, 1995: 105–129.
14. Stanley MA, Chambers MA, Coleman N. Immunology of human papillomavirus infection. In: Mindel A, ed. Genital Warts. Human Papillomavirus Infection. London, Boston, Melbourne, Auckland: Edward Arnold, 1995: 252–270.
15. Benton C, Shahidullah H, Hunter JAA. Human papillomavirus in the immunosuppressed. Papillomavirus Report 1992; 3: 23.
16. Palefsky JM. Anal papillomavirus infection and anal cancer in HIV-positive individuals: an emerging problem. AIDS 1994; 8: 283–295.
17. Ho GYF, Burk RD, Fleming I, Klein RS. Risk of genital human papillomavirus infection in women with human immunodeficiency virus-induced immunosuppression. Int J Cancer 1994; 56: 788–792.
18. Ogunbiyi OA, Scholefield JH, Raftery AT, et al. Prevalence of anal human papillomavirus infection and intraepithelial neoplasia in renal allograft recipients. Br J Surg 1994; 81: 365–367.

19. Majewski S, Jablonska S. Epidermodysplasia verruciformis as a model of human papillomavirus-induced genetic cancers: the role of local immunosurveillance. Am J Med Sci 1992; 304: 174–182.
20. Bernard C, Mougin C, Lab M. New approaches to the understanding of the pathogenesis of human papillomavirus induced anogenital lesions. The role of co-factors and co-infection. J Eur Acad Dermatol Venereol 1994; 3: 237–244.
21. Mittal R, Tsutsumi K, Pater A, Pater M. Human papillomavirus type 16 expression in cervical keratinocytes: role of progesterone and glucocorticoid hormones. Obstet Gynecol 1993; 81: 5–12.
22. Kemp EA, Hakenewerth AM, Laurent SL, et al. Human papillomavirus prevalence in pregnancy. Obstet Gynecol 1992; 79: 649–656.
23. von Krogh G, Syrjänen SM, Syrjänen KJ. Advantage of human papillomavirus typing in the clinical evaluation of genitoanal warts. Experience with the in situ deoxyribonucleic acid hybridization technique applied on paraffin sections. J Am Acad Dermatol 1988; 18: 495–502.
24. Lassus J, Niemi KM, Syrjänen S, et al. A comparison of histopathologic diagnosis and the demonstration of human papillomavirus-specific DNA and proteins in penile warts. Sex Transm Dis 1992; 19: 127–132.
25. Voog E, Löwhagen G-B. Follow-up of men with genital papilloma virus infection. Acta Derm Venereol 1992; 72: 185–189.
26. Filiberti A, Tamburini A, Stefanon B, et al. Psychological aspects of genital human papillomavirus infection: a preliminary report. J Psychosom Gynaecol 1993; 14: 145–152.
27. American Social Health Association. Survey shows how we live with HPV. HPV News 1993; 3: 1–9.
28. Goodkin K, Antoni MH, Helder L, Sevin B. Psychoneuroimmunological aspects of disease progression among women with human papillomavirus-associated cervical dysplasia and human immunodeficiency virus type 1 co-infection. Int J Psychiatry Med 1993; 23: 119–148.
29. Krebs H-B, Helmkamp BF. Does the treatment of genital condylomata in men decrease the treatment failure rate of cervical dysplasia in the female sexual partner? Obstet Gynecol 1990; 76: 660–663.
30. Ward BG, Thomas H. Randomized prospective intervention study of human cervical wart virus infection. Aust NZ J Obstet Gynecol 1994; 34: 182–185.
31. American Academy of Dermatology Task Force on Pediatric Dermatology: Genital warts and sexual abuse in children. J Am Acad Dermatol 1984; 11: 529–530.
32. Lacey CJN. Genital warts in children. Papilloma Virus Report 1991; 2: 31–33.
33. Handley J, Dinsmore E, Maw R, et al. Anogenital warts in prepubertal children: sexual abuse or not? Int J STD AIDS 1993; 4: 271–279.
34. Gross G. Treatment of human papillomavirus infection. In: Mindel A, ed. Genital Warts Human papillomavirus infection. London, Boston, Melbourne, Auckland: Edward Arnold, 1995: 198–236.

35. von Krogh G, Wikström A. Efficacy of chemical and/or surgical therapy against condylomata acuminata: a retrospective evaluation. Int J STD AIDS 1991; 2: 333–338.

36. Genital human papillomavirus infections and cancer: memorandum from a WHO meeting. Bull WHO. 1987; 64: 817–827.

37. Kaplan JW. Condylomata acuminata. New Orleans Med 1942; 94: 388–390.

38. von Krogh G. Podophyllotoxin for condylomata acuminata eradication. Clinical and experimental comparative studies on Podophyllum lignans, colchicine and 5-Fluorouracil. Acta Derm Venereol (Suppl 98) 1981 (Thesis).

39. Bashi SA. Cryotherapy versus podophyllin in the treatment of genital warts. Int J Dermatol 1985; 24: 535–536.

40. Jensen SL. Comparison of podophyllin application with simple excision in clearance and recurrence of perianal condylomata acuminata. Lancet 1985; 2: 1146–1148.

41. Lassus A. Comparison of podophyllotoxin and podophyllin in treatment of genital warts. Lancet 1987; 2: 512–513.

42. Mazurkiewicz W, Jablonska S. Comparison between the therapeutic efficacy of 0.5% podophyllotoxin preparation and 20% podophyllin ethanol solution in condylomata acuminata. Z Hautkr 1986; 61: 1387–1395.

43. Edwards A, Atma-Ram A, Thin RN. Podophyllotoxin 0.5 versus podophyllin 20% to treat penile warts. Genitourin Med 1988; 64: 263–265.

44. Mazurkiewicz W, Jablonska S. Clinical efficacy of condyline (0.5% podophyllotoxin) solution and cream versus podophyllin in the treatment of external condylomata acuminata. J Derm Treat 1990; 1: 123–125.

45. von Krogh G. Topical treatment of HPV lesions of the external genitalia. The Cervix 1992; 10: 125–131.

46. Cassidy DE, Drewry J, Fanning JP. Podophyllum toxicity: a review of a fatal case and a review of the literature. J Toxicol Clin Toxicol 1982; 19: 35–44.

47. Filley CM, Graff-Radford NR, Lacy R, et al. Neurological manifestations of podophyllin toxicity. Neurology 1982; 32: 308–311.

48. von Krogh G. Podophyllotoxin in serum: absorption subsequent to three-day repeated application of a 0.5% ethanolic preparation on condylomata acuminata. Sex Transm Dis 1982; 9: 26–33.

49. West WM, Ridgeway NA, Morris AJ, Sides PJ. Fatal podophyllin ingestion. South Med J 1982; 75: 1269–1270.

50. Sand Peterson C, Weissmann K. Quercentin and Kaempherol: an argument against the use of podophyllin? Geniturin Med 1995; 71: 92–93.

51. Cairney M, Campo MS. The synergism between bovine papillomavirus type 4 and quercetin is dependent on the timing of exposure. Carcinogenis 1995; 16: 1997–2001.

52. Mansono-Martinez R. Podophyllotoxin poisoning of microtubules of steady-state. Effect of substoichiometric and superstoichiometric concentrations of the drug. Mol Cell Biochem 1982; 45: 3–11.

53. von Krogh G. Penile condylomata acuminata: an experimental model for evaluation of topical treatment with 0.5%-1.0% ethanolic preparations of podophyllotoxin for three days. Sex Transm Dis 1981; 8: 179–186.
54. Kraus SJ, Stone KM. Management of genital infection caused by human papillomaviruses. Rev Infect Dis 1990; 12(suppl 6): S620–663.
55. Mohanty KC. The cost effectiveness of treatment of genital warts with podophyllotoxin. Int J STD AIDS 1994; 5: 253–256.
56. Loike JD, Horowitz SB. Effects of podophyllotoxin and VP-16-213 on microtubule assembly in vitro and nucleoside transport in HeLa cells. Biochemistry 1976; 15: 5435–5442.
57. von Krogh G, Maibach HI. Cutaneous cytodestructive potency of lignans. I. A comparative evaluation of influence on epidermal and dermal DNA synthesis and on dermal microcirculation in the hairless mouse. Arch Dermatol Res 1982; 274: 9–20.
58. von Krogh G, Maibach HI. Cutaneous cytodestructive potency of lignans. II. A comparative evaluation of macroscopic-toxic influence on rabbit skin subsequent to repeated 10-day applications. Dermatologica 1983; 167: 70–77.
59. Sullivan M, King L. Effects of resin of podophyllin on normal skin, condylomata acuminata and verrucae vulgares. Arch Dermatol Syph 1947; 56: 30–32.
60. Pickering RW. The treatment of condylomata acuminata—results of a questionnaire survey. Br J Sex Med 1989: 210–213.
61. Beutner KR, Conant MA, Friedman-Kien A. Patient-applied podofilox for treatment of genital warts. Lancet 1989; 1: 831–834.
62. Kirby P, Dunne A, King DH, Corey L. Double-blind randomized clinical trial of self-administered podofilox solution vehicle in the treatment of genital warts. Am J Med 1990; 88: 465–469.
63. Beutner KR, von Krogh G. Current status of podophyllotoxin for the treatment of genital warts. Semin Dermatol 1990; 9: 148–151.
64. Ljunghall K. Podophyllotoxin for treatment of genital warts in females. In: von Krogh G, Rylander E, eds. Genital Papilloma Virus Infection. A Survey for the Clinician. Karlstad Sweden: Conpharm AB, 1989: 127–177.
65. von Krogh G, Szpak E, Andersson M, Bergelin I. Self-treatment using 0.25%-0.5% podophyllotoxin ethanol solutions against penil condylomata acuminata: a placebo-controlled comparative study. Genitourin Med 1994; 70: 105–109.
66. von Krogh G, Hellberg D. Self-treatment using a 0.5% podophyllotoxin cream of external genital condylomata acuminata in women. A placebo controlled double-blind study. Sex Transm Dis 1992, 19: 170–174.
67. Hellberg D, Svarrer T, Nilsson S, Valentin J. Self-treatment of female external warts with 0.5% podophyllotoxin cream (Condyline®) vs weekly application of 20% podophyllin solution. Int J STD AIDS 1995; 6: 257–261.
68. von Krogh G, Rosén B. Wartec Cream Clinical Expert Report (Conpharm AB, Glunten, 751 83 Uppsala). Unpublished Manuscript.
69. Strand A, Brinkeborn R-M, Siboulet A. Topical treatment of genital warts in men, an open study of podophyllotoxin cream compared with solution. Genitourin Med 1995; 71: 387–390.

70. Malvija VK, Deppe G, Pluszczynski R, Boike G. Trichloracetic acid in the treatment of human papillomavirus infection of the cervix without associated dysplasia. Obstet Gynecol 1987; 70: 72–74.
71. von Krogh G. 5-Fluoro-uracil cream in the successful treatment of therapeutically refractory condylomata acuminata of the urinary meatus. Acta Derm Venereol 1976; 56: 297–300.
72. Ferenczy A. Comparison of 5-Fluoro-uracil and CO_2 laser for treatment of vaginal condylomata. Obstet Gynecol 1984; 64: 773–778.
73. Krebs HB. Treatment of extensive condylomata acuminata with topical 5-fluorouracil. South Med J 1990; 83: 761–764.
74. Pride GL. Treatment of large lower genital tract condylomata acuminata with topical 5-fluorouracil. J Reprod Med 1990; 35: 384–387.
75. Krebs HB. Prophylactic topical 5-fluorouracil following treatment of human papillomavirus-associated lesions of the vulva and vagina. Obstet Gynecol 1986; 68: 837–841.
76. Reid R, Greenberg MD, Lorincz AT, et al. Superficial laser vaporization and adjunctive 5-fluorouracil therapy of human papillomavirus-associated vulvar disease. Obstet Gynecol 1990; 76: 439–448.
77. Cetti NE. Condyloma acuminatum of the urethra: problems in eradication. Br J Surg 1984; 71: 57.
78. Wein AJ, Benson GS. Treatment of urethral condylomata acuminata with 5-FU cream. J Urol 1977; 9: 413–415.
79. Handley J, Dinsmore W. Treatment of anogenital warts. J Eur Acad Dermatol Venerol 1994; 3: 251–265.
80. Thompson JP. Perianal and anal condylomata acuminata. In: Todd IP, ed. Operative Surgery Colon Rectum and Anus. London: Butterworths, 1977: 376–377.
81. Thomson JPS, Grace RH. The treatment of perianal and anal condyloma acuminata: a new operative technique. J R Soc Med 1978; 71: 180–185.
82. Rylander E, Sjöberg I, Lilleborg S. Local anaesthesia of the genital mucosa with a lidocaine/prilocaine cream (EMLA®) for laser treatment of condylomata acuminata. A placebo-controlled study. Obstet Gynecol 1990; 75: 302–306.
83. Samenius B. Perianal and ano-rectal condyloma acuminata. Schweiz Rundsch Med Prac 1983; 72: 1009–1014.
84. McMillan A, Scott GR. Outpatient treatment of perianal warts by scissor excision. Genitourin Med 1987; 63: 114–115.
85. Scoular A. Choosing equipment for treating genital warts in genitourinary medicine clinics. Genitourin Med 1991; 67: 413–419.
86. Luchtfedl MA. Perianal condylomata acuminata. Surg Clin North Am 1994; 74: 1327–1338.
87. McKenna JG, McMillan A. Management of intrameatal warts in men. Int J STD AIDS 1990; 1: 259–263.
88. Wright TC, Ganon S, Richart R, et al. Treatment of CIN using the loop surgical excision procedure. Obstet Gynecol 1992; 79: 173–178.

89. Prendiville W, Cullimore J, Norman S. Large loop excision of the transformation zone (LETZ). A method of management for women with cervical intraepithelial neoplasia. Br J Obstet Gynecol 1989; 96: 1055–1060.
90. Luesley DM, Cullimore J, Redman CWE. Loop diathermy excision of the cervical transformation zone in patients with abnormal cervical smears. Br Med J 1990; 300: 1690–1693.
91. Wright TC, Richart RM, Ferenczy A. Comparison of specimens removed by CO2 laser conisation and the loop electrosurgical excision procedure. Obstet Gynecol 1992; 79: 147–153.
92. Torre D, In Zacarian SA, ed. Instrumentation and Monitoring Devices in Cryosurgery. Cryosurgery for Skin Cancer and Cutaneous Disorders. St Louis: Mosby, 1985: 31–40.
93. Bergman A, Matsunaga J, Bhatia NN. Cervical cryotherapy for condylomata acuminata during pregnancy. Obstet Gynecol 1987; 69: 47–50.
94. Matsunaga J, Bergman A, Bhatia NN. Genital condylomata acuminata in pregnancy: effectiveness, safety and pregnancy outcome following cryotherapy. Br J Obstet Gynecol 1987; 94: 168–172.
95. Ferenczy A. Comparison of cryo- and carbon dioxide laser therapy for cervical intraepithelial neoplasia. Obstet Gynecol 1985; 66: 793–797.
96. Ferenczy A. Epidemiology and clinical pathophysiology of condylomata acuminata. Am J Obstet Gynecol 1995; 172: 1331–1339.
97. Baggish MS. Improved laser techniques for the elimination of genital and extragenital warts. Am J Obstet Gynecol 1985; 153: 545–550.
98. Levavi H, Ovadia J. Swift lase scanner—a new modality in laser treatment of the vulva: effect on postoperative pain. Presented at the 8th World Congress of Cervical Pathology and Colposcopy, Chicago, May 1993.
99. Anderson MC, Hartley RB. Cervical crypt involvement by intraepithelial neoplasia. Obstet Gynecol 1980; 55: 546–550.
100. Larsson G, Alm P, Grundsell H. Laser conization versus cold knife conization. Surg Gynecol Obstet 1982; 154: 59–62.
101. Townsend DE, Levine RU, Crum DP, Richart RM. Treatment of vaginal carcinoma in situ with the carbon dioxide laser. Am J Obstet Gynecol 1982; 143: 546–547.
102. Baggish MS, Dorsey JH. Carbon dioxide laser for combination excisional-vaporization conization. Am J Obstet Gynecol 1985; 151: 23–27.
103. Stanhope CR, Phibbs GD, Stuart GC, Reid R. Carbon dioxide laser surgery. Obstet Gynecol 1983; 61: 624–647.
104. Landthaler M, Haina D, Brunner R, et al. Laser therapy of bowenoid papulosis and Bowen's disease. J Derm Surg Oncol 1986; 12: 1253–1257.
105. Ferenczy A. Laser therapy of genital condylomata acuminata. Obstet Gynecol 1984; 63: 703–707.
106. Garden JM, O'Banion MK, Shelnitz LS, et al. Papillomavirus in the vapor of carbondioxide laser-treated verrucae. JAMA 1988; 259: 1199–1202.

107. Abrahamson AL, Dilorenzo TP, Steinberg BM. Is papillomavirus detectable in the plume of laser-treated laryngeal papilloma? Arch Otolaryngol Head Neck Surg 1990; 116: 604–607.
108. Ferenczy A, Bergeron C. Richart RM. Human papillomavirus DNA in CO_2-laser-generated plume of smoke and its consequences to sugeon. Obstet Gynecol 1990; 75: 114–118.
109. Friedman-Kien A. Management of condylomata acuminata with Alferon N injection, interferon alpha-N3 (human leucyte derived). Am J Obstet Gynecol 1995; 172: 1359–1368.
110. Vesterinen E, Meyer B, Cantell K, et al. Topical treatment of flat vaginal condyloma with human leukocyte interferon. Obstet Gynecol 1984; 64: 535–538.
111. Keay S, Teng N, Eisenberg M, et al. Topical interferon for treating condylomata acuminata in women. J Infect Dis 1988; 185: 934–939.
112. Eron LJ, Judson F, Tucker S, et al. Interferon therapy for condylomata acuminata. N Engl J Med 1986; 315: 1059–1069.
113. Vance JC, Bart BJ, Hausen PC, et al. Intralesional recombinant alpha-2 interferon for the treatment of patients with condylomata acuminatum or verruca plantaris. Arch Dermatol 1986; 122: 272–277.
114. Frideman-Kien A, Eron LJ, Conant M, et al. Natural interferon alfa for treatment of condylomata acuminata. JAMA 1988; 259: 533–538.
115. Reichmann RC, Oakes D, Bonnez W, et al. Treatment of condyloma acuminatum with three different interferons administered intralesionally. A double-blind placebo-controlled trial. Ann Int Med 1988; 108: 675–679.
116. Welander LE, Homesley HD, Smiles KA, Peets EA. Intralesional interferon alfa-2b for the treatment of genital warts. Am J Obstet Gynecol 1990; 162: 348–354.
117. Gross G. Interferons in genital HPV disease. In: Gross G, Jablonska S, Pfister H, Stegner HE, eds. Genital Papillomavirus Infections. Berlin, Heidelberg, New York: Springer-Verlag, 1990: 393–412.
118. Eron LJ, Alder MB, O'Rourke JM, et al. Recurrence of condylomata acuminata following cryotherapy is not prevented by systemically administered interferon. Genitourin Med 1993; 69: 91–93.
119. Hohenleutner U, Landthaler U, Braun-Falco O. Postoperative adjuvante Therapie mit Interferon-Alfa-2b nach Laserchirurgie von Condylomata acuminata. Hautarzt. 1990; 41: 545–548.
120. Vance JC, Davis D. Interferon alpha-2b injections used as an adjuvant therapy to carbon dioxide laser vaporization of recalcitrant anogenital condylomata acuminata. J Invest Dermatol 1990; 955: 146–148.
121. Petersen CS, Bjerring P, Larsen J, et al. Systemic interferon alpha-2b increases the cure rate in laser-treated patients with multiple persistent genital warts: a placebo-controlled study. Genitourin Med 1991; 67: 99–102.
122. Davis BE, Noble MJ. Initial experience with combined interferon alpha and carbon dioxide laser for the treatment of condylomata acuminata. J Urol 1992; 197: 627–629.

123. The Condylomata International Collaborative Study Group. Randomized placebo-controlled double-blind combined therapy with laser surgery and systemic interferon-alpha 2a in the treatment of anogenital condylomata acuminata. J Infect Dis 1993; 167: 824–829.
124. Reid R, Greenberg MD, Petzzuti DJ, et al. Superficial laser vulvectomy V. Surgical debulking is enhanced by adjuvant systemic interferon. Am J Obstet Gynecol 1992; 166: 815–820.

26
Herpes Simplex Virus Vaccines

David I. Bernstein
Children's Hospital Medical Center, Cincinnati, Ohio

BACKGROUND

Herpes simplex virus (HSV) infections are extremely common throughout the world (1), and studies evaluating vaccines date back to the 1920s (2). Since then, there have been many attempts to prepare a safe and effective vaccine. Earliest trials used whole virus preparations inactivated by ultraviolet light, heat, or chemicals or were based on the erroneous assumption that cross protection could be achieved by vaccination with vaccinia (reviewed in 3). More recently, advances in molecular biology have allowed the development of newer, safer vaccines.

This chapter outlines the goals for an HSV vaccine and relates them to the pathophysiology of HSV disease. Various vaccine strategies are presented, with an emphasis on subunit glycoprotein vaccines, as these are the furthest along in development. Both prophylactic and therapeutic vaccines are discussed.

GOALS

The goals for an HSV vaccines are different than those applied to other commonly used vaccines because the main concern for HSV disease is not the acute episode, but the recurrent nature of the infection (Table 1). A prophylactic vaccine, therefore, should not only reduce or eliminate the acute disease produced by initial infection, but also prevent or reduce the establishment of latent virus, the source for recurrent episodes. The

Table 1 Goals for HSV Vaccines

Prophylactic Vaccine
- Prevent acute clinical disease
- Prevent infection
- Prevent or reduce establishment of latency
- Prevent or reduce subsequent recurrences
  (symptomatic and asymptomatic)

Therapeutic Vaccine
- Reduce clinical recurrences
- Reduce viral shedding

Committee on Issues and Promotion for New Vaccine Development of the National Academy of Sciences of the USA suggested that a successful vaccine should provide a 50% reduction in the number of symptomatic primary infections, with an approximate 60% reduction in the severity of disease and a 75% reduction in the number of recurrences (4).

The immunity produced by a successful vaccine could alter the course of an HSV infection in a number of targets (Figure 1). If the immune system can eliminate the initial infection that occurs at the skin or mucous membrane, then the acute disease will be prevented and virus will not enter the nerves and reach the dorsal root ganglia, the site of latency. This is the most difficult goal for a vaccine to achieve, as protection of mucosal surfaces is notoriously hard to achieve. It may be necessary for a vaccine to induce mucosal immunity for a vaccine to be active against this initial replication.

A second site that is often overlooked is preventing virus from entering the nerve. Because the virus most likely becomes extracellular at this point, it presents an opportunity for the immune system to neutralize the virus. If virus does not enter the nerve, the acute disease will be reduced because most of the lesions develop from virus completing the neural arc (i.e., returning from the dorsal root ganglia). Further, the number of latently infected neurons will also be reduced, as virus will not reach the dorsal root ganglia. For a vaccine to be active at this site may also require the induction of local (mucosal) immunity.

Vaccine-induced immunity could also work at the level of the ganglia by reducing the virus replication that occurs in neurons and/or supporting cells. This could also reduce the amount of virus that is available to return to the skin to form lesions or to become latent.

Virus exiting the neurons to form lesions also presents a likely target.

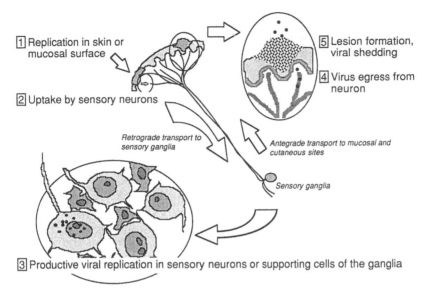

1 Replication in skin or mucosal surface

2 Uptake by sensory neurons

5 Lesion formation, viral shedding

4 Virus egress from neuron

Retrograde transport to sensory ganglia

Antegrade transport to mucosal and cutaneous sites

Sensory ganglia

3 Productive viral replication in sensory neurons or supporting cells of the ganglia

Figure 1 Pathogenesis of HSV infection. The five possible intervention points for an HSV vaccine are illustrated.

The immune system could intervene and prevent or reduce the number of lesions forming by eliminating virus before infection of the skin or reducing the magnitude of replication after. If the initial replication at the skin or mucosal surface boosts vaccine-induced immunity, which is only effective at this last site, it may be that only the acute disease is affected, but not the magnitude of latent virus. Therefore, the natural history of recurrences may not be altered.

The goals of a therapeutic vaccine—that is, a vaccine given to a patient with recurrent genital herpes in an attempt to boost immunity and decrease recurrences—are different (Table 1). A therapeutic vaccine, therefore, may need to induce or boost different immune functions than a prophylactic vaccine because the mechanisms for prevention of the initial infection are likely different from the ones responsible for controlling recurrent disease. A therapeutic vaccine could induce or enhance immune mechanisms that will eliminate or reduce viral replication in the ganglia after reactivation, or prevent or reduce viral replication after egress from the nerves as described previously. Thus, the goals of an immunotherapeutic vaccine are to decrease viral replication and the development of recurrent lesions. A therapeutic vaccine should reduce both recurrent disease and asymptomatic viral shedding. A vaccine that converted symptomatic disease to asymptomatic shedding might only increase the pool of individuals that unwittingly spread HSV.

VACCINE STRATEGIES

Viral vaccines, including HSV vaccines, have historically been divided into live (replicating) or killed (nonreplicating) vaccines (Table 2). Killed vaccines are often considered safer, but live vaccines more closely mimic natural disease and are more likely to induce long-lasting protection and especially cytolytic T-cell (CTL) responses. Recombinant DNA technology has extended the possible approaches to vaccine development to include cloned subunit vaccines, genetically engineered viral and bacterial vectors, and nucleic acid–based vaccines.

Killed Virus Vaccines

The traditional approach, using inactivated vaccines that contain crude or purified proteins derived from virus-infected cells, has several shortcoming for an HSV vaccine. There are difficulties in providing consistent concentrations of the important immunogens, problems of ensuring complete inactivation and eliminating contaminating viral DNA that may be potentially oncogenic, as well as the problem of cost. Subsequent vaccine

Table 2 Types of HSV Vaccines

Nonreplicating
1) Killed virus
      whole or subunit
2) Subunit vaccines
      purified
      genetically engineered
Replicating
1) Live attenuated
2) Live vectored
      -vaccinia
      -adenovirus
      -salmonella
      -varicella
3) Replication incompetent
4) Genetic immunization

strategies applied to HSV vaccines attempted to purify the protein of interest, creating subunit vaccines (5,6). This approach has been largely supplanted by newer techniques in molecular biology whereby the genes encoding the protein of interest are cloned, expressed, and purified, thereby overcoming the disadvantages listed previously.

Much of the research evaluating subunit vaccines has centered on the use of the HSV glycoproteins as immunogens. The glycoproteins of HSV, especially glycoproteins B and D (gB and gD), are attractive choices because they are targets for both humoral (neutralizing and antibody-dependent cell-medicated cytotoxicity (ADCC)) and cell-mediated immunity (class I and class II restricted). Both proteins also have a high degree of identity comparing HSV-1 and HSV-2 and, therefore, may provide protection against both HSV-1 and HSV-2. Further, there is an even higher degree of conservation between strains of the same type. Both animal and human trials evaluating these vaccines are discussed later in the chapter.

Replicating (Live) Viral Vaccines

The use of live viral vaccines offers certain advantages over killed or subunit vaccines, as well as disadvantages relating largely to the problems of safety. Approaches to immunization with live virus include the use of live attenuated (avirulent) HSV vaccines, live viral or bacterial vectors expressing HSV proteins, replication-defective viruses, and, although not really a live vaccine, genetic immunization (Table 2). The latter is included because, although not a live vaccine, the protein encoded is produced within a cell over a long time.

Live Attenuated Vaccines

Live attenuated HSV vaccines have been developed and tested in animal models by several groups (7–9). The approach is based on defining and eliminating genes involved in neurovirulence, latency, or reactivation (10). This work originally centered on the thymidase kinase (Tk) gene and more recently γ-34.5. The vaccine candidates furthest along were developed by Roizman et al. (10). The original candidates, R7017 and R7020, were derived from HSV-1 strain F (8,9). Both contain a deletion of the Tk gene and a second deletion in the junction region of UL and US in order to excise some of the genes responsible for neurovirulence. A segment from the HSV-2 genome encoding gD, gG, and gI was then inserted. For R7020 a Tk gene was reinserted. This candidate was considerably attenuated in animal models, including Aotus monkeys, and was also protective (8,9). In small phase I studies, this candidate was poorly immunogenic and appears to be overly attenuated (11).

More recently, this group and others have presented data on a more specific deletion, a γ 34.5 deletion mutant (12–14). This gene is believed to play a role in neurovirulence. This deletion appears to decrease the virulence of HSV and has decreased, but perhaps not eliminated, the ability of the virus to become latent and reactivate (12,14,15). Human trials for the vaccine may begin shortly (personal communication, Richard Whitley).

Live Vectors

Several groups have explored the possibility of using live viral and bacterial vectors to express HSV proteins (Table 2). In animal models, vaccinia, adenovirus, and varicella-expressing HSV glycoproteins have been shown to be protective (16–20). Although vaccinia is a potentially useful vector, it is unclear whether it will ever be acceptable as a vaccine candidate. Both salmonella and adenovirus have an advantage in that they could be given at a mucosal site and, therefore, induce mucosal immunity. Varicella has an advantage because it is already a licensed vaccine.

Replication Incompetent Viruses

This approach is intriguing because it combines some of the advantages of live and killed vaccines. These vaccines contain a mutation in an essential gene, that is, one required for replication (21–23). The vaccine virus is grown in a helper cell line that constitutively expresses the gene encoding this protein; thus the vaccine virus is infectious. Progeny viruses, however, cannot produce this protein and are not infectious. In other words, the virus can only undergo a simple round of replication. The leading candidate in this field is a gH-deleted mutant. The question remains, however, whether this single round can induce protective immune responses.

Genetic Immunization

The newest innovation in vaccine development is genetic immunization. It has recently been shown that direct inoculation of DNA or RNA encoding a protein leads to production of that protein and the induction of an immune response (24). Because the protein is made internally and is produced over an extended period, it offers some of the benefits of live vector immunization without concerns for attenuation.

This work has recently been extended to HSV in several laboratories (25,26). We have shown in guinea pigs and mice that inoculation of a plasmid encoding the gD2 protein under the promoter of an immediate early gene of cytomegalovirus (CMV) is immunogenic and protects mice and guinea pigs following intravaginal challenge (26, unpublished). In guinea pigs, three immunizations of 50 to 250 μg of DNA decreased the number of animals developing acute disease, the severity of the disease, and vaginal viral replication (26). In addition, fewer vaccinated animals developed recurrences, and those that did had a reduced number of recurrent lesion days.

ANIMAL AND HUMAN EVALUATIONS OF SUBUNIT VACCINES

Subunit vaccines are the furthest along in development and, therefore, are discussed in some detail. In the initial animal trials, we and others showed that subunit vaccines either purified as glycoprotein preparations or cloned and expressed in bacteria, yeast, baculovirus, or mammalian cells were protective (27–30). The initial approach using gD-expressed in *Escherichia coli* (31) was improved by the insertion of truncated viral genes into mammalian expressing vectors engineered so that the anchor portion of the protein was deleted (32). In this way, mammalian cells synthesize a glycosylated HSV glycoprotein that is secreted. Both subunit vaccines currently in large human trials have been developed using expression in Chinese hamster ovary (CHO) cells.

Animal Trials

We performed initial animal experiences to evaluate the potential of a subunit vaccine to achieve the goals previously outlined. We used the guinea pig model of genital herpes because after intravaginal inoculation of HSV-2, the disease that develops closely mimics human disease (33). Animals develop a self-limited vesiculoulcerative acute disease, which resolves by 14 days after inoculation and is followed by the development of spontaneous recurrences. Thus, using the guinea pig model of genital herpes, the assessment of the incidence, and severity of the acute disease, vaginal viral replication and the incidence and magnitude of recurrent genital disease and latency can be measured.

In our initial studies, we showed that cloned HSV-1 glycoprotein, either gD1 expressed in yeast or gB1 expressed in CHO cells supplied by Chiron Corporation, provided protection similar to that of a mixture of glycoproteins purified by lentil lectin chromatography (27). The incidence and severity of the acute disease, vaginal viral replication, and recurrent disease were all decreased. Later, Berman et al. (29) showed a decrease in latent infection, thus providing evidence that these vaccines could achieve all the goals discussed for an HSV vaccine. Later, experiments demonstrated the importance of maintaining the natural protein conformation, adjuvants, and the increased protection afforded by homotypic vs heterotypic (HSV-1 vs HSV-2) protection (28,29,34,35).

The results of an experiment demonstrating this protection with another vaccine currently in human trials (SmithKline Beecham, Rixensart, Belgium) is shown in Table 3. Guinea pigs received 5 µg of gD2 + alum or alum monophosphoryl lipid A (MPL) by subcutaneous injection 99, 64, and 15 days before intravaginal challenge with either HSV-1 or HSV-2. Vaccination decreased the acute and recurrent disease, as well as viral replication, but not the incidence of infection as assessed by isolation of HSV from the vagina. Interestingly, the only major difference seen with the addition of MPL was a decrease in the number of animals with recurrent HSV-2 disease.

Human Trials

In 1986, Mertz et al. performed an evaluation of a Merck, Sharp & Dohme vaccine (36). This was the first well-designed, placebo-controlled study using the experimental design now being used in two other large trials;

Table 3 Effects of Vaccination on Either HSV-1 or HSV-2 Vaginal Challenge

Vaccine	HSV-1 Challenge		Peak viral titers[a]	Animals with recurrence	Recurrent lesion days[b]
	Acute disease	Viral shedding			
None	10/12	12/12	6.7	7/14	2.1
gD2 + alum	0/8	8/15	4.6	1/8	1.0
gD + alum MPL	0/12	12/15	3.8	1/12	1.0
	HSV-2 Challenge				
None	10/12	12/12	7.7	3/5	10.7
gD + alum	1/15	15/15	5.8	9/15	3.6
gD + alum MPL	1/15	13/15	4.0	1/13	4.0

[a]Viral titers measured as geometric mean $\log_{10}$ from vaginal swabs.
[b]Number of days with recurrent lesions in those animals developing recurrences.

that is, discordant couples where one has genital HSV-2 disease and one is seronegative for HSV-2. Subjects received 50 µg of lectin purified HSV-2 glycoprotein plus alum at 0, 4, and 22 weeks. The results of this trial showed that the vaccine was ineffective, with HSV infection documented in 9/82 (11%) vaccine recipients vs 5/70 (7%) control subjects. This lack of effect, however, could be explained by the poor immunogenicity of the vaccine preparation used. In initially seronegative vaccines, antibody titers to gB and gD were one-third to less than one-twentieth of the titer of HSV-infected individuals. Further, antibody failed to persist and by 12 months was undetectable in the majority of vaccinees.

Two large trials of subunit HSV vaccines are either recently completed or underway. Chiron Corporation is conducting two large trials using either discordant couples as discussed previously or subjects with multiple partners. The vaccine consists of 30 µg each of cloned gB2 and gD2 derived from CHO cells with MF59, a squalene adjuvant. Subjects are immunized at 0, 1, and 6 months. This vaccine preparation was recently shown to be safe and highly immunogenic (37,38).

The neutralizing titers to HSV-2 described by Langenberg et al. (38) are shown in Figure 2. In seronegative subjects, neutralizing titers to HSV-2 were detected at or above the medium titer of HSV-2 infected patients (133) in 18 of 25 (72%) subjects after three immunizations. Neutralizing titers remained detectable (>1:12) in 20 of 23 patients (87%) at 1 year. In HSV-1 seropositive subjects, titers rose rapidly after the first dose and were ≥133 in 93% of subjects. Titers decreased by 37% at 1 year. Similarly, high antibody titers to gB2 and gD2 were achieved after three immunizations in seronegative subjects. gB2 titers of at least 3600 and gD2 titers of at least 1200 (the mean serum titer of HSV-2 infected patients) were detected in 21 of 23 (91%) of subjects. Among HSV-1 seropositive subjects, one immunization produced large increases in gB2 and gD2 titers that were three to five times higher than those with naturally acquired HSV-2 infection.

The ability of the vaccine to elicit cell-mediated immune response was also evaluated by assessing the number of T cells per million peripheral blood mononuclear cells (PBMC) that responded to gB2 or gD2. Before vaccination, few if any cells were detected in seronegative subjects. After the third dose of vaccine, a precursor frequency of 31.6 to gD and 26.0 to gB per million PBMC was detected. This compares favorably with that found following natural HSV-2 infection 34.1 and 12.9, respectively.

The second large trial is being conducted by SmithKline Beecham in discordant couples. Subject receive 20 µg of cloned gD2 expressed from CHO cells. The adjuvant is alum MPL (monophosphoryl lipid A). Subjects

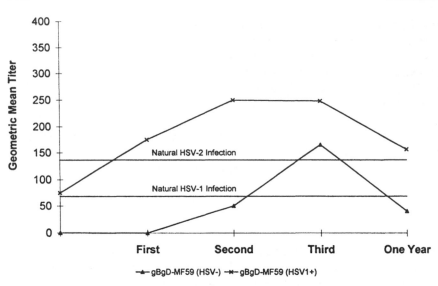

Figure 2 Neutralizing antibody titers in subjects receiving cloned HSV-2 glycoproteins B and D (gB and gD) vaccine. Subjects were either HSV seronegative (negative for both HSV-1 and HSV-2 antibody) or HSV-1 seropositive (positive for HSV-1 but negative for HSV-2 antibody). They were immunized at 0, 1, and 6 months with 30 µg each of gB and gD. The antibody titers are compared to the mean of subjects with natural HSV-1 or HSV-2 infections (Ref. 38.).

receive three doses of vaccine or adjuvant alone at 0, 1, and 6 months. In preliminary studies, this vaccine was immunogenic and, like the Chiron vaccine, produced titers similar to natural infection (39,40, unreported). In preliminary evaluations, neutralizing titers in seronegative HSV subjects were slightly greater than natural HSV infection. Titers in patients with previous HSV infection rose rapidly and achieved levels that were over twice the mean of preimmunization titers. Similarly, gD2 titers in seronegative recipients were greater than in HSV-infected patients, whereas gD2 titers rose rapidly in HSV-1 seropositive subjects. The ability of this vaccine to induce cell-mediated immunity was shown by the ability of lymphocytes from previously immunized subjects to recognize gD, proliferate, and produce IL-2 and γ interferon.

The results from the vaccine studies using these two vaccines are anxiously awaited. The improved immunogenicity of these preparations compared to previous vaccines offers great hope that an effective formulation will be developed. It is still clear, however, what proteins should be included to induce maximum humoral and cell-mediated immunity or what adjuvant will prove the most beneficial.

IMMUNOTHERAPY

The idea that immunization of patients with frequently recurring herpes infection could boost immunity and reduce recurrence has a long history. Previous attempts have included the nonspecific stimulation of the immune system by live vectors such as vaccinia or bacille Calmette-Guérin (BCG) (41–44), augmentation of the hosts immunity by autoinoculation with the subject's own strain (45,46), and specific enhancement of host immunity using inactivated HSV vaccines (47,48). Most early studies were poorly designed and produced uninterpretable results (49).

More recently, we and others have used the guinea pig model to test the concept that HSV immunization could reduce recurrences (33). These studies provided the first controlled experimental evidence that administration of HSV glycoproteins with adjuvants could reduce recurrent HSV disease (50–52). We initially reported a reduction of recurrences between 5% and 47% with HSV glycoproteins and various adjuvants (50,51). Using the immunomodulator imiquimod, we have been able to detect a peak reduction of about 75% in the weeks following a second dose of vaccine (53). Similarly, Ho et al. (52) observed that administration of gD in a liposome formulation reduced recurrence by 75%, and immunization with gD in an oil emulsion produced a 40% to 50% reduction. Vaccination not only reduced clinical recurrence, but also asymptomatic shedding (54), thus fulfilling one of the objectives for an immunotherapeutic vaccine. The efficacy of vaccination appears to be affected by adjuvants, timing of immunization in relation to infection, and the route of vaccine administration (51). Subsequent experiments suggested that augmentation of specific cell-mediated immune responses rather than humoral responses were most important for vaccine efficacy (52,55).

The success of immunotherapy in this animal model has led to further human trials. Most recently, the moderate success of immunotherapy has been reported in small human trials. Using 100 µg of gD2 plus alum, Straus et al. (56) reported that after two immunizations, recurrences were reduced from 0.55/month in controls to 0.42/month in vaccinees ($P = .06$), and virologically confirmed recurrences were reduced from 0.28 to 0.18 ($P = .02$). The median number of recurrences was reduced from six to four per patient over the 1-year observation period ($P = .04$). The decrease in recurrences appeared to be greatest in the first 4 months of the study.

Similarly, Benson et al. (57) recently reported that immunization with a mixed HSV-1 glycoprotein vaccine at 0, 1, and 2 months reduced the frequency and severity of recurrences. The proportion of vaccine recipients for whom the time of the first genital recurrence was > 60 days after immunization was significantly increased and although there was a reduction in the mean number of recurrences after vaccination, this did not reach significance. The severity of recurrences measured by the number of lesions and the number of associated systemic or local symptoms, however, were significantly reduced. In both studies, immunization increased the immune response to HSV. In one there was a significant correlation with cell-mediated immune response and modulation of disease severity (57).

These results may be viewed as particularly encouraging because, although only modest reductions were seen, these trials were conducted with adjuvants that were poorly effective in animal trials. If more potent adjuvants, especially those that induce cell-mediated immune responses, are evaluated, they may provide better protection. The most effective vaccine may also need to include other viral proteins that are targets for cell-mediated immunity.

SUMMARY

The strategies being applied to the development of effective HSV vaccines are taking advantage of modern methodologies. The subunit vaccines now in large clinical trials offer greater promise than previous vaccines based on their improved immunogenicity. The optimum combination of viral proteins and adjuvants for these subunit vaccines, however, have yet to be defined. Further improvements in HSV vaccines also may come from other immunization strategies including live attenuated, vectored, replication-incompetent, or DNA-based vaccines, which could move rapidly into human trials.

REFERENCES

1. Nahmias AJ, Lee FK, Beckman-Nahmias S. Sero-epidemiological and sociological patterns of herpes simplex virus infection in the world. Scand J Infect Dis 1990; 69(suppl): 19–36.
2. Lipchutz B. Untersuchungen über die Atiologie der krankheiten der Herpesgruppe. Arch Dermatol Syphilol 1921; 136: 428.

3. Hall MJ, Katrak K. The quest for a herpes simplex virus vaccine: background and recent developments. Vaccine 1986; 4: 138–150.

4. Committee on Issues and Priorities for New Vaccine Development: Appendix I: Prospects for immunizing against herpes simplex viruses 1 and 2, in New Vaccine Development: Establishing Priorities. Washington, DC: National Academy Press, 1985: 280–312.

5. Mertz GJ, Peterman G, Ashley R, et al. Herpes simplex virus type 2 glycoprotein-subunit vaccine: tolerance and humoral and cellular responses in humans. J Infect Dis 1984; 150: 242–249.

6. Frenkel LM, Dillon M, Garratty E, et al. A randomized double-blind, placebo-controlled phase I trial of a herpes simplex virus purified glycoprotein (gD1) vaccine (abstr 721). Proceedings of the 29th Interscience Conference on Antimicrobial Agents and Chemotherapy (ICAAC), Washington, DC, 1990.

7. Thompson RL, Nakashizuka M, Stevens JG. Vaccine potential of a live avirulent herpes simplex virus. Microb Pathog 1986; 1: 409–416.

8. Meignier B, Longnecker R, Roizman B. In vivo behavior of genetically engineered herpes simplex virus R7017 and R7020: Construction and evaluation in rodents. J Infect Dis 1988; 158: 602–613.

9. Meignier B, Martin B, Whitley RJ, et al. In vivo behavior of genetically engineered herpes simplex viruses R7017 and R7020. II. Studies in immuno-competent and immunosuppressed owl monkeys (Aotus trivirgatus). J Infect Dis 1990; 162: 313–321.

10. Roizman B, Warren J, Thuning CA, et al. Application of molecular genetics to the design of live herpes simplex virus vaccines. Dev Biol Stand 1982; 52: 287–304.

11. Cadoz M, Micoud M, Seigneurin JM, et al. Phase I trial of R7020: a live attenuated recombinant herpes simplex virus (HSV) candidate vaccine (abstr 341). Presented at the 32nd Interscience Conference on Antimicrobial Agents and Chemotherapy (ICAAC), Anaheim, California 1992: 167.

12. Whitley RJ, Kern ER, Chatterjee S, et al. Replication, establishment of latency, and induced reactivation of herpes simplex virus gamma 1 34.5 deletion mutants in rodent models. J Clin Invest 1993; 91: 2837–2843.

13. Valyi-Nagy T, Fareed MU, O'Keefe JS, et al. The herpes simples virus type 1 strain 17+ gamma 34.5 deletion mutant 1716 is avirulent in SCID mice. J Gen Virol 1994; 75: 2059–2063.

14. Spivack JG, Fareed MU, Valyi-Nagy T, et al. Replication, establishment of latent infection, expression of the latency-associated transcripts and explant reactivation of herpes simplex virus type 1 gamma 34.5 mutants in a mouse eye model. J Gen Virol 1995; 76: 321–332.

15. Perng GC, Thompson RL, Sawtell NM, et al. An avirulent ICP34.5 deletion mutant of herpes simplex virus type 1 is capable of *in vivo* spontaneous reactivation. J Virol 1995; 69: 3033–3041.

16. Cremer KJ, Mackett M, Wohlengerg C, et al. Vaccinia virus recombinant expressing herpes simplex virus type 1 glycoprotein D prevents latent herpes in mice. Science 1985; 228: 737–740.

17. Cantin EM, Eberle R, Baldick J, et al. Expression of herpes simplex virus 1 glycoprotein B by a recombinant vaccinia virus and protection of mice against lethal HSV-1 challenge. Proc Natl Acad Soc USA 1987; 80: 7155–7159.
18. McDermott MR, Graham FL, Hanke T, et al. Protection of mice against lethal challenge with herpes simplex virus by vaccination with an adenovirus vector expressing HSV glycoprotein B. Virology 1989; 169: 244–247.
19. Gallichan WS, Johnson DC, Graham FL, et al. Mucosal immunity and protection after intranasal immunization with recombinant adenovirus expressing herpes simplex virus glycoprotein B. J Infect Dis 1993; 168: 622–629.
20. Heineman TC, Connelly BC, Bourne N, et al. Immunization with recombinant varicella zoster virus expressing herpes simplex virus type 2 glycoprotein D reduces the severity of genital herpes in guinea pigs. J Virol 1995; 69: 8109–8113.
21. Nguyen LH, Knipe DM, Finbert RW. Replication-defective mutants of herpes simplex virus (HSV) induce cellular immunity and protect against lethal HSV infection. J Virol 1992; 66: 7067–7072.
22. Farrell HE, McLean CS, Harley C, et al. Vaccine potential of a herpes simplex virus type 1 mutant with an essential glycoprotein deleted. J Virol 1994, 68: 927–932.
23. Morrison LA, Knipe DM. Immunization with replication-defective mutants of herpes simplex virus type 1: sites of immune intervention in pathogenesis of challenge virus infection. J Virol 1994; 68: 689–696.
24. Ulmer JB, Donnelly JJ, Parker SE, et al. Heterologous protection against influenza by injection of DNA encoding a viral protein. Science 1993; 259: 1745–1749.
25. Manicken E, Rouse RJD, Yu A, et al. Genetic immunization against herpes simplex virus. J Immunol 1995; 155: 259–265.
26. Bourne N, Stanberry LR, Bernstein DI, Lew D. DNA vaccination against experimental genital herpes simplex virus infection. J Infect Dis 1996; 173: 800–807.
27. Stanberry LR, Bernstein DI, Burke RL, et al. Vaccination with recombinant herpes simplex virus glycoproteins: protection against initial and recurrent genital herpes. J Infect Dis 1987; 155: 914–920.
28. Sanchez-Pescador L, Burke RL, Ott G, et al. The effect of adjuvants on the efficacy of a recombinant herpes simplex virus glycoprotein vaccine. J Immunol 1988; 141: 1720–1727.
29. Berman PW, Gregory T, Crase D, et al. Protection from genital herpes simplex virus type 2 infection by vaccination with cloned type 1 glycoprotein D. Science 1985; 227: 1490–1491.
30. Ghiasi H, Kaiwar R, Nesburn AB, et al. Expression of seven herpes simplex virus type 1 glycoproteins (gB, gC, gD, gE, gG, gH, and gI): comparative protection against lethal challenge in mice. J Virol 1994; 68: 2118–2126.
31. Watson RJ, Weis JH, Salstrom JS, et al. Herpes simplex virus type-1 glycoprotein D gene: nucleotide sequence and expression in *Escherichia coli*. Science 1982; 218: 381–384.
32. Pachl C, Burke RL, Struve LL, et al. Expression of cell-associated and secreted forms of herpes simplex virus type 1 glycoprotein B in mammalian cells. J Virol 1987; 61: 315–325.

33. Stanberry LR. Evaluation of herpes simplex virus vaccine in animals: the guinea pig vaginal model. Rev Infect Dis 1991; 11(suppl): S920–S923.
34. Burke RL. Development of a herpes simplex virus subunit glycoprotein vaccine for prophylactic and therapeutic use. Rev Infect Dis 1991; 13: S906–S911.
35. Stanberry LR, Myers MG, Stephanopoulos DE, et al. Preinfection prophylaxis with herpes simplex virus immunogens: factors influencing efficacy. J Gen Virol 1989; 70: 3177–3185.
36. Mertz GJ, Ashley R, Burke RL, et al. Double-blind, placebo-controlled trial of a herpes simplex virus type 2 glycoprotein vaccine in persons at high risk for genital herpes infection. J Infect Dis 1990; 161: 653–660.
37. Straus SE, Savarese B, Tigges M, et al. Induction and enhancement of immune responses to herpes simplex virus type 2 in humans by use of a recombinant glycoprotein D vaccine. J Infect Dis 1993; 167: 1045–1052.
38. Langenberg GM, Burke RL, Adair SF, et al. A recombinant glycoprotein vaccine for herpes simplex type 2: safety and efficacy. Ann Intern Med 1995; 122: 889–898.
39. Leroux-Roels G, Moreau E, Verhasselt B, et al. Immunogenicity and reactogenicity of recombinant herpes simplex virus type-2 (HSV-2) glycoprotein D vaccine with monophosphoryl lipid A in HSV-seronegative and seropositive subjects (abstr 1209). Proceedings of the 32nd Interscience Conference on Antimicrobial Agents and Chemotherapy (ICAAC), New Orleans, 1993: 64.
40. Leroux-Roels G, Moreau E, Desombere I, et al. Persistence of humoral and cellular immune response and booster effect following vaccination either herpes simplex (gD2t) candidate vaccine with MPL. Presented at the 34th Annual Interscience Conference on Antimicrobial Agents and Chemotherapy, Orlando, Florida, October 4-7, 1994.
41. Schiff BL, Kern AB. Multiple smallpox vaccinations in the treatment of recurrent herpes simplex. Postgrad Med 1954; 15: 32–36.
42. Foster PD, Abshier AB. Smallpox vaccine in treatment of recurrent herpes. Arch Dermatol Syphilol 1937; 36: 294.
43. Bierman SM. BCG immunoprophylaxis of recurrent herpes genitalis. Arch Dermatol 1976; 112: 1410–1415.
44. Anderson FD, Ushijima RN, Larson CL. Recurrent herpes genitalis: treatment with Mycobacterium bovis (BCG). Obstet Gynecol 1974; 43: 797–805.
45. Lazar MP. Vaccination for recurrent herpes simplex infection: initiation of a new disease site following the use of unmodified material containing the live virus. Arch Dermatol 1956; 73: 70–71.
46. Goldman L. Reactions of an autoinoculation for recurrent herpes simplex. Arch Dermatol 1961; 84: 1025–1026.
47. Woodman CBJ, Buchan A, Fuller A, et al. Efficacy of vaccine Ac NFU₁ (S⁻) MRC5 given after an initial clinical episode in the prevention of herpes genitalis. Br J Vener Dis 1983; 59: 311–313.
48. Kutinova L, Benda R, Kalos Z, et al. Placebo-controlled study with subunit herpes simplex virus vaccine in subjects suffering from frequent herpetic recurrences. Vaccine 1988; 6: 223–228.

49. Stanberry LR. Herpes simplex virus vaccines. Semin Pediatr Infect Dis 1991; 2: 178–185.
50. Stanberry LR, Burke RL, Myers MG. Herpes simplex virus treatment of recurrent genital herpes. J Infect Dis 1988; 156: 156–163.
51. Stanberry LR, Harrison CJ, Bernstein DI, et al. Herpes simplex virus glycoprotein immunotherapy of recurrent genital herpes: factors influencing efficacy. Antiviral Res 1989; 11: 203–214.
52. Ho RJY, Burke RL, Merigan TC. Antigen-presenting liposomes are effective in the treatment of recurrent herpes simplex virus genitalis in guinea pigs. J Virol 1989; 63: 2951–2958.
53. Bernstein DI, Harrison CJ, Tepe E, et al. Effect of imiquimod as an adjuvant for immunotherapy of genital HSV in guinea pigs. Vaccine 1995, 13: 72–76.
54. Myers MG, Bernstein DI, Harrison CJ, et al. Herpes simplex virus glycoprotein treatment of recurrent genital herpes reduces cervicovaginal virus shedding in guinea pigs. Antiviral Res 1988; 10: 83–88.
55. Bernstein DI, Harrison CJ, Jenski LJ, et al. Cell-mediated immunologic responses and recurrent genital herpes in the guinea pig. J Immunol 1991; 146: 3571–3577.
56. Straus SE, Corey L, Burke RL, et al. Placebo-controlled trial of vaccination with recombinant glycoprotein D of herpes simplex virus type 2 for immunotherapy of genital herpes. Lancet 1994; 343: 1460–1463.
57. Benson CA, Turyk ME, Wilbanks GD, et al. A placebo-controlled trial of vaccination with a mixed glycoprotein herpes simplex virus type 1 vaccine for the modulation of recurrent genital herpes. Presented at the 33rd Annual Meeting of Infectious Diseases Society of America, San Francisco, California, September 16-18, 1995.

27

Varicella Zoster Virus Neuralgia: Diagnosis and Treatment

Michael C. Rowbotham and Grace Forde
University of California School of Medicine, San Francisco, California

ORIGIN AND EPIDEMIOLOGY OF HERPES ZOSTER

Herpes zoster is one of the most common of all neurological disorders (42,61). The unilateral, erythematous rash is well described by pairing the Greek term *herpes*, meaning "something that creeps," with the Greek term for the belt a warrior used to secure his armor, *zoster* (1). A neural origin for zoster pain was suspected by the earliest investigators; Bright noted the spread matched peripheral nerve territories in 1831, von Barensprung found necrosis in the corresponding dorsal root ganglion in 1862, and Head and Campbell's dermatomal map in 1900 was based on postmortem study of acute zoster eruptions with postmodern changes in a series of cases (1,46). Lewis and Marvin (64) briefly proposed in 1927 that "the virus causing the mischief in the root ganglion spreads along the sensory tract to the skin, there setting up a distinct inflammatory change." Straus et al. (103) finally proved Hope-Simpson's theories (52) of reactivation of latent virus as the origin of zoster by showing in 1984 that virus isolates during varicella and zoster outbreaks are identical.

During acute zoster, infectious virus and its antigens are present in neurons, nerve-associated satellite cells, peripheral nerves, and skin. The dorsal root ganglion and peripheral nerve of the involved spinal or trigeminal segment, portions of the skin served by that ganglion, and occasionally extending rostral into the spinal cord even beyond the dorsal horn become intensively inflamed (5,28,46,104,115). Most of the complications of herpes zoster are related to the destructive intensity of the

333

inflammation, including cranial nerve palsies, eye destruction, and myelitis (52,86,89).

Cell-mediated immunity specifically to varicella zoster virus (VZV) declines with age, especially after the age of 60 (5,45). The incidence of zoster rises tenfold with advancing age, to an incidence of 4.5 to 10.1 cases per 1000 person-years (13,42,43,52,89). Overall, about 15% of people who have had varicella develop zoster. Of those surviving to the age of 80, roughly one-third will have had an episode of zoster. The risk of developing a second attack of zoster is unclear (52,76). Immune system compromise resulting from drugs or HIV infection and cancer (particularly leukemia) greatly increase the risk of developing zoster (37,38,43,45).

SPECTRUM OF ZOSTER-ASSOCIATED PAIN: PREHERPETIC NEURALGIA, ZOSTER SINE HERPETE, ACUTE HERPES ZOSTER, AND POSTHERPETIC NEURALGIA

Subclinical zoster (i.e., viral reactivation without pain, neurological deficit, or rash) can occur. In 102 patients evaluated before and after bone marrow transplantation, 36% developed clinical zoster, and another 26% had sub-clinical reactivation based on either a fourfold or greater rise in VZV antibody titers or development of a positive lymphocyte transformation response (65). In another study, 19% of bone marrow transplantation patients developed subclinical zoster based on a polymerase chain reaction demonstration of viremia (117). Varicella zoster virus antibody titers in renal transplantation patients also fluctuate (68). Why subclinical zoster is painless is unknown, but one may speculate that zoster-related disorders with pain have tissue inflammation and/or destruction during the acute phase. In chronic postherpetic neuralgia, pain is thought to continue secondary to the injury sustained by the peripheral nervous system.

A brief period of preherpetic neuralgia, typically consisting of radicular pain, itching, and paresthesias for 2 to 4 days before the first lesions become apparent, is common. In an elderly patient presenting with unexplained acute and severe chest or abdominal pain, incipient zoster is high on the differential diagnosis list. Preherpetic neuralgia lasting up to 100 days has been described by Gilden et al. (39). Perhaps the reactivation is kept in check for a prolonged period by the immune system before viral transport finally progresses all the way to the skin.

Lewis (63) hypothesized zoster could be the etiology of otherwise unexplained unilateral segmental pain with or without visceral disturbances, painful unilateral muscle paresis, ophthalmic disturbances with eyeball or ocular muscle involvement, and otalgia with palsies or taste loss. He described several cases of what he felt was acute zoster without the rash, or "zoster sine herpete." In zoster sine herpete, the pain is presumably due to inflammation and destruction of neural and nonneural tissue, but since the virus never reaches the skin, the diagnosis is particularly difficult. By either VZV isolation, intrathecal VZV antibody production, high VZV titers in blood or cerebrospinal fluid, VZV DNA extraction from cerebrospinal fluid, or diagnostic titer rises, zoster sine herpete has been documented in immunocompetent patients with diverse disorders including transverse myelitis, cranial or peripheral polyneuritis, chronic radicular pain, asceptic meningitis, and encephalitis (27,29,41,47,73).

Acute herpes zoster is rarely a diagnostic dilemma. The pain results from inflammation and destruction that can be spread along the entire peripheral nerve apparatus and peripheral tissues including the skin and the nociceptive afferents of the nervi nervorum located in the dural sheath of peripheral nerve trunks (6). Inflammation, tissue destruction, nerve irritation, and nerve destruction combine to produce a severe burning, itching, dysesthetic pain, with extreme pain from any skin contact (13,52,86). Only 10% will have little or no acute zoster pain, and many describe the pain of acute herpes zoster as the most severe pain they have ever experienced.

Because patients with pain at 6 months after crusting of the skin lesions are likely to continue to have pain 1 or more years later, a conservative definition of postherpetic neuralgia (PHN) would be pain in the region affected by zoster lasting longer than 3 to 6 months. However, most clinicians and many clinical trials have used 1 month after crusting of the skin lesions to define the start of PHN (86). Postherpetic neuralgia occurs in about 10% to 15% of all herpes zoster patients, with an approximate prevalence of 180,000 persons in the United States (13,23,52,61,89). The elderly are at greatly increased risk not only for developing herpes zoster (HZ), but also for PHN (including PHN pain lasting more than 1 year) (13,23,52,89). Zoster at the age of 60 has an incidence of PHN of 47%, and by the age of 80, up to 80% will develop PHN. Other risk factors for development of PHN include trigeminal location, more severe pain during acute zoster, more severe rash, and sensory loss to thermal stimuli during and after acute HZ (79,80).

THERAPY OF ACUTE ZOSTER PAIN

There is agreement among published trials that acyclovir at the onset of HZ reduces pain in the short term (5). Although a meta-analysis of four acyclovir trials claimed a 42% reduction in PHN, most large trials indicate acyclovir to have little effect on the likelihood of developing long-lasting postherpetic pain (5,18,53,74,119,120). Studies of two newer antivirals, famciclovir and valacyclovir, provide encouraging data by showing faster rates of pain resolution when compared to placebo or acyclovir (7,107). There have been five trials of steroids for prevention of PHN (32,88,116,120). Two early studies showed benefit in reducing the incidence of PHN (88). Later studies, including comparisons of steroids plus acyclovir, indicate steroids reduce early pain without a definite impact on long-term pain (32,116,120). At this time, steroid therapy seems to have little use in the treatment of acute zoster.

What about the patient with uncontrolled pain who is already on antiviral therapy? Local anesthetic nerve blocks can be dramatically effective in alleviating the pain of acute zoster. No other treatment modality, including systemic opioids, is as routinely effective. Technique of administration varies with the location of zoster and the skill and experience of the physician. For trigeminal zoster, sympathetic blocks of the stellate ganglion and trigeminal branch blocks are used frequently. For zoster in the second to fourth cervical dermatomes, stellate ganglion blocks, nerve root blocks, and nerve branch blocks are all possible. For zoster in the fifth cervical dermatome and caudal, epidural nerve blocks are used most often, followed by peripheral nerve blocks (including intercostal nerve blocks). Some anesthesiologists prefer to leave an epidural catheter in place for intermittent injection; in hospitalized patients and selected outpatients, a continuous epidural administration system is used. A combination of local anesthetic and an opioid is preferred by some over local anesthetic alone. Administering steroid plus local anesthetic by the epidural route is a frequent clinical practice; how this compares with a tapering course of oral steroids is unknown. Simple subcutaneous infiltration of the area of lesions and pain with local anesthetic, or local anesthetic plus steroid, is another popular practice. Intravenous local anesthetic infusion has been reported to reduce acute zoster pain, but is not commonly used in clinical practice compared to the other techniques described. The relative efficacy of the different nerve block options has not been subjected to rigorous scrutiny.

Anecdotally, nerve blocks early in the course of HZ have long been thought to prevent PHN, but not all reports agree (15,19,35,48,50,91,

106,118,123). There is a strong emphasis on beginning nerve blocks as soon as possible after the onset of zoster in order to have the best chance of preventing PHN. How nerve blocks would prevent PHN is unclear. It is logical to assume that eliminating acute pain will reduce the likelihood of long-term pain; however, no properly controlled studies of adequate size have tested the hypothesis. Tenicela et al. (106) attempted a double-blind, crossover study of sympathetic blocks, but their sample size of 20 was far too small to overcome the effect of the natural history of the disorder. Both c-nociceptor primary afferents and sympathetic efferents are unmyelinated fibers and both are affected by epidural blocks. Furthermore, electrophysiological studies do not support an association between fiber size and concentration dependence (36). The strongest case for a sympathetic nervous system component to acute zoster pain is the relief of trigeminal zoster pain by stellate ganglion block. In addition, primary afferent nociceptors are known to develop a response to local release of norepinephrine after nerve injury and increased numbers of alpha receptors are synthesized (25,85,108). However, even local anesthetic blocks of the stellate ganglion for cranial pain are not completely selective for the sympathetic nervous system. Systemic lidocaine has been shown to block nerve injury-induced hyperalgesia and nociceptor-driven spinal sensitization in animal models (2). In humans, systemically administered local anesthetics relieve a variety of pains, including zoster and PHN pain, and vascular uptake from the region of the stellate ganglion is so rapid that peak venous blood levels occur within 5 minutes (95,101,122). Regional sympathetic blocks for neck, arm, and leg involvement by zoster carry the possibility of pain relief by spread to nearby sensory nerves, especially when larger volumes are used (22). Controlled studies of alternative techniques for blocking the actions of the sympathetic nervous system, such as intravenous phentolamine, have not been reported.

PATHOPHYSIOLOGY OF POSTHERPETIC PAIN

It has been proposed that persistent low level virus replication could be responsible for some cases of PHN. Viewed this way, unilateral segmental pain would be related to VZV replication in four ways: (a) preherpetic neuralgia, in which pain is present, but the virus has not yet reached the skin to produce the characteristic rash; (b) acute zoster, in which viral replication and transport has extended from dorsal root ganglion neurons to affected skin; (c) zoster sine herpete, in which viral replication occurs but rash never appears; and (d) postherpetic neuralgia, in which viral replication and transport for a limited period of time affects the skin, but pain persists because viral replication never completely ceases. In only a few cases, however, has persistent viral replication been demonstrated in immunocompetent patients with PHN (40). In a few published cases, inflammatory cell infiltrates were present 100 days and longer after rash resolution (115). This suggests that prolonged inflammation is associated with some cases of postherpetic pain. Whether or not the inflammation is related to persistent viral expression in these cases is unknown. Anecdotally, treatment of chronic PHN patients with acyclovir does not appear to provide much benefit.

Immune system competence does not seem to be a factor in development of PHN (3,37,38,100). Trigeminal zoster (especially when the eye is involved) nearly doubles the risk of developing PHN, especially longlasting PHN (52). Severe skin lesions and a large rise in VZV antibody titers are markers of a more severe outbreak and also increase the risk of PHN (48). Not surprisingly, severe acute herpetic pain seems to predispose a patient to suffer from PHN. Patients experiencing psychosocial stress at the time of the zoster outbreak are more likely to have more severe zoster pain and view their habits and activities as changed negatively because of PHN (31).

The most widely accepted view is that PHN is a neuropathic pain, resulting from damage to or abnormal functioning of the nervous system (79,86). Postmortem studies have shown that in nearly every case, only one dorsal root ganglion and its connections are affected (115). During acute zoster, inflammation and destruction of the neural apparatus extend from the dorsal root to the skin (5,6,28,46,52,86,89,104). In the chronic state, nerve cell loss in the dorsal root ganglion, fibrosis of the dorsal root, peripheral nerve and skin, and thinly myelinated axons consistent with remyelination have been reported (24,46,78,112,115). Postmortem studies by Watson and Deck (115) have shown that the dorsal horn of the spinal cord may be atrophic in chronic PHN.

Patients with PHN collectively describe three components to their discomfort: (a) a *constant*, deep, aching, "bruised," or burning sensation; (b) a spontaneous, recurrent, *neuralgic*, shooting or electric shocklike pain; and (c) an *allodynic*, superficial, sharp, radiating, burning, tender, dysesthetic, or itchlike sensation evoked by wearing clothing, very light touch, or gentle pressure on the skin (94,112). The mechanism(s) behind each of these complaints is not certain. Noordenbos (79) reported that patients who did not develop PHN after zoster had no sensory deficits on clinical examination, but patients who developed PHN had sensory deficits. Noordenbos noted the presence of allodynia, including the production of pain by stimuli at the threshold for detection. He felt, based in part on pathological study of intercostal nerves by light microscopy, that zoster produced preferential loss of large-diameter myelinated sensory fibers in some patients and that the pain was due to the loss of the normal inhibitory function of these fibers on central nervous system (CNS) pain transmission neurons. Unfortunately, his methods could not distinguish between large-diameter fibers attempting to regenerate and unmyelinated c-fibers. Many subsequent investigators have believed that the pain of PHN is due to deafferentation and central reorganization (10,81,82,115).

Nurmikko and Bowsher (81) compared 42 patients presenting for treatment of PHN with a group of 20 patients who had previously been seen for therapy of acute zoster but had not developed PHN. Consistent with Noordenbos' and Watson's reports, they found that there were significant sensory deficits in the area of pain in the PHN patients, but examination of the area of the herpetic outbreak in 90% of the patients who had not developed PHN revealed normal sensation (79,112). In the PHN patients, the group means for all sensory modalities tested (warm, cold, and heat pain thresholds; tactile, pinprick, 2-point discrimination, and vibration thresholds) were abnormal compared to the unaffected mirror image area. Allodynia to gently brushing the skin was present in 87% of their sample of PHN patients. The authors postulated that the allodynia was a result of central reorganization consequent to deafferentation such that second order pain transmission neurons became capable of responding to A-beta low threshold mechanoreceptors. Bowsher (10) later concluded that the degree of pain in PHN Is determined by the extent of loss of unmyelinated and small myelinated primary afferent function and is due to changes in the spinal cord resulting from deafferentation.

Based on a study of 10 patients with PHN and allodynia on examination compared to 3 patients who did not experience PHN after zoster and 10 healthy controls, Baron and Saguer (4) concluded that c-nociceptors were not involved in the signalling and maintenance of allodynia. Skin temperature, skin resistance, resting blood flow, and thermally evoked blood flow were the same in PHN skin and contralateral uninvolved skin. The flare reaction to iontophoresed histamine was significantly impaired in allodynic PHN skin, and little pain or itch was provoked. The severity of the defect in flare response was strongly correlated with the severity of spontaneous pain complaint, which they felt supported central deafferentation as the major mechanism for the pain. Although iontophoresis of histamine does stimulate a c-fiber-mediated axon flare response, this is an indirect measure of c-nociceptor function, and corroborating evidence in the form of detailed baseline sensory findings was not provided. Jancso et al. (55) previously reported defects in the flare response to capsaicin in both PHN and zoster. LeVasseur et al. (62) and colleagues reported defects in the flare response to capsaicin in PHN skin compared to control sites distant from the area, but found no correlation of pain and capsaicin-induced flare response.

Rowbotham and Fields (94) reported their analysis of the sensory features of PHN in 1989, based on a clinical study of 12 patients with PHN. Although the area of greatest sensory loss and scarring was generally included in the area of maximum pain, the most severe pain correlated best with the area of most severe allodynia. Areas of severe allodynia often had minor or no clinical sensory deficit. Areas of perceived abnormal sensation (including allodynia) sometimes extended far beyond the borders of visible scarring and beyond the borders of the original rash. Using an infrared device for determining skin temperature that does not require skin contact, they reported that allodynic skin was sometimes asymmetrically warm, and that extensively deafferented areas without allodynia were sometimes asymmetrically cool. Infiltrating the most severely allodynic skin with dilute lidocaine frequently produced a dramatic reduction in pain severity. The findings suggested that afferent input was critical for maintaining PHN pain in most cases and that abnormal c-nociceptor activity arising in fibers that were still functionally connected to their peripheral and central targets could account for the sensory and thermographic findings and the response to local anesthetic skin infiltration.

More than one pain mechanism may thus be necessary to account for the continuing pain of PHN (34). A subset of patients have severe sensory deficits, little or no allodynia, and little or no pain relief from peripheral neural blockade (94). In such patients, the precise mechanism of pain is obscure, but is possibly related to enduring changes in the CNS induced by deafferentation (6,67,121). In contrast, patients with prominent allodynia may have important pain generators located in the skin. As primary afferents of all types, including nociceptors, are damaged during acute zoster, there is a source for increased primary afferent activity via ectopic impulse generation, as has been demonstrated in both animal models of experimental nerve injury and humans with peripheral nerve injury (14,25,60,108). The intensely painful stimulus of acute herpes zoster could produce sensitization of spinal cord neurons maintained by continuing input from damaged c-nociceptors in the area of pain. Instead of rewiring in the dorsal horn of the spinal cord to produce pain from innocuous mechanoreceptor stimulation, the mechanism of allodynia in some PHN patients could thus be analogous to areas of secondary hyperalgesia observed after experimental capsaicin injection (60,121). In this situation, continuing c-nociceptor input is required to maintain pain and allodynia as cuff block of A-beta fibers blocks allodynia but not pain, whereas c-fiber block eliminates both allodynia and ongoing burning pain.

THERAPY OF POSTHERPETIC NEURALGIA

Perspective

In essence, established PHN is chronic and resistant to therapy (86). Social isolation, depression, and even suicide occur. The only therapy proven effective for PHN in *multiple* and *independent* controlled studies are the tricyclic antidepressants (58,70,72,86,109,110,112,113). Beyond that, the number of options with any proof of efficacy is quite limited. Opioids and anticonvulsant or antiarrhythmic medications may be of substantial benefit in selected patients, although long-term benefit has not been proven in prospective, controlled trials (83,87,95,97,112). Transcutaneous electrical nerve stimulation (TENS) presents almost no risks and is occasionally of benefit (86). Topical medications containing capsaicin, local anesthetics, or aspirinlike compounds hold significant promise (96). Patients with PHN in the C4 to T4 dermatomes (affecting the shoulder) and L1 and S2 dermatomes (hip and knee) may develop limitation of joint movement because of pain and can benefit from physical therapy.

Patients refractory to widely accepted interventions should be referred to a pain management center, preferably a multidisciplinary treatment program, that is experienced in managing difficult cases of PHN. This is particularly important if more invasive therapies are being considered, such as intrathecal opioid infusion pumps, spinal cord stimulation, deep brain stimulation, surgical destructive lesions, and neurolytic nerve blocks. Psychological intervention, including education about pain physiology, can address depression, concern over chronic fatigue, and perceived global loss of ability to function at the preillness level. Counseling, combined with biofeedback or relaxation therapies, can occasionally be helpful.

Antidepressants

The tricyclic antidepressants amitriptyline and desipramine have been effective in well-designed, controlled clinical trials (58,70,109,110,113). Antidepressants remain the oral medication treatment of first choice for

PHN. Although desipramine appears to have fewer side effects than amitriptyline, all tricyclic antidepressants have unpleasant and potentially dangerous adverse effects, including altered cardiac conduction, orthostatic hypotension, dry mouth, constipation, urinary retention, confusion and memory impairment, and seizures (16,44). Alternatives exist, such as serotonin-specific reuptake inhibitors (SSRI) antidepressants such as fluoxetine, sertraline, paroxetine, and trazodone, and mixed serotonin–norepinephrine antidepressants such as maprotiline, nefazodone, and venlafaxine. Compared to the newer antidepressants, tricyclic antidepressants present greater hazards in patients who may intentionally or accidentally take an overdose. *All* antidepressants, however, have the potential for significant side effects. Fluoxetine alters serum levels of some other drugs and may cause troublesome nausea, diarrhea, anxiety, tremor, insomnia, symptomatic hyponatremia, and suicidal ideation; but it is essentially free of changes in cardiac conduction and blood pressure. Trazodone may be sedating and can cause significant orthostatic hypotension and priapism in men. Maprotiline has a higher incidence of seizures than other antidepressants. Venlafaxine may produce hypertension.

At present, the mechanism of antidepressant analgesia is incompletely understood. One obvious possibility is that antidepressants act within the CNS by enhancing neurotransmission at biogenic amine links of the well-described brain stem to dorsal horn nociceptive modulating system (33). Serotonin (5HT) and norepinephrine (NE) projections have been demonstrated between brain stem nuclei implicated in nociceptive modulation as well as from these nuclei to the dorsal horn. The action of either or both transmitters may be critical to the function of this endogenous system. Nearly all antidepressants have been shown to have analgesic activity in a variety of animal pain models (54). It remains to be determined whether differences in the characteristics of analgesic activity between the different antidepressants relate to their differences in effects on biogenic amine systems, but the studies reported to date with fluoxetine and zimelidine indicate lower analgesic activity for serotonin selective drugs (71,110). A trial of the relatively selective noradrenergic drug maprotiline, however, also showed it was not as effective as amitriptyline (113).

Differences among antidepressants in binding to neurotransmitter receptors of human brain and rat brain synaptosomes may explain the clinical side effect profiles of these drugs (90). Alpha-adrenergic receptor blockade is associated with orthostatic hypotension, histamine receptor effects with sedation and possibly weight gain, acetylcholine receptor effects with constipation, dry mouth, blurred vision, nightmares, confusional states, and impaired memory. Amitriptyline affects a large number of neurotransmitter systems; 5HT, NE, and dopamine reuptake are inhibited; and histamine H-1, acetylcholine, and α-1 and α-2 adrenergic receptor antagonism is significant. Relative to amitriptyline, desipramine only weakly affects histamine and α-1 and α-2 receptors, and is less potent at blocking acetylcholine receptors, but potently blocks NE reuptake. Fluoxetine is a potent and selective inhibitor of serotonin reuptake. Relative to both amitriptyline and desipramine, fluoxetine has almost no effect on histamine H-1, muscarinic acetylcholine, and α-1 and α-2 receptors, but potently blocks 5HT reuptake. Studies that have examined the relationship between dose or blood level and clinical analgesic response have produced conflicting results (58,69–72,109,110,113).

A common misconception among patients is that antidepressants are of no value in treating pain unless associated with depression because their pain-reducing effect is only a by-product of mood elevation. The animal literature is unequivocal with regard to a direct analgesic action of antidepressants (54). In addition, studies by Max et al. (69), using amitriptyline clearly show that pain relief is independent of the presence or absence of depression. The analgesic effects of antidepressants are variably expressed. Some patients report they feel better and tolerate their discomfort more easily, but the underlying pain is unchanged. Others note significant qualitative changes in their pain pattern, such as the cessation of lancinating pain and allodynia (58). In a fortunate few, the pain and dysthesias disappear altogether. Overall, controlled studies show that the majority of PHN patients treated with tricyclic antidepressants report at least partial pain relief, with continued pain or return of pain during treatment periods with placebo (72).

Unfortunately, in clinical practice the results are not as good (112). Elderly patients with PHN who already have other significant health problems, especially cognitive impairment, are particularly difficult to treat with antidepressants. To increase the likelihood of successful completion of the medication trial, the patient must understand that side effects appear immediately, and the benefit may be subtle at first and slow to develop. Commitment to giving the medication a fair chance is crucial. Unless the patient's medical condition indicates otherwise, the literature supports starting with a tricyclic antidepressant, particularly desipramine or amitriptyline. It is best to start with a dose low enough so that the patient is likely to tolerate it initially and then slowly increase the dose every 3 to 5 days. The dose should be increased until pain relief occurs, intolerable side effects develop, or blood levels well into the therapeutic range are documented. An adequate trial would be 2 weeks at minimum, 75 mg/day, of a tricyclic antidepressant, or better yet, 2 weeks at a dose that produces blood levels in the antidepressant range. If the trial fails to relieve pain or is not tolerated, a trial of an alternate antidepressant is warranted, either another tricyclic, an SSRI, or one of the newer mixed 5HT-NE reuptake blocking antidepressants. When the first agent fails to relieve PHN pain, however, the response rate to subsequent antidepressant trials is uncertain.

Opioids

One obvious approach is to use opioid analgesics; there is ample anecdotal evidence that many patients achieve satisfactory long-term control of their pain without untoward effects (83,87,95,97,112). A placebo-controlled study showed intravenous morphine reduced the pain of PHN (95). Although longer term controlled trials have not been completed, Pappagallo and Campbell (83) has recently reported excellent results after 6 months of treatment in 16 of 20 consecutive cases using slow release morphine or oxycodone. In individual patients, opioids may succeed even when multiple trials of antidepressants have failed; in others, opioids may provide equivalent relief with fewer side effects (97,112).

Other Oral Medications

Despite the prominence and severity of the pain in PHN, there are few controlled trials of other therapeutic agents. A variety of other medications have been tried, including anticonvulsants such as carbamazepine and valproate, neuroleptics such as chlorprothixene and phenothiazines, and histamine-receptor blockers such as cimetidine (86). None have proved effective compared to placebo and cannot be recommended until a thorough trial of antidepressants has been completed. Although intravenous lidocaine has been shown in a controlled trial to relieve PHN pain, prospective controlled trials of the oral congener, mexiletine, have not been reported (95). Anticonvulsants have been anecdotally recommended, especially for lancinating, electric shocklike pains in PHN, but antidepressants are also effective for this subtype of PHN pain (58,70). Recently released anticonvulsants such as gabapentin have a favorable side effect profile, but have not been studied in large scale, open label, or controlled studies. Benzodiazepines are used with some frequency in clinical practice, even though the study by Max et al. (70) showed lorazepam ineffective compared to amitriptyline. Neuroleptics present particular problems with side effects in elderly persons. There is no convincing proof of efficacy for neuroleptics as monotherapy or combined with an antidepressant. NMDA-blocking agents, such as ketamine, have been reported to reduce PHN pain when given intravenously, and orally in one case report, but their role in long-term management of this condition has not been determined (30,49).

Topical Agents

Three types of topically applied medications have been intensively studied in recent years: capsaicin, local anesthetic preparations, and aspirin and nonsteroidal antiinflammatory drugs (NSAIDS) (96). Because the disease begins with a skin rash that leads to scarring and hypersensitive skin, therapy directed at cutaneous nerves is logical. Although the original outbreak of HZ may be extensive, most PHN patients have only limited areas of affected skin that they feel is the source of their pain (79,94,112). Only a modest amount of an effective preparation would need to be applied to produce pain relief. Unlike antidepressants, topical therapies have few systemic side effects. Nearly all patients are potential candidates for topical therapy, and for some there are no other practical alternatives. It seems logical, although unproven, that patients with prominent superficial pain and allodynia would be more likely to respond to topicals than those with deep pain and no allodynia.

Capsaicin-containing preparations have received much attention in recent years. Capsaicin selectively stimulates and then blocks unmyelinated primary afferents with eventual depletion of substance P and other peptide transmitters from nociceptive primary afferents (51). These afferents release the same transmitter both peripherally (where they help promote neurogenic inflammation) and at their CNS termination in the dorsal horn. Repeated application of capsaicin on normal skin produces a sensory deficit to thermal stimuli, loss of flare response from intradermal histamine, and other changes expected from depletion of peptide transmitters.

Several studies of topical capsaicin for PHN have been carried out, with mixed results (7,9,11,17,26,84,111,112,114). Controversy has surrounded clinical trials of capsaicin because blinding such studies is nearly impossible, as a high percentage of patients report significant warmth or a burning sensation on application (17). When all the PHN patients could recognize capsaicin effects, Bjerring et al. (9) abandoned use of blinding and placebo controls in their study of capsaicin-induced sensory changes using argon laser stimuli. Although five of their eight patients reported pain relief during the 5-week trial, none were still using the cream in open label follow-up 1 month later. Even at the 0.025% concentration, 66% to

79% of patients have reported burning with application in the uncontrolled studies of Peikert et al. (84) and Watson et al. (111). The controlled study by Drake et al. (26) of 30 patients using a 0.025% concentration showed no benefit compared to placebo. Two controlled studies showed benefit using 0.030% and 0.075% concentrations in a total of 91 subjects (7,11). Significant differences from placebo appear after 4 or more weeks of therapy, and subjects are instructed to apply the compound four or more times a day. In Peikert's uncontrolled study of 39 patients, although 19 of 39 reported improvement, only 33% continued to use the drug at follow-up (84). The largest double-blind, vehicle-controlled study is that of Watson et al. (114), who reported efficacy in a group of 143 patients using the 0.075% cream. By the end of the 6-week study, 39% reported pain relief with capsaicin compared to 11% with vehicle. The magnitude of the pain reduction was not large, only a 15% reduction from baseline. In addition to the 6-week blinded trial, 77 subjects were followed for up to 2 years and experienced stable or improved pain relief in more than 80% of cases.

Local anesthetic preparations in five different vehicles have been reported effective for PHN, two of which have shown efficacy in double-blind, vehicle-controlled studies. In one, 39 subjects treated with 5% lidocaine in a gel vehicle using a three-session crossover design, which included application on the contralateral, mirror-image skin as an additional control, showed both efficacy and a local site of action (98). In the other, efficacy was shown in 35 patients using lidocaine, 5%, in a soft, self-adherent patch compared with both vehicle and no-treatment controls (99). In uncontrolled studies, 5% lidocaine-prilocaine cream (EMLA), 5% lidocaine in a liquid base containing mostly isopropyl alcohol, 10% lidocaine base in an enhancing gel vehicle, and 9% lidocaine in petrolatum have all been effective (59,92,93,102). Placebo-controlled, longer-term efficacy studies have not been reported for any local anesthetic preparations.

There has been significant interest in topical application of aspirin and antiinflammatory medications mixed in chloroform or diethyl ether (20,21,57,96). The solution is daubed onto the painful skin. As the solvent evaporates, the active drug is left behind to penetrate to cutaneous nerve endings. In a recent uncontrolled study, King (57) reported excellent results in both acute herpetic pain and PHN in 42 consecutive patients treated this way. Similar to King's method, De Benedittis et al. (20) reported benefit from the use of 750 to 1500 mg of acetylsalicylic acid crushed to a fine powder and mixed into 20 to 30 ml of diethyl ether in 25 patients with either acute zoster or PHN. In a follow-up study, both acute herpetic pain and PHN were relieved with daily use of aspirin in diethyl ether (21). Single-session comparative studies of aspirin, diclofenac, and indomethacin have shown benefit compared to placebo (21). Morimoto et al. (77) reported that both indomethacin (in self-adherent poultice form) and a chloroform-aspirin combination were effective, but the poultice was much easier to use. Kassirer (56) reported anecdotally that aspirin in a cream base was also effective. The only negative study is that of McQuay et al. (75) who carried out a carefully designed, multiple-dose, placebo-controlled crossover study of benzydamine in 23 patients.

Theoretical advantages of local anesthetic preparations and aspirin/ NSAID preparations over capsaicin would be efficacy with the first few applications, a lower incidence of burning sensations, and possibly a lower frequency of application. All three types of topical preparations presumably share modulation of cutaneous sensory fiber function, especially that of small diameter nerve fibers, as their mechanism of action (96). No studies directly comparing the different types of topical therapies have been reported.

INVASIVE THERAPIES FOR REFRACTORY PHN

Unfortunately, some patients with PHN continue to have intolerable pain despite multiple antidepressant trials, anticonvulsant and antiarrhythmic trials, a variety of opioids, several different topical agents, transcutaneous electrical stimulation (TENS) units, physical therapy, psychological intervention, repetitive local anesthetic nerve block, and continuous epidural local anesthetic plus narcotic for several days. Neurolytic nerve blocks, nerve sectioning, and other ablative procedures such as DREZ lesions (usually described by the requesting physician or patient as a "*permanent nerve block*") are then proposed as treatment. The majority of the literature on surgical ablative therapies is more than a decade old, predating the widespread use of antidepressants and topical therapies (12,66). The number of cases treated with any particular procedure has been small and reports are entirely anecdotal. Should refractory patients be offered destructive therapies? The case of trigeminal PHN reported by Sugar and Bucy (105) in 1951 is especially instructive as a spectacular failure and argues against destructive therapy for refractory cases. Their patient continued to report pain despite treatment that included alcohol injection into the supraorbital nerve, division of the sensory root, alcohol injection into the trigeminal ganglion, stellate ganglion block, electroconvulsive therapy, extirpation of the contralateral then ipsilateral sensory cortex, and finally, prefrontal lobotomy.

Anecdotally, neuromodulatory procedures such as deep brain and spinal stimulation and placement of intrathecal infusion pumps help some patients. Implanted opioid pumps and stimulators offer the advantages of a trial period before permanent implantation and do not compound the preexisting neural injury by damaging more neural tissue. Long-term outcome of pumps and stimulators for PHN remains uncertain. As they are very expensive and require considerable ongoing care, widespread acceptance will require an objective and prospective demonstration of benefit in cases refractory to simpler interventions.

FUTURE RESEARCH

Postherpetic neuralgia is a painful disorder uniquely suited for clinical research. Much can be learned about the mechanisms and management of neuropathic pain in general from well-designed studies of patients with PHN. Zoster and PHN are common, typically strike otherwise healthy persons in a relatively restricted age distribution, are unilateral and in one nerve root territory, have a clearly defined onset, and consistent symptomatology. Can PHN be prevented by antivirals, nerve blocks, or combinations of the two? Recent postmortem studies by Watson and Deck (115) have shown that the dorsal horn of the spinal cord may be significantly atrophied in chronic PHN. Do CNS changes alter the response to therapy, making PHN more like a central myelopathic pain than a peripheral nerve pain? What role does the extent and severity of sensory disturbance play in ongoing symptomatology and response to therapy? Finally, what is the best therapy or combination of therapies?

REFERENCES

1. Abraham N, Murray J. The belt of roses from hell: historical aspects of herpes zoster and post-herpetic neuralgia. In: Watson CPN, ed. Herpes Zoster and Postherpetic Neuralgia, Amsterdam: Elsevier, 1993: 1–6.
2. Abram SE, Yaksh TL. Systemic lidocaine blocks nerve injury-induced hyperalgesia and nociceptor-driven spinal sensitization in the rat. Anesthesiology 1994; 80: 383–391.
3. Balfour HH. Varicella zoster virus infections in immunocompromised hosts. A review of the natural history and management. Am J Med 1988; 85: 68–73.
4. Baron R, Saguer M. Postherpetic neuralgia: are C-nociceptors involved in signalling and maintenance of tactile allodynia? Brain 1993; 116: 1477–1496.

5. Bean B, Deamant C, Aeppli D. Acute zoster: course, complications and treatment in the immunocompetent host. In: Watson CPN, ed. Herpes Zoster and Postherpetic Neuralgia. Amsterdam: Elsevier, 1993: 37–58.
6. Bennett GJ. Hypotheses on the pathogenesis of herpes zoster-associated pain. Ann Neurol 1994; 35(suppl): S38–S41.
7. Bernstein JE, Korman NJ, Bickers DR, et al. Topical capsaicin treatment of chronic postherpetic neuralgia. J Am Acad Dermatol 1989; 21: 265–270.
8. Beutner KR, Friedman DJ, Forszpaniak C, et al. Improved therapy for herpes zoster in immunocompetent adults: valacyclovir HCL compared with acyclovir. Antimicrob Agents Chemother 1995; in press.
9. Bjerring P, Arendt-Nielsen L, Soderberg U. Argon laser induced cutaneous sensory and pain thresholds in post-herpetic neuralgia: quantitative modulation by topical capsaicin. Acta Derm Venereol 1990; 70: 121–125.
10. Bowsher D. Sensory change in postherpetic neuralgia. In: Watson CPN, ed. Herpes Zoster and Postherpetic Neuralgia. Amsterdam: Elsevier, 1993: 97–108.
11. Bruxelle J, Luu M, Kong-a-Siou D. Randomized double-blind study of topical capsaicin for treatment of post-herpetic neuralgia. In: Congress Abstracts, 7th World Congress on Pain. Seattle: IASP Publications, 1993: 187.
12. Burchiel KJ. Deafferentation syndromes and dorsal root entry zone lesions. In: Fields HL, ed. Pain Syndromes in Neurology. London: Butterworths, 1990: 201–222.
13. Burgoon C, Burgoon J, Baldridge G. The natural history of herpes zoster. JAMA 1957; 164: 265–269.
14. Coderre TJ, Katz J, Vaccarino AL, Melzack R. Contribution of central neuroplasticity to pathological pain: review of clinical and experimental evidence. Pain 1993; 52: 259–285.
15. Colding A. Treatment of pain: organization of a pain clinic: treatment of acute herpes zoster. Proc R Soc Med 1971; 66: 541–543.
16. Cookson J. Side-effects of antidepressants. Br J Psychiatry 1993; 20(suppl): 20–24.
17. Cotton P. Compliance problems, placebo effect cloud trials of topical analgesic. JAMA 1990; 264: 13–14.
18. Crooks RJ, Jones DA, Fiddian A. Zoster-associated chronic pain: an overview of clinical trials with acyclovir. Scand J Infect 1991; 80: 62–68.
19. Dan K, Higa K, Noda B. Nerve block for herpetic pain. In: Fields HL, Cervero F, Dubner R. Advances in Pain Research and Therapy, Vol. 9. New York: Raven Press, 1985: 831–838.
20. DeBenedittis G, Lorenzetti A, Besana F. A new topical treatment for acute herpetic neuralgia and postherpetic neuralgia. Pain 1990; (suppl 5): S57.
21. DeBenedittis G, Besana F, Lorenzetti A. A new topical treatment for acute herpetic neuralgia and postherpetic neuralgia: the aspirin/diethyl ether mixture. An open-label study plus a double-blind controlled clinical trial. Pain 1992; 48: 383–390.
22. Dellemijn PLI, Fields HL, Allen RR, et al. The interpretation of pain relief and sensory changes following sympathetic blockade. Brain 1994; 117: 1475–1487.

23. DeMoragas J, Kierland R. The outcome of patients with herpes zoster. Arch Dermatol 1957; 75: 193–196.
24. Denny-Brown D, Adams R, Fitzgerald P. Pathologic features of herpes zoster: a note on geniculate herpes. Arch Neurol Psychiatry 1994; 51: 216–231.
25. Devor M, Rappaport ZH. Pain and the pathophysiology of damaged nerve. In: Fields HL, ed. Pain Syndromes in Neurology. London: Butterworths, 1990: 47–84.
26. Drake HF, Harries AJ, Gamester RE, et al. Randomised double-blind study of topical capsaicin for treatment of post-herpetic neuralgia (abstr). Pain 1990; (supplement 5): S58.
27. Easton HG. Zoster sine herpete causing acute trigeminal neuralgia. Lancet 1970; ii: 1065–1066.
28. Ebert M. Histologic changes in sensory nerves of the skin in herpes zoster. Arch Dermatol 1949; 60: 641–648.
29. Echevarria JM, Martinez-Martin P, Tellez A, et al. Aseptic meningitis due to varicella-zoster virus: serum antibody levels and local synthesis of specific IgG, IgM, and IgA. J Infect Dis 1987; 155: 959–967.
30. Eide PK, Jorum E, Stubhaug A, et al. Relief of post-herpetic neuralgia with the N-methyl-D-aspartic acid receptor antagonist ketamine: a double-blind, cross-over comparison with morphine and placebo. Pain 1994; 58: 347–354.
31. Engberg IB, Grondahl GB, Thibom K. Patients' experiences of herpes zoster and postherpetic neuralgia. J Adv Nurs 1995; 21: 427–433.
32. Esmann V, Kroon S, Peterslund NA, et al. Prednisolone does not prevent post-herpetic neuralgia. Lancet 1987; 2: 126–129.
33. Fields HL, Heinricher MM, Mason P. Neurotransmitters in nociceptive modulatory circuits. Annu Rev Neurosci 1991; 14: 219–245.
34. Fields HL, Rowbotham MC. Multiple mechanisms of neuropathic pain: a clinical perspective. In Gebhart GF, Hammond DL, Jensen TS, eds. Proceedings of the 7th World Congress on Pain, Progress in Pain Research and Management, Vol. 2, Seattle: IASP Press, 1994: 437–454.
35. Fine PG. Nerve blocks, herpes zoster, and postherpetic neuralgia. In: Watson CPN, ed. Herpes Zoster and Postherpetic Neuralgia. Amsterdam: Elsevier, 1993: 173–183.
36. Fink B, Cairns A. Lack of size-related differential sensitivity to equilibrium conduction block among mammalian myelinated axons exposed to lidocaine. Anesth Analg 1987; 66: 948.
37. Freidman-Kein AE, Lafleur FL, Gendler E, et al. Herpes zoster: a possible early clinical sign for development of acquired immunodeficiency syndrome. J Am Acad Dermatol 1986; 14: 1023–1028.
38. Gershon A. Zoster in immunosuppressed patients. In: Watson CPN, ed. Herpes Zoster and Postherpetic Neuralgia. Amsterdam: Elsevier, 1993: 73–86.
39. Gilden DH, Dueland AN, Cohrs R, et al. Preherpetic neuralgia. Neurology 1991; 41: 1215–1218.
40. Gilden DH. Herpes zoster with postherpetic neuralgia—persisting pain and frustration. N Engl J Med 1994; 330: 932–934.

41. Gilden DH, Wright RR, Schneck SA, et al. Zoster sine herpete, a clinical variant. Ann Neurol 1994; 35: 530–533.
42. Glynn C, Crockford G, Gavaghan D, et al. Epidemiology of shingles. Proc R Soc Med 1990; 83: 617–619.
43. Guess HA, Broughton DD, Melton LJ, Kurland LT. Epidemiology of herpes zoster in children and adolescents: a population-based study. Pediatrics 1985; 76: 512–517.
44. Halper JP, Mann JJ. Cardiovascular effects of antidepressant medications. Br J Psychiatry 1988; 153(suppl 3): 87–98.
45. Hardy I, Gershon AA, Steinberg SP, LaRuss P. The incidence of zoster after immunization with live attenuated varicella vaccine. N Engl J Med 1991; 325: 1545–1550.
46. Head H, Campbell A. The pathology of herpes zoster and its bearing on sensory localization. Brain 1990; 23: 353–523.
47. Heller HM, Carnevale NT, Steigbigel RT. Varicella zoster virus transverse myelitis without cutaneous rash. Am J Med 1990; 88: 550–551.
48. Higa K, Dan K, Manabe H, Noda B. Factors influencing the duration of treatment of acute herpetic pain with sympathetic nerve block: importance of severity of herpes zoster assessed by the maximum antibody titers to varicella-zoster virus in otherwise healthy patients. Pain 1988; 32: 147–157.
49. Hoffmann V, Coppejans H, Vercauteren M, Adriaensen H. Successful treatment of postherpetic neuralgia with oral ketamine. Clin J Pain 1994; 10: 240–242.
50. Hogan QH. The sympathetic nervous system in post-herpetic neuralgia. Reg Anaesth 1993; 18: 271–273.
51. Holzer P. Local effector functions of capsaicin-sensitive sensory nerve endings: involvement of tachykinins, calcitonin gene-related peptide and other neuropeptides. Neuroscience 1988; 24: 739–768.
52. Hope-Simpson R. The nature of herpes zoster: a long term study and a new hypothesis. Proc R Soc Lond B Biol Sci 1965; 58: 9–20.
53. Huff JC, Bean B, Balfour HH Jr, et al. Therapy of herpes zoster with oral acyclovir. Am J Med 1988; 85(suppl): 84–89.
54. Hwant AS, Wilcox GL. Analgesic properties of intrathecally administered heterocyclic antidepressants. Pain 1987; 28: 343–355.
55. Jancso G, Husz S, Simon N. Impairment of axon reflex vasodilatation after herpes zoster. Clin Exp Dermatol 1983; 8: 27–31.
56. Kassirer MR. King and Robert, concerning the management of pain associated with herpes zoster and of post-herpetic neuralgia. Pain 1988; 35: 368–369.
57. King RB. Topical aspirin in chloroform and the relief of pain due to herpes zoster and postherpetic neuralgia. Arch Neurol 1993; 50: 1046–1053.
58. Kishore-Kumar R, Max MB, Schafer SC, et al. Desipramine relieves post-herpetic neuralgia. Clin Pharmacol Ther 1990; 47: 305–312.
59. Kissin I, McDanal J, Xavier AV. Topical lidocaine for relief of superficial pain in postherpetic neuralgia. Neurology 1989; 39: 1132–1133.

60. Koltzenburg M, Torebjork HE, Wahren LK. Nociceptor modulated central sensitization causes mechanical hyperalgesia in acute chemogenic and chronic neuropathic pain. Brain 1994; 117: 579–591.
61. Kurtzke JF. Neuroepidemiology. Ann Neurol 1984; 16: 265–277.
62. LeVasseur SA, Gibson SJ, Helme RD. The measurement of capsaicin-sensitive sensory nerve fiber function in elderly patients with pain. Pain 1990; 41: 19–25.
63. Lewis GW. Zoster sine herpete. Br Med J 1958; 2: 418–419.
64. Lewis T, Marvin HM. Observations relating to vasodilatation arising from antidromic impulses, to herpes zoster and tropic effects. Heart 1927; 14: 27–47.
65. Ljungman P, Lonnqvist B, Gahrton G, et al. Clinical and subclinical reactivations of varicella-zoster virus in immunocompromised patients. J Infect Dis 1986; 153: 840–847.
66. Loeser JD. Surgery for postherpetic neuralgia. In: Watson CPN, ed. Herpes Zoster and Postherpetic Neuralgia. Amsterdam: Elsevier 1993: 221–238.
67. Lombard MC, Larabi Y. Electrophysiological study of cervical dorsal horn cells in partially deafferented rats. In: Bonica JJ, Lindblom U, Iggo A, eds. Advances in Pain Research and Therapy, Vol. 5. New York: Raven Press, 1983: 147–154.
68. Luby J, Ramirez-Ronda C, Rinner S, et al. A longitudinal study of varicella zoster virus in renal transport recipients. J Infect Dis 1977; 135: 659–663.
69. Max MB, Culnane M, Schafer SC, et al. Amitriptyline relieves diabetic neuropathy pain in patients with normal or depressed mood. Neurology 1987; 37: 589–596.
70. Max M, Schafer S, Culnane M, et al. Amitriptyline, but not lorazepam, relieves postherpetic neuralgia. Neurology 1988; 38: 1427–1432.
71. Max MB, Lynch SA, Muir J, et al. Effects of desipramine, amitriptyline, and fluoxetine on pain in diabetic neuropathy. N Engl J Med 1992; 326: 1250–1256.
72. Max MB. Treatment of post-herpetic neuralgia: antidepressants. Ann Neurol 1994; 35(suppl): S50–S53.
73. Mayo DR, Boos J. Varicella zoster-associated neurologic disease without skin lesions. Arch Neurol 1989; 46: 313–315.
74. McKendrick MW, McGill JI, Wood MJ. Lack of effect of acyclovir on postherpetic neuralgia. Br Med J 1989; 298: 431.
75. McQuay HJ, Carroll D, Moxon A, et al. Benzydamine cream for the treatment of post-herpetic neuralgia: minimum duration of treatment periods in a cross-over trial. Pain 1990; 40: 131–135.
76. Molin L. Aspects of the natural history of herpes zoster. Acta Derm Venereol 1969; 49: 569–583.
77. Morimoto M, Inamori K, Hyodo M. The effect of indomethacin stupe for post-herpetic neuralgia particularly in comparison with chloroform-aspirin solution (abstr). Pain 1990; (suppl 5): S59.
78. Muller S, Winkelmann R. Cutaneous nerve changes in zoster. J Invest Dermatol 1969; 52: 71–77.
79. Noordenbos W. Pain. Amsterdam: Elsevier, 1959.
80. Nurmikko TJ, Räsänen A, Häkkinen V. Clinical and neurophysiological observations on acute herpes zoster. Clin J Pain 1990; 6: 284–290.

81. Nurmikko T, Bowsher D. Somatosensory findings in postherpetic neuralgia. J Neurol Neurosurg Psychiatry 1990; 53: 135–141.
82. Nurmikko T. Sensory dysfunction in postherpetic neuralgia. In: Boivie J, Hansson P, Lindblom U, eds. Touch, Temperature, and Pain Health and Disease: Mechanisms and Assessments. Progress in Pain Research and Management, Vol. 3, Seattle: IASP Press, 1994: 133–141.
83. Pappagallo M, Campbell JN. Chronic opioid therapy as alternative treatment for post-herpetic neuralgia. Ann Neurol 1994; 35(suppl): S54–6.
84. Peikert A, Hentrich M, Ochs G. Topical 0.025% capsaicin in chronic postherpetic neuralgia: efficacy, predictors of response and long-term course. J Neurol 1991; 238: 452–456.
85. Perl ER. Causalgia and reflex sympathetic dystrophy revisited. In: Boivie J, Hansson P, Lindblom U, eds. Touch, Temperature, and Pain Health and Disease. Progress in Pain Research and Management, Vol. 3, Seattle: IASP Press, 1994: 231–248.
86. Portenoy R, Duma C, Foley K. Acute herpetic and postherpetic neuralgia: clinical review and current management. Ann Neurol 1986; 20: 651–664.
87. Portenoy R, Foley K. Chronic use of opioid analgesics in non-malignant pain: report of 38 cases. Pain 1986; 25: 171–186.
88. Post BT, Philbrick JT. Prevention of postherpetic neuralgia by corticosteroids. In: Watson CPN, eds. Herpes Zoster and Postherpetic Neuralgia. Amsterdam: Elsevier, 1993: 159–172.
89. Ragozzino M, Melton L, Kurland L, et al. Population based study of herpes zoster and its sequelae. Medicine 1982; 61: 310–316.
90. Richelson E. Antidepressants and brain neurochemistry. Mayo Clin Proc 1990; 65: 1227–1236.
91. Riopelle JM, Naraghi M, Grush K. Chronic neuralgia incidence following local anesthetic therapy for herpes zoster. Arch Dermatol 1984; 120: 747–750.
92. Riopelle J, Lopez-Anaya A, Cork RC, et al. Treatment of the cutaneous pain of acute herpes zoster with 9% lidocaine (base) in petrolatum/paraffin ointment. J Am Acad Dermatol 1994; 30(5 Pt 1): 757–767.
93. Rowbotham M, Fields H. Topical lidocaine reduces pain in post-herpetic neuralgia. Pain 1989; 38: 297–302.
94. Rowbotham MC, Fields HL. Post-herpetic neuralgia: the relation of pain complainant, sensory disturbance, and skin temperature. Pain 1989; 39: 129–144.
95. Rowbotham MC, Reisner LA, Fields HL. Both intravenous lidocaine and morphine reduce the pain of post-herpetic neuralgia. Neurology 1991; 41: 1024–1028.
96. Rowbotham MC. Topical agents for post-herpetic neuralgia. In: Watson CPN, ed. Herpes Zoster and Postherpetic Neuralgia. Amsterdam: Elsevier, 1993: 185–203.
97. Rowbotham MC Managing post-herpetic neuralgia with opioids and local anesthetics. Ann Neurol 1994; 35(suppl): S46–S49.
98. Rowbotham MC, Davies PS, Fields HL. Topical lidocaine gel relieves postherpetic neuralgia. Ann Neurol 1995; 37: 246–253.

99. Rowbotham MC, Davies PS, Verkempinck C, Galer BS. Lidocaine patch: double-blind controlled study of a new treatment method for post-herpetic neuralgia. Pain 1995; in press.
100. Rusthoven JJ, Ahlgren P, Elhakim T, et al. Varicella-zoster infection in adult cancer patients. Arch Intern Med 1988; 148: 1561–1566.
101. Shanbrom E. Treatment of herpetic pain and postherpetic neuralgia with intravenous procaine. JAMA 1961; 176: 1041–1043.
102. Stow PJ, Glynn CJ, Minor B. EMLA cream in the treatment of post-herpetic neuralgia: efficacy and pharmacokinetic profile. Pain 1989; 39: 301–305.
103. Straus SE, Smith HA, Ruyechen WT, et al. Endonuclease analysis of viral DNA from varicella and subsequent zoster infections in the same patient. N Engl J Med 1984; 311: 1362–1364.
104. Straus S. Varicella-zoster virus infections: biology, natural history, treatment, and prevention. Ann Intern Med 1988; 108: 221–237.
105. Sugar O, Bucy P. Postherpetic trigeminal neuralgia. Arch Neurol Psychiatry 1951; 65: 131–145.
106. Tenicela R, Lovasik D, Eaglestein W. Treatment of herpes zoster with sympathetic blocks. Clin J Pain 1985; 1: 63–67.
107. Tyring S, Barbarash RA, Nahlik JE, et al. Famciclovir for the treatment of acute herpes zoster: effects on acute disease and postherpetic neuralgia. Ann Intern Med 1995; in press.
108. Wall PD, Gutnick M. Ongoing activity in peripheral nerves: the physiology and pharmacology of impulses originating form a neuroma. Exp Neurol 1974; 43: 580–593.
109. Watson C, Evans R, Reed K, et al. Amitriptyline vs placebo in postherpetic neuralgia. Neurology 1982; 32: 671–673.
110. Watson CPN, Evans RJ. A comparative trial of amitriptyline and zimelidine in postherpetic neuralgia. Pain 1985; 23: 387–394.
111. Watson C, Evans R, Watt V. Postherpetic neuralgia and topical capsaicin. Pain 1988; 33: 333–340.
112. Watson CPN, Evans RJ, Watt VR, Birkett N. Post-herpetic neuralgia: 208 cases. Pain 1988; 35: 289–297.
113. Watson CPN, Chipman M, Reed K, et al. Amitriptyline versus maprotiline in postherpetic neuralgia: a randomized, double-blind, crossover trial. Pain 1982; 48(1): 29–36.
114. Watson CPN, Tyler KL, Bickers DR, et al. A randomized vehicle-controlled trial of topical capsaicin in the treatment of postherpetic neuralgia. Clin Ther 1993; 15: 510–526.
115. Watson CPN, Deck JH. The neuropathology of herpes zoster with particular reference to postherpetic neuralgia and its pathogenesis. In: Watson CPN, ed. Herpes Zoster and Postherpetic Neuralgia. Amsterdam: Elsevier, 1993: 139–158.
116. Whitley RJ, Weiss H, Gnann J, et al. The efficacy of steroid and acyclovir therapy of herpes zoster in the elderly. J Invest Med 1995; 43: A114.

117. Wilson A, Sharp M, Koropchak C, et al. Subclinical varicella-zoster virus viremia, herpes zoster, and T lymphocyte immunity to varicella-zoster viral antigens after bone marrow transplantation. J Infect Dis 1992; 165: 119–126.
118. Winnie AP, Hartwell PW. Relationship between time of treatment of acute herpes zoster with sympathetic blockade and prevention of post-herpetic neuralgia: clinical support for a new theory of the mechanism by which sympathetic blockade provides therapeutic benefit. Reg Anesth 1993; 18: 277–282.
119. Wood MJ, Ogan PH, McKendrick MW, et al. Efficacy of oral acyclovir treatment of acute herpes zoster. Am J Med 1988; 85: 79–83.
120. Wood MJ, Johnson RW, McKendrick MW, et al. A randomized trial of acyclovir for 7 days or 21 days with and without prednisolone for treatment of acute herpes zoster. N Engl J Med 1994; 330: 896–900.
121. Woolf CJ, Shortland P, Coggeshall RE. Peripheral nerve injury triggers central spouting of myelinated afferents. Nature 1992; 355: 75–78.
122. Wulf H, Maier C, Schele HA, Wabbel W. Plasma concentration of bupivacaine after stellate ganlion blockade. Anesth Analg 1991; 72: 546–548.
123. Yanagida H, Suwa K, Corssen G. No prophylactic effect of early sympathetic blockade on postherpetic neuralgia. Anesthesiology 1987; 66: 73–76.

28
Management of Herpes Simplex Labialis

Spotswood L. Spruance
University of Utah School of Medicine, Salt Lake City, Utah

Multiple trials of drugs for recurrent herpes labialis in immunocompetent hosts have been undertaken in the last 30 years (1). Unfortunately for the patients, these studies have yielded largely negative results, and only a few compounds have been approved by regulatory authorities. Idoxuridine (IDU) in dimethyl sulfoxide (DMSO) and acyclovir (ACV) cream are commercially available in Europe. There are no Food and Drug Administration–approved treatments in the United States. Acyclovir ointment is used by practitioners for this indication, but the evidence from multiple clinical trials shows little or no therapeutic effect (2–4). The approval of ACV ointment in the United States was based on its activity in primary genital herpes (5) and herpes labialis in immunocompromised patients (6).

Intravenous foscarnet is effective for the treatment of herpes simplex virus (HSV) infections in immunocompromised patients (7). Topical foscarnet cream had a major effect on clinical and virological measures of lesion severity in the dorsal cutaneous guinea pig model of cutaneous HSV-1 disease (8). Unfortunately, a large Canadian trial of foscarnet cream for the treatment of herpes labialis found tantalizing but only marginal evidence of efficacy.

Assessment of the reasons for treatment failure in herpes labialis trials has identified issues of drug formulation and protocol design, which can be corrected and will increase our chances of finding effective therapy (9). Geometric increases in skin penetration can be accomplished by antiviral

358   Spruance

drug formulation in compounds that effect a major disruption in the
biochemistry of the stratum corneum, such as DMSO or laurocapram
(Azone) (10,11). Among patients who began treatment of herpes labialis
in the prodromal or erythema lesion stages, topical 15% IDU in DMSO
reduced the time to loss of crust by 3.3 days (38%, $P < .001$) and the
duration of pain by 1.8 days (42%, $P = .08$) in comparison to vehicle-treated
controls (12).

Delivery of drug by peroral administration can ensure lesion drug
concentrations roughly equivalent to serum levels. Raborn et al. (13)
reported a 12% to 17% decrease in the healing time of herpes labialis
among patients treated with peroral ACV. The duration of secondary
lesions was reduced by 30% to 40%, demonstrating the greater activity of
ACV when early treatment is ensured. Our study with peroral ACV confirmed Raborn's results and again demonstrated the importance of
patient-initiated treatment starting in the prodromal or erythema stage of
an incipient episode. When these conditions were met, time to loss of crust
was reduced by 2.1 days (27%, $P = .03$) and the duration of pain by 1.4 days
(36%, $P = .02$) in comparison to placebo-treated controls (14).

The poor bioavailability of peroral ACV likely contributes to its limited
efficacy, and clinical studies with the well-absorbed prodrug of ACV,
valaciclovir, and another acyclic nucleoside, famciclovir, are awaited with
interest. A preliminary dose-ranging trial of peroral famciclovir for treatment of experimental ultraviolet radiation–induced herpes labialis has
been described in abstract form (15). Patients were given 125, 250, or 500
mg of famciclovir or placebo three times a day by mouth for 5 days,
beginning 2 days after irradiation. There was evidence of a dose-response
effect on the duration of the induced lesions. Famciclovir, 125 and 250 mg
three times a day, healed lesions one day faster, and 500 mg three times a
day healed lesions 3 days faster and the improvement was statistically
significant. These results provide important additional evidence that
herpes labialis is a treatable disease and show the need for high doses of
antiviral drug to maximize clinical benefit.

High-dose peroral famciclovir treatment of experimental herpes
labialis and aggressive topical therapy with IDU in DMSO (12) both
reduced lesion duration to the same degree (3 days). This amount of
clinical effect could be near the maximum achievable benefit of episodic
antiviral therapy for this disease.

In the last 13 years, 11 studies have evaluated prophylactic ACV
for suppression of herpes labialis (16). Four studies evaluating the efficacy
of topical ACV showed inconsistent efficacy, including "escape" lesions
outside the zone of application. We found no efficacy with 8×/day

application when ACV cream was used to suppress experimental ultraviolet radiation–induced lesions (17). In contrast to the experience with topical ACV, seven studies in which prophylactic peroral ACV was evaluated all reported positive results. The degree of reduction in lesion frequency changed from 50% to 78%. Systemic prophylactic therapy may have been more effective than topical therapy because virus replication was suppressed in the neural ganglia, as well as in the periphery (18).

Considerable clinical investigation is in progress to develop a vaccine for herpes genitalis. Goals include both primary vaccination (protection of seronegative persons from infection) and therapeutic vaccination (augmentation or alteration of the immunity of persons already infected). A recent report has shown that intramuscular administration of recombinant glycoprotein D to patients with recurrent herpes genitalis reduced the frequency of recurrences by 24% over 12 months of observation compared to placebo-vaccinated control subjects (19).

An "alternative" herpes simplex treatment is a substance or procedure advocated by someone for which the mechanism of action is illogical or unknown and that usually has not been subjected to a rigorous large-scale, placebo-controlled clinical trial. Individual alternative medications have occasionally received attention in the medical literature, but the general subject of alternative therapies has only occasionally been reviewed (20). Alternative treatments include substances that lyse or inactivate free virus (virus unassociated with cells), a mode of action considered to be of limited value for an agent that replicates within cells (21,22), and vaccines that have a general immunomodulatory activity or are composed of antigens from a different virus (smallpox, influenza).

Although there is considerable justified skepticism about alternative treatments, several potentially important areas of therapeutics have not been thoroughly investigated: symptomatic therapy, antiinflammatory therapy, and acceleration of wound healing. Many alternative strategies that seem effective to patients probably act through relief of symptoms. We have routinely advised patients to use nonsteroidal antiinflammatory agents and local application of ice or refrigerant packs to reduce pain and inflammation.

REFERENCES

1. Overall JC Jr. Dermatologic viral diseases. In: Galasso GJ, Merigan TC, Buchanan RA, eds. Antiviral Agents and Viral Diseases of Man. 2nd ed. New York: Raven Press, 1984: 247–312.

2. Raborn GW, McGaw WT, Grace M, Houle L. Herpes labialis treatment with acyclovir 5 per cent ointment. Can Dent Assoc J 1989; 55: 135–137.

3. Spruance SL, Crumpacker CS, Schnipper LE, et al. Early, patient-initiated treatment of herpes labialis with topical 10% acyclovir. Antimicrob Agents Chemother 1984; 25: 553–555.

4. Spruance SL, Schnipper LE, Overall Jr JC, et al. Treatment of herpes simplex labialis with topical acyclovir in polyethylene glycol. J Infect Dis 1982; 146: 85–90.

5. Corey L, Nahmias AJ, Guinan ME, et al. A trial of topical acyclovir in genital herpes simplex virus infections. N Engl J Med 1982; 2: 1313–1319.

6. Whitley RJ, Levin M, Barton N, et al. Infections caused by herpes simplex virus in the immunocompromised host: natural history and topical acyclovir therapy. J Infect Dis 1984; 150: 323–329.

7. Safrin S, Crumpacker C, Chatis P, et al. A controlled trial comparing foscarnet with vidarabine for acyclovir-resistant herpes simplex in the acquired immunodeficiency syndrome. N Engl J Med 1991; 325: 551–555.

8. Spruance SL, Freeman DJ, Sheth NV. Comparison of topical foscarnet, acyclovir (ACV) cream and ACV ointment in the treatment of experimental cutaneous herpes simplex virus (HSV) infection. Antimicrob Agents Chemother 1986; 30: 196–198.

9. Spruance SL. The natural history of recurrent oral-facial herpes simplex virus infection. Semin Dermatol 1992; 11: 200–206.

10. Freeman DJ, Sheth NV, Spruance NL. Failure of topical acyclovir (ACV) in ointment to penetrate human skin. Antimicrob Agents Chemother 1986; 29: 730–732.

11. Sheth NV, Freeman DJ, Higuchi WI, Spruance SL. The influence of Azone, propylene glycol and polyethylene glycol on the in vitro skin penetration of trifluorothymidine. Int J Pharmaceut 1986; 28: 201–209.

12. Spruance SL, Stewart JCB, Freeman DJ, et al. Early application of topical 15% idoxuridine in dimethyl sulfoxide shortens the course of herpes simplex labialis: a multicenter placebo-controlled trial. J Infect Dis 1990; 161: 191–197.

13. Raborn GW, McGaw WT, Grace M, et al. Oral acyclovir and herpes labialis: a randomized, double-blind, placebo-controlled study. J Am Dent Assoc 1987; 115: 38–42.

14. Spruance SL, Stewart JCB, Rowe NH, et al. Treatment of recurrent herpes simplex labialis with oral acyclovir. J Infect Dis 1990; 161: 185–190.

15. Spruance SL, Rowe N, Raborn GW, et al. Oral famciclovir in the treatment of experimental ultraviolet radiation-induced herpes labialis: a double-blind, dose-ranging, placebo-controlled multi-centered trial (abstr). Proc Intersci Conf Antimicrob Agents Chemother 1995; 35: 205.

16. Spruance SL. Prophylactic chemotherapy with acyclovir for recurrent herpes simplex labialis. J Med Virol 1993; 41(suppl 1): 27–32.

17. Spruance SL, Freeman DJ, Stewart JCB, et al. The natural history of ultraviolet radiation-induced herpes simplex labialis and responses to therapy with peroral and topical formulations of acyclovir. J Infect Dis 1991; 163: 728–734.

18. Demangone M, Hill JM, Kwon BS. Effects of acyclovir therapy during simultaneous reactivation of latent HSV-1 in rabbits. Antiviral Res 1987; 7: 237–243.
19. Straus SE, Corey L, Burke RL, et al. Placebo-controlled trial of vaccination with recombinant glycoprotein D of herpes simplex virus type 2 for immunotherapy of genital herpes. Lancet 1994; 343: 1460–1463.
20. Spruance SL. Herpes simplex labialis. In: Sacks SL, Straus SE, Whitley RJ, Griffiths PD, eds. Clinical Management of Herpes Viruses. Amsterdam: IOS Press, 1995: 3–42.
21. Lodmell DL, Niwa A, Hayashi K, Notkins AL. Prevention of cell-to-cell spread of herpes simplex virus by leukocytes. J Exp Med 1973; 137: 706–720.
22. Guinan ME, MacCalman J, Kern ER, et al. Topical ether and herpes simplex labialis. JAMA 1980; 243: 1059–1061.

29

Cidofovir Therapy for Cutaneous Viral Infections

H. S. Jaffe and Brian William McGuire
Gilead Sciences, Inc., Foster City, California

INTRODUCTION

Cidofovir (1-[(S)-3-hydroxy-2-(phosphonomethoxy)propyl]cytosine dihydrate or HPMPC) is a nucleotide analog with potent activity against a broad spectrum of human DNA viruses, including herpesviruses (cytomegalovirus [CMV], herpes simplex virus [HSV] types 1 and 2, varicella-zoster virus [VZV], and Epstein-Barr virus [EBV], adenovirus, and human papillomaviruses.

Current herpesvirus therapies include nucleoside analogs such as acyclovir, famciclovir, or ganciclovir and the phosophonacetic acid analog, foscarnet. Most nucleoside analogs rely on viral enzymes (e.g., thymidine kinase) for activation. Many viruses, however, may become drug-resistant because of an acquired deficiency or alteration in such enzymes. Certain available antiviral agents are also associated with significant toxicities. Because of these limitations, other strategies have emerged over the last decade for creating agents with broader spectra of antiviral activity and improved toxicity profiles (1–3).

One such strategy favored the development of nucleoside monophosphate (nucleotide) analogs as opposed to unphosphorylated nucleosides such as acyclovir and ganciclovir. It was evident that it would not be possible to merely phosphorylate a nucleoside derivative, because the phosphorus–oxygen bond is labile in vivo. To produce a stable nucleotide analog, the oxygen in the phosphoester bond was exchanged with the proximate carbon in the nucleotide, creating a class of compounds termed phosphonomethylethers (1–3). Of these compounds, cidofovir was selected for clinical development because of its high in vivo potency and advantageous therapeutic index. The chemical structure is as follows:

NH$_2$

$\overset{O}{\underset{||}{\text{OCH}_2\text{P(OH)}_2}}$

OH   • 2 H$_2$O

The active intracellular metabolite is cidofovir diphosphate, which inhibits HSV-1 and HSV-2 DNA polymerases at concentrations about 50-fold, 120-fold, and 600-fold lower than that needed to inhibit human DNA polymerases α, β, and γ, respectively. Unlike acyclovir and ganciclovir, which require intracellular activation by virally encoded enzymes (thymidine kinase and protein kinase, respectively), phosphorylation of cidofovir in cells to cidofovir diphosphate is independent of virus infection. Cidofovir diphosphate persists in cells with a half-life of 17 to 65 hours. Cidofovir diphosphate in uninfected cells, therefore, may prime them to resist replication when subsequently infected. Additionally, the long intracellular half-life might allow for efficacy with infrequent dosing (4–7).

As a topical agent in vivo, cidofovir is active against HSV-1 and HSV-2 infection in mice, guinea pigs, and rabbits and against cottontail rabbit papillomavirus (CRPV) disease in rabbits. Toxicology evaluation in rabbits demonstrates dose- and schedule-dependent localized dermatitis with high or prolonged doses, which is reversible after discontinuation of treatment. Pharmacokinetic data from guinea pigs and rabbits indicate a low to undetectable degree of systemic absorption of cidofovir applied topically to unbroken skin.

Cidofovir intravenous injection is currently in Phase II/III clinical studies for the systemic treatment of CMV infection in patients with AIDS. Phase I/II clinical studies of a topical gel formulation of cidofovir have been initiated in the treatment of cutaneous viral diseases caused by herpes simplex and human papillomavirus.

IN VITRO STUDIES

The activity of cidofovir against HSV-1 and HSV-2 has been evaluated using a variety of virus strains and cell types (1,2). Isolates of HSV-1, which have become resistant to acyclovir because of a thymidine kinase (TK) mutation, are not cross-resistant to cidofovir. In fact, the 50% inhibitory dose (ID_{50}) of cidofovir in vitro has been shown to be lower for acyclovir-resistant than for acyclovir-sensitive strains. This further supports the observation that cidofovir does not rely on viral TK for activation.

Retention of intracellular metabolites of cidofovir suggests that antiviral effects may persist after removal of cidofovir from treated cells (7). Three intracellular cidofovir metabolites have been found: cidofovir phosphate, cidofovir diphosphate, and cidofovir phosphate-choline (5). These cidofovir metabolites were shown to have long intra-cellular half-lives in comparison with other antiviral nucleoside analogs: ~6, 17 to 65, and 87 hours, respectively. This feature of cidofovir pharmacology is thought to be the reason for the long duration of the antiviral effect.

Cidofovir diphosphate, the putative active antiviral metabolite, is a potent inhibitor of HSV-1, HSV-2, and HCMV DNA polymerases, with Ki values of 0.86 μM, 1.4 μM, and 6.6 μM, respectively (5,7). The incorporation of a single cidofovir molecule caused the DNA synthesis to slow down by approximately 31%. The incorporation of two consecutive cidofovir molecules, or two cidofovir molecules separated by one molecule of dAMP, dCMP, or dTMP, caused the DNA synthesis to cease (7).

The Ki value of cidofovir against human DNA polymerase α was 51 μM versus a Km value of 4.7 μM for dCTP (5). This indicates that cidofovir diphosphate is a poor inhibitor of human DNA polymerase α.

The mechanism of action for the anti-HPV activity of cidofovir is not as well understood as that for herpesviruses, which encode their own DNA polymerase. Papillomaviruses in contrast use the DNA polymerase of the host cell. It has been shown that HPV infection causes enhanced expression of nucleotide kinases in the host cell by approximately 10-fold (7) and increased expression of DNA polymerase. The enhancement of host nucleotide kinases and DNA polymerase activities would be expected to increase the formation of cidofovir diphosphate and its subsequent incorporation into HPV DNA, which in turn would disrupt DNA chain elongation and inhibit viral replication.

IN VIVO STUDIES

The antiviral activity of topical cidofovir has been evaluated in mice and guinea pigs for the treatment of infection with HSV and in rabbits for infection with CPRV, a close relative of HPV.

Models of HSV Infection

In a study of hairless mice infected intracutaneously with HSV-1 or HSV-2, topical cidofovir at concentrations of 0.1%, 0.3%, or 1% applied four times a day for 5 days completely suppressed all manifestations of disease; control animals developed skin lesions and hind leg paralysis followed by death in all cases (8). Similarly, in athymic nude mice, topical cidofovir at strengths of 0.1%, 0.3%, or 1% completely suppressed HSV-1 infection by TK-minus strains. None of the treated animals showed evidence of disease, whereas all control and acyclovir-treated animals developed fulminant disease and died. No cidofovir-associated toxicity was observed.

In a murine genital model of primary HSV-2 infection, topical cidofovir at concentrations of 0.5%, 1%, or 5% applied three times a day for 5 days beginning 24 hours after virus inoculation reduced vaginal viral replication by 100-fold relative to controls and by 5-fold relative to 5% acyclovir (9). A 100-fold reduction in viral titer was also seen with once daily application of cidofovir 6 hours after inoculation, a statistically significant reduction compared with control or acyclovir-treated animals. Again, there was no evidence of cidofovir-associated toxicity.

The effect of topical cidofovir has also been evaluated in a guinea pig model of primary genital HSV (9). Treatment with 0.3% or 1% cidofovir applied intravaginally either once a day or three times a day for 7 days beginning 24 hours after inoculation reduced viral titer as well as lesion scores to a statistically significant degree when compared to placebo.

Data from a guinea pig model have demonstrated the activity of single doses of cidofovir in genital HSV-2 infection (7). Twenty-four hours postintravaginal inoculation, topical therapy was initiated with either placebo gel or 0.3%, 1%, or 3% cidofovir gel given once a day for 1, 3, or 5 days. Suppression of viral replication by a single-dose application of cidofovir at all strengths was statistically significant compared with placebo; additionally, single-dose therapy appeared to be as effective as multiple doses.

Models of Papillomavirus Infection

Topically applied cidofovir effectively induced regression of papillomas in a CRPV model (10,11). Rabbits with established papillomas were treated with 0.1% or 1% cidofovir, or 5% podofilox twice a day 5 days a week for 8 weeks. Application of 0.1% cidofovir reduced papilloma size by 50% to 70% compared with untreated control subjects. Seventy percent of papillomas treated with 1% cidofovir disappeared.

A comparison of antipapilloma activity between cidofovir topical gel and podofilox was conducted in Dutch-belted rabbits (12). Rabbits were infected on their backs with a high and low inoculum of papillomavirus and received either placebo gel, 0.1%, 0.3%, or 1% cidofovir, or 0.5% podofilox, all given topically twice a day 5 days a week for 8 weeks, beginning 4 weeks postinfection. Treatment with cidofovir displayed a dose-dependent effect on papilloma growth. Cidofovir at 1% completely suppressed papilloma growth compared to placebo, and the lesions cleared. Notably, in the animals who received 1% cidofovir, seven of nine animals showed no recurrence. In contrast, podofilox at the high inoculum sites cleared the papilloma in only one of five animals; this animal showed recurrence 4 weeks later. At the low inoculum sites, although all four sites resolved with podofilox, three of four recurred.

Preclinical Pharmacokinetics

A pharmacokinetic study in guinea pigs was conducted to compare the systemic exposure to cidofovir given topically or intravenously (7). ^{14}C-Cidofovir was given intravenously at a dose of 1 mg/kg or topically in the genital area at a dose of 1 mg per animal as a 1% gel. Plasma cidofovir levels were undetectable in all animals after topical administration. Based on recovered ^{14}C isotope, mean urinary excretion over 48 hours was 3.5 ± 1.6% of the topical dose (n = 9), yielding an approximate 3.9% bioavailability of topical cidofovir.

In a bioavailability and tissue distribution study conducted in rabbits, groups of animals were given either a single intravenous dose of ^{14}C-cidofovir (1 mg/kg), 1% ^{14}C-cidofovir gel (2 mg) applied to experimentally abraded skin, or 1% ^{14}C-cidofovir gel (2 mg) applied to normal intact skin (7). Absolute bioavailability of the topical formulation was 2.1% for normal intact skin and 41% for abraded skin. Radioactivity present in kidney and testes after topical application to intact skin was <1% and <4% of those after intravenous administration, respectively, and following application to abraded skin was 47% and 52% of the intravenous values. These results demonstrated that in the setting of intact skin, bioavailability of topically applied cidofovir is low, as are the resulting concentrations in kidney and testes.

CLINICAL STUDIES

Extensive clinical experience has been obtained with cidofovir intravenous injection in the setting of CMV retinitis in patients with AIDS. More than 200 patients have been treated to date. The emergent dose-limiting toxicity from these studies is renal, as evidenced by increases in proteinuria, which are generally subclinical.

Clinical experience with cidofovir injection has also been reported on the intralesional treatment of a woman with recurrent hypopharyngeal and esophageal papillomatous lesions of HPV types 16 and 18 (13,14). The patient presented with squamous papillomatosis extending 8 cm across and displaying at biopsy malignant degeneration. Despite surgical resection and several courses of laser photocoagulation with α-interferon treatment, the lesion progressed to the point of eliciting dysphagia. The patient was then given multiple local injections of cidofovir at a dosage of 1.25 mg/kg a week for 4 weeks then every 3 to 5 weeks for an additional 3 weeks. Complete resolution of the hypopharyngeal lesions was achieved; small residual lesions were observed in the esophagus, which also resolved after three additional treatments of cidofovir. The response has been maintained for 2 years. No side effects to treatment were observed.

Lalezari et al. (15) reported a case study on the response of an acyclovir-resistant mucocutaneous herpes simplex infection to intravenous cidofovir in a patient with AIDS. The patient entered a Phase I/II trial of intravenous cidofovir for asymptomatic CMV shedding with concurrent perineal HSV-2 lesions, which had demonstrated in vitro resistance to acyclovir and clinical nonresponse to both high-dose oral acyclovir and trifluridine. The patient received 4 weekly infusions of intravenous cidofovir at 5 mg/kg a week and displayed a 95% healing of HSV lesions.

Snoeck et al. have published their clinical experience with the topical application of cidofovir from two patients (16). One was a patient with AIDS and severe persistent HSV-2 perineal ulceration. The other was a patient with chronic myelogenous leukemia who had received a bone marrow transplantation in conjunction with myeloablative therapy and subsequently developed severe oral HSV-1 mucositis during the period of profound myelosuppression. The first patient, who had failed previous acyclovir, foscarnet, and ganciclovir therapy, was given a total of eight courses, each consisting of 3 or 4 days of topical application of 1% cidofovir. Each course resulted in either notable improvement or complete clearing of lesions. The second patient had failed acyclovir (given both orally and intravenously), foscarnet, and α-interferon. He received a 3-day course of 1% topical cidofovir, which resulted in complete resolution of lesions. In response to new lesions that subsequently developed, an additional 3-day course was given as before, which, followed by oral acyclovir, was associated with complete clearance.

Snoeck et al. (14) also reported three case studies of the topical administration of cidofovir to immunocompromised patients with severe relapsing anogenital papillomavirus infections. One was a male with biopsy-proven Bowenoid papulosis, another was a male with recurrent exophytic perigenital and intraanal condyloma acuminatum, and the third a female with cervical and vulvar condyloma acuminatum. Each case was refractory to standard treatment. The patients received cidofovir 1% in Beeler base daily for 5 days, 11 days, and 5 weeks, respectively. Each patient experienced a complete cure of the treated lesions, with response durations of 12+, 6+, and 6+ months, respectively.

Clinical experience with cidofovir topical gel is presently being obtained from three multicenter Phase I/II studies, which are described below.

In Protocol GS-93-301, patients with AIDS who possess acyclovir-resistant mucocutaneous HSV lesions are randomized to receive 5 days of once a day double-blinded therapy with one of three topical gel formulations: 0% (placebo), 0.3%, or 1% cidofovir. Patients are observed for a 2-week study period. Patients who do not display significant toxicity are eligible to receive subsequent cycles of open-label treatment with 1% gel. Primary end points of the study include safety, healing of lesions, and time to cessation of viral shedding. Thirty patients have been randomized into the trial. Nineteen of 27 treated patients have received between 1 and 12 additional open-label cycles of therapy for a cumulative total of 76 cycles. As the study is still blinded, no efficacy data are available.

In Protocol GS-93-302, patients who are HIV-positive and display biopsy-proven external condyloma acuminatum lesions (anogenital warts) are sequentially assigned to one of four treatment regimens: (a) 0.3% cidofovir topical gel once a day for 5 consecutive days, (b) 0.3% cidofovir topical gel once a day for 10 days (two 5-day periods), (c) 1% cidofovir topical gel once a day for 5 consecutive days, and (d) 1% cidofovir topical gel once a day for 10 days (two 5-day periods). Patients are observed throughout treatment and for an additional 2-week period. Patients who do not display significant toxicity are eligible to receive additional cycles of treatment. Primary end points of the study include safety and regression of lesions. To date, 30 patients have been enrolled into this trial: 10 each into groups A, B, and C. A total of 37 cycles of 5- or 10-days each (234 applications of gel) have been given. Preliminary analysis indicates evidence of clinical activity without significant drug-related toxicity.

In Protocol GS-94-305, patients with recurrent herpes genitalis who are otherwise healthy are stratified by gender and randomized within 12 hours of lesion appearance to either placebo or cidofovir topical gel at one of three sequential dose levels: 1%, 3%, or 5%. A single application of gel is given on day 1, and the patient is then seen twice a day until the primary end point, complete healing of treated lesions, is reached. Secondary end points include time to cessation of viral shedding and time to cessation of lesion-associated pain. This trial has recently been initiated.

Pharmacokinetic data on the systemic absorption of topically applied cidofovir have been obtained from 16 patients in study GS-93-301. Only three patients have displayed quantifiable blood levels of drug, at concentrations far below that expected to be associated with clinical or laboratory abnormalities. This is despite the often large and ulcerated lesions characteristic of acyclovir-unresponsive HSV infection in patients with AIDS.

Beyond the clinical activity described here, additional work is planned to further define the role of cidofovir in the treatment of viral cutaneous infections in humans.

REFERENCES

1. De Clercq E, Sakuma T, Baba M, et al. Antiviral activity of phosphonyl-methoxyalkyl derivatives of purines and pyrimidines. Antiviral Res 1987; 8: 261–272.
2. Bronson JJ, Ghazzouli I, Hitchcock MJM, et al. Synthesis and antiviral activity of the nucleotide analogue (S)-1-[3-hydroxy-2-(phosphonylmethoxy)propyl]-cytosine. J Med Chem 1989; 32: 1457–1463.
3. Martin JC, Hitchcock MJM. Phosphomethylether compounds as antiviral agents. Trans Proc 1991; 23: 156–158.
4. Biron KK, Stanet SC, Sorrell JB, et al. Metabolic activation of the nucleoside analog 9-[2-hydroxy-1-(hydroxymethyl)ethoxy]methylguanine in human diploid fibroblasts infected with human cytomegalovirus. Proc Natl Acad Sci USA 1985; 82: 2473–2477.

5. Ho HT, Woods KL, Bronson JJ, et al. Intracellular metabolism of the antiherpes agent (S)-1-[3-hydroxy-2-(phosphonylmethoxy)propyl]cytosine. Mol Pharmacol 1991; 41: 197–202.
6. Talarico C, Stanet S, Lambe C, et al. Mode of action studies on the anticytomegalovirus nucleoside analog [1-(2-hydroxy-1-(hydroxymethyl)ethoxymethyl)cytosine] (abstr 92). Antiviral Res 1990; S1: 87.
7. Data on file, Gilead Sciences, Inc.
8. DeClercq E, Holy A. Efficacy of (S)-1-[3-hydroxy-2-(phosphonylmethoxy)propyl]cytosine in various models of herpes simplex virus infection in mice. Antimicrob Agents Chemother 1991; 35: 801–806.
9. Bravo FJ, Stanberry LR, Kier AB, et al. Evaluation of HPMPC therapy for primary and recurrent genital herpes in mice and guinea pigs. Antiviral Res 1993; 21: 59.
10. Study GS-JWK-PAP-PVR45, Topical HPMPC suspension: eight-week treatment study in New Zealand White rabbits infected with CRPV (Data on file, Gilead Sciences, Inc.).
11. Kurtzman G, Pickel M, Christensen N, Kreider J. Phosphonate nucleoside analogs are potent anti-papillomavirus agents in animal models. Abstracts of the 33rd ICAAC #1593, 410, 1993.
12. Study GS-JWK-PAP-PVR45A, Topical Cidofovir Gel: Eight-week treatment study in Dutch-Belted rabbits infected with cottontail rabbit papillomavirus (CRPV) (Data on file, Gilead Sciences, Inc.).
13. Cutsem EV, Snoeck R, et al. Successful treatment of a squamous papilloma of the hypopharynx-esophagus by local injections of (S)-1-(3-hydroxy-2-phosphonylmethoxypropyl)cytosine. J Med Virol 1994; 45: 230–235.
14. Snoeck R, Van Ranst M, Andrei G, et al. Treatment of anogenital papillomavirus infections with an acyclic nucleoside phosphonate analogue. N Engl J Med 1995; 333: 943–944.
15. Lalezari JP, Drew L, Glutzer E, et al. Treatment with intravenous (S)-1-[3-hydroxy-2-(phosphonylmethoxy)propyl]cytosine of acyclovir-resistant mucocutaneous infection with herpes simplex virus in a patient with AIDS. J Infect Dis 1994; 170: 570–572.
16. Snoeck R, Andrei G, Gerard M, et al. Successful treatment of progressive mucocutaneous acyclovir- and foscarnet-resistant herpes simplex virus infection with (S)-1-(3-hydroxy-2-phosphonylmethoxypropyl)cytosine (HPMPC). Clin Infect Dis 1994; 18: 570–578.

30
Background and Rationale for Prescription to Over-the-Counter Switch for Zovirax (Acyclovir) Capsules

Gray Davis, Edgar L. Hill, and Theodore C. Spaulding
Glaxo Wellcome, Research Triangle Park, North Carolina

Graham Darby
Glaxo Wellcome, Stevenage, England

INTRODUCTION

Zovirax (acyclovir) capsules, 200 mg, has been widely available in the United States for more than 11 years for the management of recurrent genital herpes. Throughout this time, more than 21 million people in the United States have received prescriptions for oral Zovirax, predominantly for genital herpes. After initial diagnosis and treatment by a physician, recurrent genital herpes can be managed by treatment with Zovirax in a dose of 200 mg five times a day. This chapter provides background information on the rationale to support the conversion of Zovirax from prescription to over-the-counter (OTC) status for the treatment of recurrent genital herpes.

NATURAL HISTORY OF GENITAL HERPES

For the last 30 years, it has been recognized that two types of herpes simplex virus (HSV) cause human disease, type 1 (HSV-1) and type 2 (HSV-2). They are readily differentiated by type-specific antibodies, and characterization of virus isolates has demonstrated that they have different epidemiological features. HSV-2 usually causes genital infections, accounting for 70% to 90% of cases of genital herpes, with HSV-1 accounting for the remaining 10% to 30% of cases. In contrast, HSV-1 usually causes orolabial infections, accounting for 80% to 90% of nongenital herpes infections (1). The recent development of type-specific serological assays has facilitated a greater understanding of the epidemiology of HSV. These assays are based on the ability to detect antibodies to specific viral proteins, either by separating the proteins based on their size in an immunoblot (Western blot) assay, or by using purified viral proteins or proteins expressed by recombinant DNA techniques in enzyme immunoassays. These assays are generally based on detection of antibodies to glycoprotein G (gG), which is antigenically quite different between HSV-1 and HSV-2. Thus persons infected with HSV-1 will develop antibodies only to gG-1, and persons infected with HSV-2 will develop antibodies only to gG-2. The presence of antibodies to both gG-1 and gG-2 implies prior infection with both HSV-1 and HSV-2.

In the last 5 years, several cross-sectional seroepidemiological studies have identified the following factors to be associated with a higher prevalence of antibodies to HSV-2: increasing age, lower levels of income or education, increased numbers of sexual partners, black or Hispanic race, female gender, male homosexual activity, and HIV infection (2). In a study of serum samples collected from 1976 to 1980 in the United States, the prevalence of antibodies to HSV-2 was <1% of persons under 15 years of age, but increased to 7% in the 15- to 29-year age group, 20% in the 30- to 44-year age group, and 23% in the 60- to 74-year age group (3). The overall prevalence in the 15- to 74-year age group was 16.4% in 1976 to 1980 but rose to 21.7% in 1989 to 1991, an increase of almost one-third (National Health and Nutrition Evaluation Survey). The cumulative lifetime incidence of HSV-2 infection is approximately 20% for white men, 25% for white women, 60% for black men, and 80% for black women. It is estimated that as many as 44 million people are infected with HSV-2 and that up to 500,000 new cases occur annually.

Most infected people must endure recurrent outbreaks, some as frequently as once a month. Infected people on average experience four to six outbreaks a year. Because genital herpes is a very common sexually transmitted disease (STD) and recurs throughout life, it is believed that patients can recognize a recurrence, once diagnosed by a clinician, and can take appropriate action.

GENITAL HERPES—TREATMENT INDICATION

Zovirax OTC is intended for the treatment of recurrent genital herpes in individuals who have been previously diagnosed by their health care provider. Dosing is one 200 mg caplet taken five times a day for 5 days. Using this dosing regimen, Glaxo Wellcome (GW) has established efficacy of Zovirax in the treatment of genital herpes in placebo-controlled trials conducted in North America and Europe. Results indicated that treatment with Zovirax significantly:

> shortened healing times
> shortened the duration of pain
> shortened the duration of viral shedding
> decreased new lesion formation

LABELING

The package label and an expanded patient information have been proposed to address key issues associated with an OTC product. The external packaging (i.e., the box or carton containing the product) highlights important information that must be understood by the patient and includes:

- Use or indication—limiting the application for the treatment of *recurrent genital herpes*
- Directions—reemphasizing the indication of *recurrent genital herpes* as well as early treatment of symptoms that have been *previously diagnosed by a clinician*
- Warnings—reinforcing the need for *patient/doctor dialogue* as well as recommendations for handling common side effects, pregnancy issues, or medication overdose
- Important notice—highlighting that Zovirax *does not cure or prevent the spread of genital herpes*, reinforcing further the need for continuing *patient/doctor dialogue* on a regular basis
- *Educational information* contained in the enclosed pamphlet
- *Help line* and toll free telephone number that GW has found effective for the transmittal of important product information

HISTORY OF THE OTC SWITCH PROJECT

Glaxo Wellcome not only has undertaken extensive interactions with the federal regulatory agency (Food and Drug Administration [FDA]) but has solicited public comments about the implications of converting oral Zovirax, 200 mg, to OTC status for the management of genital herpes. This process has included an interactive dialogue between GW and leaders in the field of STD research and public policy, as well as an ongoing dialogue with the FDA.

The key issues identified and integrated into the development of the OTC indication include (a) viral resistance, (b) asymptomatic shedding, (c) misuse due to symptom recognition, (d) overall clinical safety (including safety in pregnancy), (e) product use/misuse by the general public of an OTC product (OTCness), and (f) public awareness and education about STDs. To ensure there is no risk to the patient, available information has been accumulated on each area of concern and where data were not available, programs were integrated into the development plan.

KEY ISSUES

Viral Resistance

The impact of the broader availability of Zovirax on the development of viral resistance with implications of an adverse impact on Public Health has been addressed.

- Glaxo Wellcome has an intensive program for the evaluation of in vitro drug sensitivity for clinical isolates of HSV in both the United States and the United Kingdom. The program began as a support for the clinical development of Zovirax and has collected data on more than 5000 isolates from 1973 to 1993. Most of these isolates were recovered from immunocompetent patients enrolled in the clinical trials of Zovirax including isolates obtained pretherapy, during therapy, or posttherapy for both treated and placebo patients. The database includes isolates from patients:
- before the introduction of Zovirax (as a baseline prevalence of viral resistance)
- who received at least six years of chronic suppressive therapy
- participating in clinical trials
- presenting with primary genital herpes 10 years after the availability of Zovirax.

The median EC_{50} of Zovirax for isolates from each of these groups is presented in Table 1. The data provide strong evidence that Zovirax has not caused an increase in the prevalence or emergence of herpes viruses resistant to Zovirax in the overall population.

Observations made on more than 5000 isolates recovered over the last 20 years and characterized in GW's research laboratories indicate that an increase in the prevalence of drug-resistant variants in immunocompetent individuals has not occurred since the introduction of Zovirax. A summary of the available resistance data from immunocompetent patients is presented in Table 2.

When assessing the relationship between antiviral therapy and the incidence of viral resistance, however, patients should be stratified with regard to immune status. Because the normal immune system effectively eliminates the small number of spontaneously emerging resistant mutants in most patients, it is necessary to examine isolates from patients with little or no immune function to understand fully the biological and pathogenic potential of herpes resistance in all clinical settings. Although these patients are not representative of the patient population at large, who are likely to use antimicrobials in the absence of physician advice or intervention, microbial resistance in them is well documented (e.g., Morbid Anxiety Inventory (MAI) in advanced AIDS patients), and such chronic and persistent infection is the ideal circumstance to allow development of resistance. Fortunately, unlike bacteria, which have multiple resistance mechanisms, herpes viruses exhibit resistance to acyclovir only as a result of mutation in either the thymidine kinase (TK) or the DNA polymerase genes.

Table 1 In Vitro Susceptibility of Isolates to Zovirax

				Resistance		
Population		N	Median	Resistant isolates*	Percent	P value
Pre-1980 population	Baseline	304	0.86	8	2.6	
Six-year suppression therapy population	Chronic	113	0.78	4	3.5	0.42
Post-1992 therapy population	Episodic	353	0.70	2	0.6	0.03
Previous clinical trials		1286	0.81	38	3.0	0.47

*Dye-update assay

Table 2 Prevalence of Resistance in the Immunocompetent Population

	Site	Isolates	Resistant variants	%	P value[a]
Untreated	Research Triangle Park[b]	1878	58	3.1	
	Beckenham[c]	379	0	0	
	Manchester[c]	760	3	0.4	
Treated	Research Triangle Park[b]	976	31	3.4	0.49
	Beckenham[c]	420	2	0.5	0.28
	Manchester[c]	162	1	0.6	0.54
Unknown	Manchester[c]	618	1	0.2	
Total		5193	96	1.8	
Total (plaque assay)		2339	7	0.3	

[a]One-sided Fisher's exact test
[b]Dye-update assay
[c]Plaque-reduction assay

Although Zovirax-resistant isolates have been recovered from *immunocompetent* patients, most do not cause clinically significant disease. The most common type of resistant virus recovered from patients is self-limiting in its ability to cause disease. They are attenuated, do not grow very well in the skin, and do not reactivate from latency to cause recurrent disease. To our knowledge, there has been only one documented report of a resistance virus recovered in an immunocompetent individual who failed therapy; however, this patient fully recovered.

Viruses resistant to Zovirax have resulted in refractory disease in some *immunocompromised* patients. In vitro data from GW and others indicate that the incidence of resistant virus in the *immunocompromised* population may approach 5% of treated episodes. Results of two prospective studies that assessed the emergence of resistance in individuals with profound impairment of immune function are shown in Table 3 (4,5). The incidence of resistance was consistent between groups. These studies indicated that only approximately 5% of immunocompromised patients treated with Zovirax will shed resistant virus.

A common measurement of the prevalence of resistance is to consider only those individuals who shed virus during therapy. Included in Table 4 are the results of culturable virus from 102 patients from the Wade and Englund database and 248 patients from three other databases. These show a higher prevalence of resistant variants (in the range of 4.1%

Table 3 Incidence of Resistance in Treated Immunocompromised Patients

Investigators	Patients	Resistant isolates	%
Wade et al. (4)[a]	80	3	3.8
Englund et al. (5)[b]	126	7	5.6
Total	206	10	4.9

[a]Bone marrow transplantation recipients
[b]Transplantation (N = 83), AIDS or ARC (N = 9), malignancies (N = 30), miscellaneous (N = 4)

to 10.9%) from immunocompromised patients who shed virus during treatment.

This difference in immunocompromised patient populations can be attributed to the indolent nature of the disease, the higher virus load, and the ability of resistant viruses to persist in *immunocompromised patients*. These conditions present a greater opportunity for the selection of resistant viruses, which occurs in approximately 5% of the treatment episodes, but only about 9% of these variants (0.5% overall) have a virulent phenotype. Attempts to further categorize immunocompromised patients into different subgroups according to immunostatus has not been possible because of the small numbers in each group. However, there is nothing to suggest that the incidence of resistance differs markedly between groups. In patients with HIV infection, resistant herpes isolates appear to occur only in those patients with extremely low CD4 counts (e.g., < 100/mm^3) and who have received prolonged and repeated courses of therapy. Herpes virus resistant to Zovirax have reduced virulence, and to date

Table 4 Prevalence of Resistant Variants in Isolates from Immunocompromised Patients Who Shed Virus During Treatment

Investigators	Patients	Resistant isolates	%
Wellcome US[a]	104	9	8.7
Manchester[b]	95	6	6.3
Gray et al. (6)[c]	49	2	4.1
Wade et al. (4)	38	3	7.9
Englund et al. (5)	64	7	10.9
Total	350	27	7.7

[a]Bone marrow transplantation recipients
[b]Oncology patients (N = 46), transplant recipients (N = 20), HIV positive (N = 29)
[c]Organ transplantations (N = 10), radiotherapy (N = 4), chemotherapy (N = 35)

there are no documented cases of transmission of resistant viruses in any patient population.

The proposed package labeling states that Zovirax OTC should *not* be taken by individuals who are immunocompromised. This restriction was clearly understood by participants in a *label comprehension study*.

Asymptomatic Shedding

Several studies have found that asymptomatic transmission may be the primary mode of viral transfer. For example, Mertz et al. (7) found that among 66 persons identified as having transmitted herpes to a sex partner, 49 (74%) denied a history of genital herpes. A further study was published assessing 144 heterosexual couples in whom one partner had recurrent genital herpes and the other did not (8). The couples were followed for an average of 11 months, during which 14 of the 144 (9.7%) unaffected partners acquired genital herpes as evidenced by a positive culture or the development of type-specific antibodies. Transmission resulted from sexual contact when the partner was lesion-free in 9 of 13 couples in whom the data were available. These include one occurrence related to sexual contact during the prodrome and three related to sexual contact a few hours before the lesions were noted.

The pattern of asymptomatic shedding and transmission of genital herpes has been further defined (9,10). These studies show patients at greatest risk of asymptomatic shedding are those with primary HSV-2 infections. In women with primary HSV-2 infection, the risk of asymptomatic shedding is greatest in the early months after the first episode.

To determine whether acyclovir had an effect on asymptomatic shedding, a double-blind, placebo-controlled, crossover study was conducted to evaluate the effectiveness of oral acyclovir in preventing asymptomatic shedding of HSV-2 in women with recurrent genital herpes (11). Doses of acyclovir, 400 mg twice a day for 70 days, decreased the frequency of asymptomatic shedding of HSV-2 from 6.9% of days to 0.3% of days—a 96% reduction in 34 women. Using a paired analysis (N = 26), viral shedding rates at all anatomical sites were significantly reduced for both subclinical shedding (89% to 97%) and symptomatic shedding (92% to 100%). When secretions from these same women were examined by polymerase chain reaction (PCR), acyclovir reduced HSV-PCR positivity from 27.9% to 8% of days, a 71% reduction.

Because acyclovir significantly reduces but does not completely eradicate HSV shedding, its impact on transmission is unknown. Therefore, this risk, coupled with the risk of acquisition of other sexually transmitted diseases, including HIV, is compelling evidence that safer sex practices should always be used. The lack of information will be emphasized in the patient materials, and the patient will be instructed to always use safer sex practices. In addition, the indication in the package labeling will be only for episodic treatment of genital herpes. In conjunction with the educational pamphlet and package size, this treatment will reduce the possibility of patients taking Zovirax OTC suppressively to prevent HSV-2 transmission.

Misuse—Symptom Recognition

Patients once diagnosed with recurrent genital herpes can recognize recurrent symptoms. In two controlled clinical trials sponsored by GW, patients previously diagnosed were able to recognize symptoms of a recurrence more than 97% of the time (12,13). In the first study, patients diagnosed with recurrent genital herpes were enrolled into a placebo-controlled trial that evaluated response to therapy in three consecutive episodes. In the first episode, patients who were aware that they had genital herpes came to a clinic within 48 hours of an outbreak, and the physician initiated treatment. The patients were then instructed to self-initiate therapy at the earliest sign or symptom of the next two episodes. In this trial, 97% of the time that patients self-initiated placebo therapy, they developed lesions (12). In a large placebo-controlled suppression trial of 1146 patients, 98% of the patients on daily placebo therapy correctly self-diagnosed an episode of recurrent genital herpes (13). These studies suggest that patients with recurrent genital herpes previously diagnosed by a clinician can recognize disease.

Patients with previously unrecognized genital herpes can also be taught to recognize disease. In a study conducted between 1983 and 1986, patients identified as potentially having "asymptomatic" genital herpes were enrolled in a trial in which they were instructed on how to recognize disease and asked to return to the clinic either whenever they suspected they were having a recurrence or every 3 months. These patients represented those who sought care in private practices as well as in public health clinics. More than 50% of the women who were HSV-2 antibody positive were able to correctly recognize their disease and returned to the clinic with symptomatic genital herpes (14).

To assess the risk of self-misdiagnosis in patients at high risk of multiple STDs, GW conducted a Symptom Self-Recognition and Self-Treatment Study in public health clinics to determine patients' ability to recognize syphilis, chancroid, and other STDs and to initiate appropriate action. More than 3000 patients were interviewed before seeing a physician to determine what the patient thought they had and what medication they had used before coming to the clinic. The major concern was that patients with syphilis would think they had herpes and delay coming to the clinic. The specific objective was to quantify the percentage of syphilis patients who thought they had genital herpes. Other study objectives were to describe self-treatment patterns of STD patients before seeking care and to measure the time from symptom onset to seeking care to discern whether self-treatment was associated with a significant delay in seeking care. Data generated from the Symptom Self-Recognition and Self-Treatment Study showed the following:

- There is minimal confusion between syphilis and genital herpes in a population at high risk for multiple STDs.
- Persons with genital lesions who self-treat do not significantly delay medical care compared to those who do not self-treat (personal communication, D. Irwin, Glaxo Wellcome).

Overall Safety

The safety of Zovirax has been established in clinical trials, epidemiological safety studies, and spontaneous reports. More than 7500 patients have been evaluated in clinical trials. Doses ranging from 200 mg twice a day to 800 mg five times a day for durations of 5 days to 10 years have been evaluated. Almost 4000 patients with genital herpes, more than 2200 patients with herpes zoster, and almost 1400 patients with chickenpox were studied. The most common adverse experiences were nausea/vomiting, headache, diarrhea, and abdominal pain (Table 5).

In epidemiological safety studies, more than 72,000 patients have been evaluated under conditions of general use and no evidence of safety risks were reported. There were no cases of serious but rare adverse experiences possibly attributable to acyclovir and no increase in the frequency of serious events that could be attributable to acyclovir therapy. Of these, 847 were acyclovir exposures during pregnancy (578 in the first trimester). The incidence of birth defects (3.3% in the first trimester) does not differ from that reported in the general population (Table 6).

A total of 2256 spontaneous reports have occurred out of 32.5 million people treated worldwide through December 1994. This represents an extremely low rate of reporting adverse events. Additionally, the most commonly reported events were similar to those seen in clinical trials. The

Table 5 Adverse Experiences—Clinical Trials of Oral Zovirax (Genital Herpes, Herpes Zoster, Chickenpox)

	Zovirax	Placebo
Nausea/vomiting	0.4–11.3%	0.2–14.0%
Headache	0–7.4%	0–9.5%
Diarrhea	1.0–3.6%	0.3–2.9%
Abdominal pain	0.4–0.8%	0.2–0.4%

five most commonly noted adverse events were rash, nausea, pain, headache, and pruritus.

Product Use/Misuse by General Public

Appropriate candidates for OTC therapy should have a simple pharmacokinetic profile. Important characteristics relate to the timing of dosing and food consumption, excretion patterns, and disease interactions. Zovirax has no important food or drug or disease interactions. Severe renal failure (CrCl < 10 ml/min/1.73m^2) is the only disease in which a dose reduction is suggested. Therefore, there are no contraindications for Zovirax in any patient group.

Any drug being considered for broad availability should be evaluated for the risk of misuse. Namely, if Zovirax were used for another disease, would it mask its symptoms. Zovirax has a limited number of pharmacological effects. It is effective only against herpes group infections with no effect on any other STD or infectious agent. Therefore, if a patient takes Zovirax for an infection other than that caused by a herpes virus, it will not mask the symptoms of another disease.

Table 6 Acyclovir Pregnancy Registry June 1984–June 1995

Trimester of exposure	Birth defects	Live births	Spontaneous abortion	Induced abortion	Total
First	14	427	64	73	578
Second	2	110	0	0	112
Third	3	153	1	0	157
Total	19	690	65	73	847

Only the oral capsule formulation will be available over the counter, and labeling and packaging will be specific for recurrent genital herpes. These deterrents coupled with the lack of third party coverage should discourage Zovirax use for chickenpox, shingles, cold sores, or immune disorders.

Public Awareness and Education About STDs

Numerous meetings with experts in infectious diseases, obstetrics and gynecology, dermatology, family practice, nursing, and pharmacy have been held to determine potential needs of the community if Zovirax were available without a prescription. In addition, consumer groups representing family planning, the HIV community, minority health interests, STD education, and women's health were also consulted. The common theme throughout each meeting was the need for education. The consumer's desire and need for education were also identified in extensive market research studies and in a national women's survey conducted by the Campaign for Women's Health and the American Medical Women's Association. Consumer research showed that patients want to be informed about diseases and told how to decrease risk. The national women's survey found that women who were more knowledgeable about diseases and risks were more likely to take measures to reduce risks.

Burroughs Wellcome (now Glaxo Wellcome) has a strong history of providing education about sexually transmitted diseases, especially genital herpes and HIV. Medical education through symposia, publications, speakers programs, innovative management resource guides, and patient education materials designed for distribution from the health care provider have been available for many years. In addition, GW is committed to supporting its products by enhancing customer education. Educational efforts currently underway support both the prescription and OTC availability of Zovirax. What would be enhanced by OTC Zovirax is the emphasis on education directed to the public. Educational efforts for prescription products are focused primarily on the health care provider. Educational efforts for OTC products must be focused toward the consumer. Over-the-counter availability greatly increases ways in which messages can be transmitted. Media that are not routinely available for prescription products are readily available for consumer products.

Strategically developed and accurately targeted health education and communication programs can have a positive effect on public health. The educational program for Zovirax OTC was designed to increase awareness of STDs, specifically genital herpes, in three audiences: the general public, patients infected with genital herpes, and health care providers. The overall objectives of education were:

- To increase people's awareness, knowledge, and acceptance of genital herpes specifically and sexually transmitted diseases (STDs) in general.
- To motivate people who may suspect they have the symptoms of genital herpes or another STD to see a health care provider for appropriate diagnosis, counseling, and treatment.
- To support the health care professional's role in effective diagnosis, counseling, and treatment.
- To promote correct and appropriate use of OTC Zovirax.

SUMMARY

Drugs that are acceptable for OTC use should be safe and efficacious, and patients should be able to recognize symptoms and initiate appropriate action. If misdiagnosed, the drug should not mask the symptoms of another disease. If a drug meets these criteria, the risk/benefit analysis should favor OTC availability.

The safety and efficacy of oral Zovirax 200 mg as a prescription product for the management of recurrent genital herpes have been thoroughly documented. The OTC consideration of Zovirax does not involve evaluation of issues relative to a new use or dose of the product. Approval would provide the consumer the option to self-treat.

Any drug being considered for OTC availability should have a safety profile compatible with broad use in many different populations. The safety of Zovirax has been evaluated in more than 7500 patients in clinical trials, over 72,000 patients in epidemiology surveillance studies, and from spontaneous reports received from an exposed population of more than 32 million people worldwide. None of these databases have signaled a safety risk for Zovirax. The prevalence of resistant isolates have been monitored for more than 20 years and found to be no different even after 15 years of widespread availability. Nevertheless, the potential of emergence of resistance in the future should still be studied.

The potential for misuse of Zovirax is likely to be small. Clinical trials have shown that patients, once diagnosed by a clinician, can recognize a recurrence of genital herpes. In addition, the potential for patients to confuse another STD with herpes has been assessed in a high-risk population and found to be small. Finally, patients should be discouraged from using the drug for chickenpox, shingles, cold sores, or immune disorders by specific labeling, packaging, and lack of third party coverage for non-approved OTC indications.

Concern has arisen that patients who take Zovirax OTC will not continue to see their physician for evaluation. Market research data from vaginal yeast symptoms indicate that this is not necessarily true. Although office visits for a vaginal yeast product initially declined, office visits for this diagnosis have been stable for the last 4 years, indicating that patients are seeking a diagnosis.

There are many potential benefits to OTC availability of Zovirax. Clinical trials have proven the efficacy of Zovirax for the treatment of recurrent genital herpes. Enabling the patient access to Zovirax OTC after a physician's diagnosis can enhance its benefits to the patient. Zovirax OTC will not only allow the patient to access the drug promptly and conveniently as needed, but also will improve efficacy through early treatment. Even though Zovirax is effective for the treatment of recurrent genital herpes when therapy is initiated by a health care practitioner or by the patient, the drug is most effective when given early in the course of an outbreak. Therapy with Zovirax significantly reduces the parameters of healing, new lesion formation, pain, and viral shedding. Therefore, having Zovirax readily accessible to patients should improve the management of recurrent genital herpes by decreasing the duration of symptomatic disease and viral shedding compared to courses of disease when therapy is physician-initiated.

Genital herpes establishes latency after the first episode and recurs periodically throughout life. Because of the recurring nature of this disease and the fact that there is no cure, genital herpes has reached epidemic proportions in the United States. It is estimated that more than 40 million people are infected with HSV-2 and that 500,000 new cases occur annually, with no evidence that the disease is decreasing in incidence. The changing demography and social mores of our culture over the last few decades have led to (a) more people in the sexually active range, (b) more people remaining single for longer time periods, (c) decreasing age at first intercourse, (d) more people having more than one sexual partner, and (e) increased recognition of sexually transmitted diseases. There is no reason to believe that the incidence of herpes will decline in the near future given these trends in American society.

Zovirax OTC may have a beneficial impact on the epidemic of genital herpes by decreasing the clinical episodes of viral shedding and increasing disease recognition.

- Viral shedding, which is believed to be necessary for transmission to occur, is shortened by therapy with Zovirax. Viral shedding during lesion episodes is shortened by 1 day when episodic therapy is initiated by the clinician and by 2 days when patients are allowed to self-initiate episodic therapy. If Zovirax decreases the amount of time that lesions are infectious, improved access to therapy, which facilitates early treatment initiation by patients, may have a beneficial impact on disease transmission.
- The educational effort that will accompany this switch will make the public more aware of the symptoms of genital herpes and precautions to prevent transmission. Labeling and educational materials will emphasize disease recognition, transmission potential, and safer sex practices. This educational effort along with availability of early therapy may act positively to decrease the incidence of a disease that has become epidemic.

Under current prescribing guidelines, Zovirax could be readily available to patients now. Physicians could write prescriptions with refill permission; however, many physicians do not prescribe Zovirax in this manner. Instead, many require patients to return to their office for refills, thus adding to health care costs both to patients and to the health care system. In addition, patients frequently experience outbreaks over a weekend, while away from their primary care physician, or in other circumstances where access to prescription medication is delayed or difficult. These patients must experience the outbreak without benefit of therapy. Having Zovirax OTC available would enable patients to treat all recurrences they deem necessary.

Assessment of the potential impact of OTC availability of Zovirax, 200 mg, has included a series of critical public policy issues that extend beyond the efficacy and safety evidence that already support expanded use. These issues have been addressed through a variety of mechanisms, including literature review, assembly of professional advice and opinion, collection of data, and external research. With such a large body of work, one would expect some diversity in outcomes. Moreover, some questions cannot be answered while the product is available only by prescription. To address these additional questions, GW has proposed an extensive monitoring program to detect early signals of problems with misuse, safety, and viral resistance. The balance of the evidence suggests more societal benefits than risk of OTC availability of oral Zovirax for management of recurrent genital herpes. Substantial benefit can reasonably be expected if a better informed public is more aware of STD symptoms, and consumers and health professionals are more likely to include STD risk assessment and counseling in their practices.

ACKNOWLEDGMENT

The authors would like to thank Dr. Sharon Srebro and Dr. Debra Irwin for their suggestions, as well as Kerry Pratt and Brenda Newkirk, CPS, for secretarial support during the preparation of the manuscript.

REFERENCES

1. Hirsch MS. Herpes simplex virus.In: Mandel GL, Douglas RG, Bennett JE, eds. Principles and Practices of Infectious Diseases, 3rd ed. New York: Churchill Livingstone, 1990: 1144–1151.
2. Mertz GJ. Epidemiology of genital herpes infections. Infect Dis Clin North Am 1993; 7: 825–839.
3. Johnson RE, Nahmias AJ, Magder LS, et al. A seroepidemiology survey of the prevalence of herpes simplex virus type 2 infection in the United States. N Engl J Med 1989; 321: 8–12.
4. Wade JC, Newton B, McLaren C, et al. Intravenous acyclovir to treat mucocutaneous herpes simplex virus infection after marrow transplantation: a double blind test. Ann Intern Med 1982; 96: 265–269.
5. Englund JA, Zimmerman ME, Swierkosz EM, et al. Herpes simplex virus resistant to acyclovir: a study in a tertiary care center. Ann Intern Med 1990; 112: 416–422.
6. Gray JJ, Wreghitt TG, Baglin TP. Susceptibility to acyclovir of herpes simplex virus: emergence of resistance in patients with lymphoid and myeloid neoplasia. J Infect Dis 1989; 19: 31–40.
7. Mertz GL, Schmidt O, Jourden JL, et al. Frequency of acquisition of first episode genital infection with herpes simplex virus from asymptomatic and asymptomatic source contacts. Sex Transm Dis 1985; 12: 33–39.
8. Mertz GL, Benedetti J, Ashley R, et al. Risk factors for the sexual transmission of genital herpes. Ann Intern Med 1992; 116: 197–202.
9. Koelle DM, Benedetti J, Langenberg A, et al. Asymptomatic reactivation of herpes simplex virus in women after the first episode of genital herpes. Ann Intern Med 1992; 116: 433–437.
10. Wald A, Barnum G, Selke S, et al. Acyclovir suppresses asymptomatic shedding of HSV2 in the genital tract. 34th International Conference on Antimicrobial Agents and Chemotherapy. Orlando, Florida, October 4–7, 1994.
11. Wald A, Zeh J, Barnum G, et al. Suppression of subclinical shedding of herpes simplex virus type 2 with acyclovir. Ann Intern Med 1996; 124: 8–15.

12. Goldberg LH, Kaufman R, Conant MA, et al. Oral acyclovir for episodic treatment of recurrent genital herpes. J Am Acad Dermatol 1986; 15: 256–264.
13. Mertz GJ, Jones CC, Mills J, et al. Long-term acyclovir suppression of frequently recurring genital herpes simplex infection. JAMA 1988; 260: 201–206.
14. Langenberg A, Benedetti J, Jenkins J, et al. Development of clinically recognizable genital lesions among women previously identified as having "asymptomatic" herpes simplex virus 2 infection. Ann Intern Med 1989; 110: 882–887.

31

Psychosocial Aspects of Genital Human Papillomavirus and Herpes Simplex Virus Infection

Peggy Clarke
American Social Health Association, Research Triangle Park, North Carolina

INTRODUCTION

A diagnosis of a sexually transmitted disease (STD) can trigger emotional and personal responses in patients that, to some health care providers, may appear disproportionate to the medical condition. When some patients are told that they have acquired their infection through sexual activity, their attention turns quickly to such personal issues as their self-image, their sexual relationships, and their perception of the stigma associated with sexual matters. In the case of a viral infection, the news is accompanied by a realization that the infection will be lifelong.

This chapter examines the psychosocial aspects of infection with genital human papillomavirus (HPV) and herpes simplex virus (HSV). Drawing on population research about the public's awareness of STDs, the cultural context against which patients perceive their infection will be explored. Research conducted among patients with HSV infections and among patients with genital HPV infection will also examine the potential impact of STDs on self-image, sexual relations, and patient/provider relationships.

Programmatic experience of the American Social Health Association (ASHA) over the last 17 years in addressing the patient needs for support and education supplements these data in suggesting implications for the health counseling appropriate to newly diagnosed individuals and those coping with the chronic nature of their conditions. Through its Herpes Resource Center and HPV Support Program, ASHA counsels more than 100,000 people each year over the agency's confidential telephone hot-lines. ASHA operates 100 patient support groups located in the United States, Canada, Mexico, and Australia. It also publishes two quarterly newsletters that address the scientific, clinical, and personal aspects of these two infections. Each year, ASHA distributes more than 300,000 educational publications about HSV and/or HPV.

Based on this overview of the psychological and emotional aspects of infection with viral STDs, the chapter concludes with a review of the literature in counseling for sexual health. A framework for counseling patients is provided along with referrals for psychosocial support systems.

CULTURAL CONTEXT OF STD AWARENESS

In an era of heightened public awareness of one sexually acquired infec-tion (HIV/AIDS) (1), it is somewhat paradoxical that awareness of other STDs is so limited. This is evidenced in the frequency and volume of media and press attention to all sexually acquired conditions, as well as inquiries from the public to the National AIDS Hotline and the National STD Hotline (2).

A survey conducted in 1995 by the Gallup Organization for ASHA examined various aspects of the public's awareness of STDs other than HIV/AIDS in six industrialized countries. One thousand individuals were randomly selected from each of the following countries: Italy, Spain, United Kingdom, France, Sweden, and the United States. Interviews were conducted either by telephone or face-to-face, with a sampling error of plus or minus 3% (3). The survey's objectives included the measurement of knowledge, awareness, and communications about STDs other than HIV/AIDS. (Because results were consistent among all countries, they are reported in the aggregate.)

Awareness was surprisingly low, with 32% unable to name at least one STD other than AIDS. When those who knew of STDs other than AIDS were asked to name them, the "traditional" STDs, such as syphilis and gonorrhea, were most often mentioned (44% and 37%, respectively). Only 17% were able to name herpes and 3% mentioned genital warts.

Using herpes as a proxy measure for awareness of the prevalence of non-AIDS STDs, the survey asked respondents to estimate how many people have genital herpes. Accurate prevalence data for all countries surveyed are unavailable; however, estimates range from 10% to 25%, translating to a 1 in 5 or a 1 in 10 estimate for infection (4). In no country did the majority of respondents accurately identify this answer. Thirty percent of all respondents were unable to venture a guess for prevalence of genital herpes infection and, of the remaining, 56% estimated at least 10 times *less* prevalence.

These findings of low awareness of sexually transmitted disease in six industrialized countries highlights a lack of public consciousness of these epidemics and creates a backdrop of isolation and ignorance against which people newly diagnosed with viral infections must consider the management of their infections.

WHAT A DIAGNOSIS MEANS TO THE INDIVIDUAL

Most health care providers who care for patients with viral infections agree that, for some people, the diagnosis of genital herpes or human papilloma infection is often accompanied by strong emotional and personal concerns. In addition to the physical implications, it is important to identify and address the potential influence of the diagnosis on patients' lives to provide adequate anticipatory guidance and satisfactory patient care.

During the last decade, studies about the emotional effects of HIV/AIDS have outnumbered those investigating the effects of other STDs. Nonetheless, a diagnosis of a non-HIV viral STD can be very upsetting as presented in investigations that have found the emotional responses to these diagnoses include fear of rejection, lowered self-esteem, anger, guilt, and depression (5,6). The fear of rejection can prevent a person from disclosing the diagnosis to friends or family members, in turn leading to isolation from potential sources of support (7,8).

To better understand the impact of viral infection on all aspects of patients' lives, ASHA undertook two studies of inquiry into patient populations of people with genital herpes infection and people with HPV infection. Strikingly similar results were seen in the areas of influence of the infection on patients' perception of self-image, on their concerns about personal or sexual relationships, and on communication patterns between patients and their diagnosing health care providers.

The populations under study were drawn from readers of the two quarterly publications of ASHA, which target patients with viral infections (*the helper* and *HPV News*). The sample size in the genital herpes survey was 2940 (of a 10,000 readership base) and 454 (of an 1800 readership base) in the survey of people with genital HPV infection. The majority of the patients with HPV had apparent genital warts, which alerted them to their condition.

Among those with genital herpes infection, 65% were female and 35% were male. Eighty percent were 30 years of age or older. Ninety-two percent were Caucasian, and 70% had graduated from college. Ninety percent reported at least one outbreak in the 12-month period before the study, and 55% had experienced their first genital herpes outbreak 6 or more years before the study.

Among those with genital HPV infection, 77% were female and 23% were male. Seventy-six percent were 30 years of age or older. Ninety-seven percent were Caucasian, and 70% had graduated from college. Nearly half (49%) reported that they had had HPV for 3 years or more. Sixty percent reported having had visible warts at some time; however, a larger proportion of the men (94%) said they had visible warts than women (49%). No attempts were made to confirm HPV infection independently or to differentiate in the analysis between people with genital warts or subclinical infection.

Caution must be taken in interpreting these data because these patients are not clearly representative of the total populations of people with HSV or HPV infection. Although these patients are likely not a representative sample, however, their experiences may be instructive with regard to the underinvestigated psychosocial effects of these infections and may provide insight for health care providers who treat people with HPV or HSV genital infection.

SELF-IMAGE

The first outbreak initiates a period of anxiety and emotional upheaval for many. In the ASHA survey, the great majority reported that they had experienced a range of negative feelings when they first learned they had a viral STD. Initial reactions included anger, depression, isolation, shame, guilt, and fear of rejection (Figure 1). Specifically, 82% of HSV patients and 76% of HPV patients reported feelings of depression, 75% with HSV and 70% with HPV reported concern or fear about potential rejection, and 69% with HSV and 70% with HPV reported feelings of isolation.

The emotional impact of many medical or personal health conditions can decrease over time because of several factors including patients' greater understanding of the condition, reduced or controlled symptoms, or perhaps simply because of people's ability to adapt or adjust to a changed condition. In an attempt to determine whether the negative

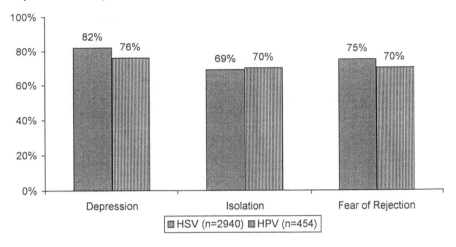

Figure 1 Influence of STD diagnosis on self-image.

emotional responses reported by people with genital viral infections continued over time, respondents to ASHA's surveys were asked about their feelings during the 12 months immediately preceding the survey. As expected, fewer respondents reported negative feelings in the more recent period as compared with the time of initial diagnosis (Figure 2). Nevertheless, between 3 in 10 and 5 in 10 people continued to report negative feelings, which they attributed to their medical condition.

PERSONAL AND SEXUAL RELATIONSHIPS

Infection from HSV or HPV can have a strong impact on the social and sexual relationships of those involved. When asked who they had told about their diagnosis, most people had disclosed this information to someone. In both surveys, 69% of those surveyed had told their current sexual partner. Fifty-eight percent of those with HPV and 61% with HSV told a friend. Family members were consulted by 48% of those with HPV and 47% with HSV. Four percent with HPV and 2% with HSV had told no one. Surprisingly, 31% with HSV and 47% with HPV had not told their current health care provider.

Perhaps not surprisingly, the diagnosis did have an effect on people's sexual feelings and behavior (Figure 3). Most noted an impact on their

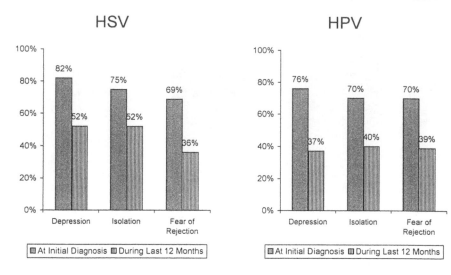

Figure 2 Reactions over time.

behavior in approaching a new sexual partner (HPV 86%, HSV 69%), their feelings of desirability (HPV 72%, HSV 76%), and frequency (HPV 72%, HSV 79%) and enjoyment (HPV 68%, HSV 66%) of sexual contact. Of people with herpes, 89% expressed concern about transmitting herpes to a sexual partner, 68% feared they would be rejected by a new sexual partner because of their infection, and 51% believed that their infection influenced their capacity to be spontaneous sexually. Twenty-six percent of people with genital HSV infection reported being rejected by a sexual partner because of their herpes infection.

PATIENT AND PROVIDER RELATIONSHIPS

Ninety-nine percent of people with HPV infection and 96% of those with HSV infection had visited a health care provider because of their condition. These experiences with providers were recounted through a series of answers to questions about service-related issues, including providers' openness to discussion and the provision of information and emotional support.

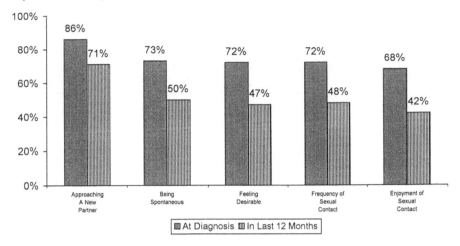

Figure 3 Negative impact of HPV on sexual feelings and behavior.

Many people were clearly dissatisfied with their diagnosing providers, specifically in the areas of providing information about their condition and in providing emotional or sexual counseling. For example, 64% of those with herpes and 59% of those with HPV rated the health care provider who diagnosed their condition as "poor" or "fair" at answering questions. Other areas of concern centered on perceived deficiencies in communication with regard to interpersonal considerations related to the infection, sexual counseling, and emotional support.

Of those who reported having a current health care provider for either their genital herpes or HPV conditions, their evaluation of the service and support they receive currently is much higher than evaluations given to diagnosing providers. Still, dissatisfaction about counseling on several personal issues remained for some people. (See Table 1 for evaluation of current health care providers by a subset of respondents in the HSV survey.)

SEXUAL COUNSELING PRACTICES

Two surveys by ASHA suggest that the expectations of patients for counseling and communication from their health care providers are higher than the services they received. Patients appear to be seeking advice on

Table 1   Satisfaction with Current Health Care Provider (N = 975)

HSV respondent satisfaction regarding provider[a]	Not applicable (%)	Poor (%)	Fair (%)	Good (%)	Excellent (%)
Answering questions	5	7	22	38	28
Providing treatment information	4	12	20	35	27
Advising on emotional issues	12	25	22	23	17
Being supportive	6	13	22	31	27
Discussing sex life	15	19	22	25	18
Asking about sexual practices	16	24	21	22	16
Welcoming questions about sexual practices/STDs	12	13	17	31	26

[a]Two percent did not answer all questions and were excluded. Percentages may not total to 100 because of rounding.

emotional issues, an avenue to discuss their sex lives, and ways to ask specific questions about their sexual practices.

The influence of communication by health care providers on their patients' well-being and health care practices can be great; yet recent studies suggest that the frequency and quality of patient-provider communication about sexual health matters could be improved.

COMMUNICATION BARRIERS

Counseling patients with STDs is difficult. These diseases are linked to numerous sensitive issues that both providers and patients are likely to feel uneasy discussing such as sexual practices, sexual orientation, partner(s) selection, patient ignorance or misconception about sexual information, and transmission and partner communication about exposure and safety.

Communications between patients and providers are subject to some of the same constraints as other interpersonal communications: verbal mismatches (e.g., differing levels of communication skills) or differing personality styles; cultural, experiential, or other outlook differences (e.g., different beliefs about health, risks, illness, religion, and morality); demographic mismatches (e.g., difficulties in communications that sometimes arise between people of differing race or age); environmental barriers (e.g., privacy, noise, and note taking); and the stability of the relationship (e.g., first encounter versus established relationship) (9,10).

Effective, two-way communication between provider and patient requires effort by both participants. The traditional roles of patient (passive and dependent) and provider (authority figure with power over patient behavior) constitute one barrier to mutual participation (11). Another is differences in knowledge, educational levels, and perspectives on the patient's condition, which make it difficult to find a common ground for communications (10).

The ASHA surveys of people with herpes and HPV infection highlight the need for increased communication between health care providers and their patients. Other recent research indicates that this communication could be improved. For example, a 1992 national survey by the Centers for Disease Control and Prevention of primary care physicians found that of those surveyed, only 49% asked new adult patients about STDs, 31% asked about condom use, 27% asked about sexual orientation, and 22% asked about the number of sexual partners. In comparison, 94% asked these same patients about cigarette smoking behavior (12). Several other studies suggest that physicians often neglect to take a sexual history of their patients, even though their patients say that they would find it appropriate for the physician to do so (13–15).

Studies assessing counseling practices between physicians and patients with STDs also suggest areas for improvement. One review of practice in five health departments found that whereas almost all patients received an STD diagnosis, about one-fourth of these did not receive any information about treatment or prevention. Only slightly more than one-half were given complete information about their condition (e.g., diagnosis, treatment, and future prevention) (15).

Why don't clinicians discuss sexual health more often with their patients? One study suggests that some physicians may omit taking a sexual history because they assume that sexual experience may be unimportant in a health assessment for selected patients (13). Other providers are reluctant to initiate discussions about sexual health because of the perceived reaction from their patients with regard to the relevance or appropriateness of the discussion.

Compounding these concerns about the patient's reactions to possibly misinterpreted questions about sexual practices are other priorities competing for the clinician's attention. These include the obvious need to address presenting symptoms, as well as managing a busy schedule that is generally not structured to permit open-ended discussions with patients.

Most office or clinic settings are busy, hectic places where discussions of personal issues might easily be interrupted.

In the case of a diagnosis of a sexually transmitted infection, the provider and the patient likely have rather differing views of the significance of the infection to the patient's overall health. For example, for the provider, the relatively benign nature of HSV infection, the often predictable and episodic nature of outbreaks, and the availability of treatment to minimize or eliminate symptoms contribute to a perception of herpes as a manageable infection that, from a strictly medical view, suggests relatively little cause for concern. Although genital warts and HPV infection present a different clinical picture, and the range of treatment options and the link of several strains of HPV infection with cervical cancer present unique challenges to health care providers, many view HPV infection in much the same way as genital herpes. For the patient who is newly diagnosed, the physical discomfort is frequently accompanied by emotional turmoil. The patient's view must be understood, and counseling should begin from the understanding and immediate concerns of the individual.

STD COUNSELING MODEL

Working with an advisory panel of medical experts, ASHA has devised a tool to assist health care providers in perhaps the most difficult part of STD management and treatment—counseling patients in the clinical setting. Counseling for STDs need not be difficult, time consuming, or intimidating. Awareness of important communication factors and the stages of the counseling process can greatly ease any pressure and quicken the process without compromising any critical element or the overall effectiveness. This model for counseling patients on various aspects of sexual health supported by patient education materials can assist the providers in educating the patient (Figure 4).

The goals of STD counseling include educating all sexually active individuals about STDs, assessing individual factors for infection, offering nonjudgmental advice about behavior changes to reduce risk of infection or reinfection, advising about treatment compliance, providing anticipatory guidance about psychological concerns related to an STD diagnosis, and ensuring partner notification and follow-up (16).

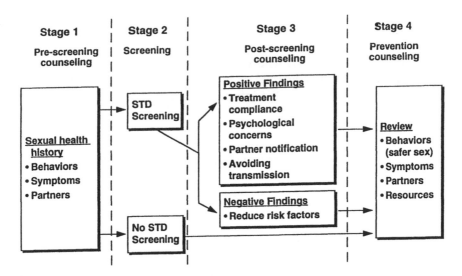

Figure 4 American Social Health Association STD counseling model.

COUNSELING A NEWLY DIAGNOSED PATIENT

Each of the four stages of STD counseling is important. Stage 3 of the ASHA STD Counseling Model addresses postscreening counseling. Applying this stage to counseling a patient newly diagnosed with a viral STD, a health care provider discusses several key topics, beginning with a full explanation of what is known about an HPV or HSV infection. This includes a description of the natural history of the disease (e.g., transmission, the nature of the virus, description of prodrome recurrences, possible locations and nature of lesions, physical discomfort, and autoinoculation).

Patients also need to be informed about available treatment regimens so they can make informed decisions about their treatment plan. Compliance with treatment, costs, and possible side effects of therapies should also be discussed, as well as the means to monitor a patient's perception of treatment success. Nonprescription therapies including improved nutrition and physical rest and stress reduction may also be appropriate.

As the ASHA patient surveys demonstrated, people with viral STDs often have psychological concerns at the time of first outbreak and diagnosis. Shame, guilt, anger, and fear are common initial emotional reactions. It is important for health care providers to acknowledge the negative emotions a patient may experience and to provide anticipatory guidance on emotional issues. Guidance may include a sample statement such as: "It is normal for some people to initially feel sad or depressed when they first learn they have an STD. This generally passes."

People who have just learned of an infection may blame their current or former sexual partner for the infection, and/or they may be fearful of letting the partner know about the infection. Counseling patients about notifying their partner (or partners) will differ with each patient. Patients need to be able to explain to their partner(s) the diagnosis and how it will affect sexual activity. Written instructions for partner notification are often helpful.

A clear understanding of the mechanism by which STDs are transmitted is essential for newly diagnosed patients. Patients need to understand the precautions necessary to avoid future infections. They must understand the potential for transmission during asymptomatic periods. Issues include the importance of safer sex practices and personal decision making. Patients with HSV need to be reminded that they remain infectious while taking antiviral medicine. The high prevalence of infection with HPV should be explained, and the need for regular Pap smears for women with HPV infection should be part of this counseling.

Finally, counseling should include referrals for more information and emotional support. Perhaps a suggested call back to a nurse or counselor in the provider's practice would be useful. HELP groups, which are support groups for people with herpes and/or genital warts, can be found throughout the United States and Canada. These listings and other referral materials for sources of emotional support and educational material about herpes or HPV are available from ASHA.

By openly discussing STDs during all routine visits and by providing supportive assistance to those diagnosed with STDs, clinicians open doors to greater communication about all facets of sexual health and help to increase awareness and practice of personal preventive behaviors. The positive impact that STD counseling can have on a patient's life and health is immeasurable.

REFERENCES

1. Gallup Jr G, Gallup AM. AIDS: 35-nation survey. Gallup Report, 1988: 273.
2. American Social Health Association 1994 Annual Report and Centers for Disease Control and Prevention, Division of STD/HIV Prevention, 1994 Annual Report.

3. Presentation of results at International Society for Sexually Transmitted Disease Research, New Orleans, August 1995.
4. Holmes K, Sparling PF, eds. Sexually Transmitted Diseases, 2nd ed. New York: McGraw-Hill, 1990.
5. VanderPlate C, Aral S. Psychosocial aspects of genital herpes virus infection. Health Psychol 1987; 6: 57–72.
6. Swanson JM, Chenitz WC. The prevention and management of genital herpes: a community health approach. J Community Health 1989; 6: 209–221.
7. Catotti DN, Clarke P, Catoe KE. Herpes revisited. J Sexually Transmitted Disease 1993; 20: 77–80.
8. Survey shows how we live with HPV. HPV News 1993; 3: 2.
9. Norton R, Schwartzbaum J, Wheat J. Language discrimination of general physicians: AIDS metaphors used in the AIDS crisis. Comm Res 1990; 17: 809–826.
10. Quill TE. Recognizing and adjusting to barriers in doctor-patient communication. Ann Intern Med 1989; 111: 51–57.
11. Brody DS. The patient's role in decision-making. Ann Intern Med 1980; 93: 718–722.
12. Loft J, Marder W, Bresolin L, Rinaldi R. HIV prevention practices of primary-care physicians—United States, 1992. MMWR 1994; 42: 988–992.
13. Ende J, Rockwell S, Glasgow M. The sexual history in general medicine practice. Arch Intern Med 1984; 144: 558–561.
14. Lewis CE, Freeman HE. The sexual history-taking and counseling practices of primary care physicians. West J Med 1987; 147: 165–167.
15. Weisman CS, Nathanson CA, Ensminger M, et al. AIDS knowledge, perceived risk and prevention among adolescent clients of a family planning clinic. Fam Plann Perspect 1989; 21: 213–217.
16. American Social Health Association. STD counseling and treatment guidelines 1994.

32
Imiquimod: In Vivo and In Vitro Characteristics and Toxicology

Mark A. Tomai, Woubalem Birmachu, Marvin T. Case,
John F. Gerster, Sheila J. Gibson, Linda M. Imbertson,
Richard L. Miller, Michael J. Reiter, and Tamara L. Wagner
3M Pharmaceuticals, St. Paul, Minnesota

CYTOKINE INDUCTION

Systemic In Vivo

Mice

Imiquimod (R-837, S-26308) (Figure 1) is a potent inducer of cytokines in a number of species including mice, rats, guinea pigs, monkeys, and humans (1–7). In mice, studies have demonstrated induction of interferon (IFN) in the serum as early as 1 hour after treatment. Concentrations of IFN generally peak 2 hours after dosing and at doses lower than 30 mg/kg return to background by 4 to 6 hours after administration. At doses higher than 30 mg/kg, peak concentrations of IFN are not any higher than those seen at the 30 mg/kg dose; however, IFN concentrations remain elevated for an extended time. Imiquimod not only induces IFN but also causes increases in tumor necrosis factor (TNF)-α and interleukin (IL)-6.

Induction of IL-1α is not seen with oral dosing of imiquimod. Kinetic studies reveal that elevation in TNF-α concentrations are seen at 30 minutes after oral administration and generally peak 1 hour after dosing. As with IFN, TNF-α concentrations return to background by 4 hours after administration. With regard to IL-6, the kinetic curve parallels that seen with IFN; levels are seen as early as 1 hour after dosing, peak at 2 hours

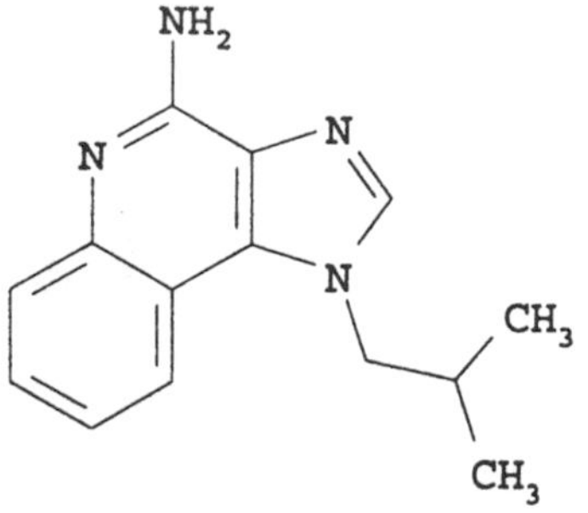

Figure 1 1-(2-Methylpropyl)-1*H*-imidazo[4,5-C]quinolin-4-amine.

after dosing, and return to background by 4 hours after dosing. Studies demonstrate that 1 to 3 mg/kg is a minimum effective dose for induction of IFN in mice. This induction can be seen by a number of routes of administration including subcutaneously, intraperitoneally, dermally and intravaginally. In addition, nude mice, which lack T cells, and severe combined immunodeficiency disease (SCID) mice, which lack both T and B cells produce high levels of cytokines in their serum in response to oral dosing of imiquimod. These results demonstrate that T and B cells are not required for cytokine induction in mice.

Rats

Imiquimod given orally is capable of inducing significant concentrations of IFN and TNF-α in the serum of rats. Kinetics are similar to those seen in mice; however, the time of induction is slightly delayed. TNF-α concentrations are seen 1 hour after dosing and generally peak by 2 hours but remain elevated for at least another 2 hours. IFN concentrations generally are seen by 1 hour after dosing, peak between 4 and 6 hours after administration and, at doses lower than 30 mg/kg, return to background by 24 hours after administration. Interestingly, multiple high doses of imiquimod given daily actually lead to a diminished IFN response. This reduced response with daily dosing is also seen in mice.

Cynomolgus Monkeys

Imiquimod, when given orally to cynomolgus monkeys, is capable of inducing detectable concentrations of IFN in the serum. A single dose of 10 mg/kg of imiquimod is capable of inducing IFN. Interestingly, multiple daily doses of imiquimod at 3 mg/kg demonstrate induction of IFN after 1 month and IFN concentrations remain elevated even after 6 months of dosing. In addition, high doses of imiquimod (30 to 100 mg/kg) after 1 month of daily dosing induce lower IFN concentrations, and after 6 months of high dose administration, the concentrations of IFN seen are even lower. Studies using antibodies to the various IFNs demonstrated that neutralizing antibody specific for IFN-α, but not IFN-β or IFN-γ, was capable of abrogating the IFN activity seen in the serum from monkeys.

Summary

A summary of IFN induction by imiquimod is presented in Table 1. The induction of IFN by imiquimod is seen in a number of species. Doses of 1 to 3 mg/kg are effective at inducing IFN in all species listed. Slightly higher single doses of imiquimod are required for IFN induction in monkeys.

Effects in Skin of Hairless Mice After Topical Application

Effects of IFN-α m-RNA Expression and Concentrations of IFN and TNF-α

A cream formulation has been evaluated for its ability to induce cytokine-specific mRNA in the skin from hairless mice. Results have demonstrated increases in IFN-α m-RNA levels in the skin of mice after topical application of imiquimod cream (unpublished data). Elevations in IFN-α m-RNA are seen as early as 1 hour after dosing with return to background by 24 hours after dosing. Other cytokine-specific m-RNAs, including TNF-α, IL-1, IL-6 and IL-12, were also measured; however, no differences were seen when compared to untreated animals.

Table 1 Minimal Effective Imiquimod Dose Required for IFN Induction

Species	Cytokines detected	Oral dose (mg/kg) required
Mouse	IFN, TNF-α, IL-6	1–3
Rat	IFN, TNF-α	3
Guinea pig	IFN	2
Monkey	IFN	3*
Human	IFN	2, 3

*Indicates multiple doses are required.

Studies have also measured IFN and TNF-α concentrations in the skin of mice after topical administration of imiquimod. Results show increased concentrations of IFN and TNF-α at the site of drug application when compared to a site where drug was not applied. These results demonstrate that topical application of imiquimod to the skin leads to the local production of cytokines.

In Vitro

Human Peripheral Blood Mononuclear Cells (PBMC) and Monocytes

Unseparated human PBMC secrete a number of cytokines in response to imiquimod (8–11). IFN, TNF-α, IL-1β, IL-6, and IL-8 are induced by imiquimod. In addition, data in Table 2 show dose-dependent induction of IL-1 receptor antagonist (RA), IL-10, granulocyte macrophage colony stimulating factor (GM-CSF), G-CSF, as well as the chemokines macrophage inflammatory protein (MIP)-1α, MIP-1β, and monocyte chemotactic protein (MCP-1). Imiquimod is ineffective at inducing the T-cell cytokines IL-2, IL-4, and IL-5 in human PBMC. Studies have also demonstrated that elimination of monocytes by a number of techniques results in significantly lower concentrations of cytokines induced by imiquimod (9). In addition, monocytes isolated by elutriation are capable of secreting high concentrations of IFN, TNF-α, and IL-6 (11). On the other hand, purified lymphocytes were unable to secrete these cytokines in response to imiquimod. Interestingly, Poly I:C was effective at inducing IFN in PBMC, monocytes, and lymphocytes. These studies demonstrate that human PBMC, and specifically monocytes, produce cytokines in response to imiquimod.

In human PBMC cultures, imiquimod is capable of inducing a number of subclasses of IFN-α including α1, α2, α5, α6 and α8, with α2 being the predominant form induced (10). Kinetic studies have revealed that cytokines, especially IFN and TNF-α, can be detected as early as 1 hour after administration of imiquimod. Concentrations of most of the cytokines plateau between 6 and 8 hours after treatment and do not increase substantially over the next 16 hours of culture. These results correlate with those seen with m-RNA levels; m-RNA for the cytokines are elevated within the first few hours of culture (9,11). The induction of m-RNA for IFN-α does not require protein synthesis, indicating that the machinery necessary for cytokine production in response to imiquimod is already present. We hypothesize that activation of these cytokines occurs through a phosphorylation/dephosphorylation event. Indeed, imiquimod

Table 2 Cytokine Induction by Imiquimod in Cultures of Human PBMC

Treatment	IFN (U/ml)	TNF (pg/ml)	IL-1α (pg/ml)	IL-1β (pg/ml)	IL-1RA (pg/ml)	IL-6 (pg/ml)	IL-8 (pg/ml)	IL-10 (pg/ml)	G-CSF (pg/ml)	GM-CSF (pg/ml)	MIP-1α (pg/ml)	MIP-1β (pg/ml)	MCP-1 (pg/ml)
Medium	<2.8	37	0	9	324	0	1350	19	3.3	0.4	65	5	52
Imiquimod (1 µg/ml)	86	67	NA	33	2467	106	10050	34	12.5	0	NA	226	4724
Imiquimod (5 µg/ml)	210	452	3	425	3566	1401	12880	127	49.3	74	2783	2036	9239
LPS (1 µg/ml)	13	1055	800	1000	9782	9748	282000	1998	6454	1221	27164	10000	6250

Blood was collected from normal volunteers and PBMCs were isolated by density gradient centrifugation. PBMC were stimulated for 24 hours with the various agents. After incubation, supernatants were collected, filter sterilized, and stored at −20°C until they were assessed for cytokine levels. IFN was measured by bioassay using A549 cells and encephalomyocarditis (EMC) virus and presented in U/ml, TNFα, IL-6 and IL-10 were measured using an ELISA kit from Biosource Intl. and IL-1α, IL-1β, IL-1RA, IL-8, G-CSF, GM-CSF, MIP-1α, MIP-1β and MCP-1 were assayed using ELISA kits from R&D Systems. NA = not available; MIP = macrophage inflammatory protein; MCP = monocyte chemotactic protein; ELISA = enzyme-linked immunosorbent assay.

is capable of activating the transcription factors of αF1, which is important for IFN-α gene expression, and NFκB, which is important in activating many of the other cytokines induced by imiquimod including TNF-α, IL-1, and IL-6.

Other Cell Populations

Imiquimod has been evaluated in a number of other cell types. In keratinocytes, Kono et al. (12) have shown induction of m-RNA for IL-6 and IL-8, but not IL-1α. Furthermore, imiquimod has been shown to induce IFN, TNF-α, and IL-6 in mouse splenic and bone marrow cultures. Concentrations as low as 0.5 μg/ml are effective in inducing IFN, TNF-α, and IL-6 (3).

The mouse macrophage cell line RAW 264.7 is also capable of secreting TNF-α in response to imiquimod (EC_{50} is 10μM). Interestingly, these cells fail to secrete IFN in response to imiquimod. This is not surprising because peritoneal macrophages and alveolar macrophages are also only capable of secreting high concentrations TNF-α and IL-6, but not IFN, in response to imiquimod. Thus, monocytes and macrophages secrete different cytokine profiles in response to imiquimod. Several other human cell lines, including a number of B cell lines, have been tested for cytokine induction in response to imiquimod; however, none are able to secrete IFN.

ANTIVIRAL ACTIVITY

Imiquimod has no direct antiviral activity in various in vitro assays; however, it is effective in several viral infection models. The models that have been evaluated are presented in Table 3.

Herpes Simplex Virus-2 Infection of Guinea Pigs

Imiquimod's antiviral activity was originally described in the guinea pig model of herpes simplex virus type-2 (HSV-2) infection (13). Imiquimod at doses of 2 to 3 mg/kg are effective at inhibiting primary HSV-2 infection. The compound was effective when given orally, parenterally, or topically and was active both prophylactically and therapeutically. As discussed in the next chapter, imiquimod is also effective at inhibiting recurrent HSV-2 in guinea pigs (14–17). This was seen both during drug treatment and after treatment was stopped, indicating a long-lasting effect most likely through up-regulation of cell-mediated immunity.

Table 3 In Vivo Antiviral Activity of Imiquimod

Species	Virus	Imiquimod effectiveness
Guinea Pig	HSV-1, Primary	+
	HSV-2, Primary	+
	Recurrent	
	CMV	+
Mouse	HSV-1,2	±
	CMV	+
	Rift Valley	+
	Banzi	+
	Influenza	+
	Rauscher leukemia	−
Monkey	Yellow fever	+

Mouse and Monkey Models of Virus Infection

In a mouse model of cytomegalovirus (CMV) infection, imiquimod at doses of 10 to 30 mg/kg and greater protected animals from CMV infection. Imiquimod was effective only when given prophylactically. If it was given at the same time or after infection, no inhibition in mortality was seen. Inhibition was also seen in a guinea pig model of CMV infection (18). Imiquimod also increases survival of mice to Rift Valley fever virus and Banzi virus infection in mice (19). Much of this antiviral activity is mediated by IFN-α because antibody to IFN-α abrogated much of the antiviral effects seen with imiquimod. In contrast, imiquimod was ineffective at inhibiting Rauscher leukemia virus infection of mice even though significant IFN was seen in the serum of these mice. Finally, in cynomolgus monkeys, imiquimod was effective at increasing the survival of these animals in response to yellow fever virus infection.

The duration of antiviral activity after imiquimod treatment generally lasts 3 to 4 days. This correlates with induction of the IFN-inducible enzyme 2'5' oligoadenylate synthetase (2'5' AS). This molecule has been implicated as a mediator in IFN's antiviral activity. Elevated 2'5' AS activity is seen in a number of species after oral administration of imiquimod, including mice, rats, guinea pigs, monkeys, and humans.

ANTITUMOR ACTIVITY OF IMIQUIMOD IN MOUSE TRANSPLANTABLE TUMORS

In mice, imiquimod has shown potent antitumor activity (20–22). A summary of the various models is presented in Table 4. Imiquimod has no direct antitumor activity in vitro. When imiquimod is given orally to mice, however, it inhibits the growth of several transplantable tumors including FCB and MBT-2 bladder tumors, B-16 melanoma tumors, Lewis lung tumor cells, RIF-1 sarcoma cells, and MC-26 colon carcinoma cells (20,22). Studies have also demonstrated activity of imiquimod against the human mammary tumor, MCF-7, in nude mice. These studies indicate that T cells are not required for the antitumor effects seen in this model. In some studies, total elimination of tumors has been seen. This is most evident in the FCB bladder tumor model (22). Tumor-specific immunity has been demonstrated in this model. Activation of natural killer (NK) cells and inhibition of tumor-induced angiogenesis are also seen with imiquimod. Mechanistically, IFN-α plays a major role in imiquimod's antitumor activity because antibodies to IFN-α abrogate much of imiquimod's antitumor activity. Imiquimod is not active in all tumor models, however, because it was ineffective at inhibiting the effect of the P388 leukemia in mice. These studies indicate that imiquimod demonstrates potent antitumor activity against a number of transplantable mouse tumors.

IMIQUIMOD TOXICOLOGY STUDIES

Several animal studies have been performed evaluating both oral and dermal safety of imiquimod. Studies in rabbits, both after a single dose

Table 4 In Vivo Antitumor Activity of Imiquimod

Model	Imiquimod effectiveness
MC-26 colon carcinoma	+
B16-F10 melanoma	+
MCF-7 human mammary tumor in nude mice	+
FCB bladder carcinoma	++
3LL Lewis lung carcinoma	+
RIF-1 Sarcoma	+
MBT-2 mouse bladder tumor	+
P388D1 leukemia	−

and after 10 daily doses, revealed only mild irritation in the skin. Dermal sensitization studies in guinea pigs using both unformulated imiquimod and imiquimod cream showed no sensitization reactions. In addition, 21-day dermal toxicity studies in mice and rats, as well as 4-month dermal studies using 25 and 45 times the human dermal dose, demonstrated no systemic toxicity. There was mild irritation in the skin of mice, which was more severe in rats. The irritation seen in these studies was confined to the epidermis.

Studies were performed to address the dermal absorption of imiquimod cream. A major metabolite, S-26704, was found in rats after 3 weeks of dosing dermally with imiquimod cream at 5 mg/kg, which is 50 times the clinical dose administered to humans. At 1 mg/kg, no S-26704 was found in rats.

Both acute and chronic toxicity studies have been performed in rats and monkeys. Six-month toxicology studies revealed immune stimulation in several lymphoid organs including the spleen and lymph nodes. At high doses, anemia, thrombocytopenia, and increased globulin levels are seen. These effects are not related to cell toxicity or necrosis, but are attributed to overexpression of cytokines. These effects are readily reversible once the animals are no longer receiving imiquimod.

The structure of imiquimod resembles that of the nucleoside adenine: however, imiquimod is not a nucleoside analog. Several studies have been performed both in vitro and in vivo demonstrating that imiquimod is not mutagenic. In vitro studies include the Ames test, a mouse lymphoma model, chromosome aberration studies in Chinese hamster ovary cells, and transformation of simian hamster embryo cultures. Results of these assays showed no effects with imiquimod. In vivo, imiquimod was evaluated in both rats and hamsters for cytogenetic effects in bone marrow cells; also a dominant lethal mouse test was performed. Again, imiquimod showed no mutagenic effects in these models. Imiquimod had no mutagenic or genotoxic effects in any of the models evaluated. In summary, toxicity studies demonstrate a wide safety margin when imiquimod is applied topically with apparently little systemic absorption.

CONCLUSIONS

Imiquimod is a potent systemic cytokine inducer in several animal species and in humans when given orally. When administered topically, imiquimod induces both IFN and TNF-α in the skin. Monocytes in blood, macrophages in tissues, and possibly keratinocytes in skin produce cytokines in response to imiquimod. The antiviral and antitumor activity seen in animal models with imiquimod is largely mediated through the production of IFN. Imiquimod is not mutagenic, and its safety has been demonstrated in animals using both oral and topical delivery.

REFERENCES

1. Miller RL, Birmachu W, Gerster JF, et al. Cytokine induction by imiquimod: preclinical results and pharmacology. Chemotherapie J 1995; 4: 148–150.
2. Miller RL, Birmachu W, Gerster JF, et al. Imiquimod: cytokine induction and antiviral activity. Antiviral News 1995; 3: 111–113.
3. Reiter MJ, Testerman TL, Miller RL, et al. Cytokine induction in mice by the immunomodulator imiquimod. J Leukoc Biol 1994; 55: 234–240.
4. Miller RL, Imbertson LM, Reiter MJ, et al. Interferon induction by antiviral S-26308 in guinea pigs. ASM, Interscience Conference on Antimicrobial Agents and Chemotherapy 1986: 168.
5. Wick KA, Kvam DC, Weeks CE, et al. Oral R-837 induces interferon in healthy volunteers. Proc Am Assoc Cancer Res 1991; 32: 257.
6. Borden E, Witt P, Kvam D, et al. An effective oral inducer of interferons in humans. J Interferon Res 1991; 11: S92.
7. Imbertson LM, Weeks C, Adams N, et al. Induction of antiviral activity and cytokines by oral imiquimod in healthy volunteers. J Interferon Res 1992; 12: S127.
8. Weeks CE, Gibson SJ. Induction of interferon and other cytokines by imiquimod and its hydroxylated metabolite R-842 in human blood cells in vitro. J Interferon Res 1993; 14: 93–97.
9. Gibson SJ, Imbertson LM, Wagner TL, et al. Cellular requirements for cytokine production in response to the immunomodulators imiquimod and S-27609. J Interferon Cytokine Res 1995; 15: 537–545.
10. Megyeri K, Au W-C, Rosztoczy I, et al. Stimulation of interferon and cytokine gene expression by imiquimod and stimulation by sendai virus utilize similar signal transduction pathways. Mol Cell Biol 1995; 15: 2207–2218.
11. Testerman TL, Imbertson LM, Reiter MJ, et al. Cytokine induction by the immunomodulators imiquimod and S-27609. J Leuk Biol 1995; 58: 365–372.
12. Kono MD, Kondo S, Shivji GM, et al. Effects of the new immunomodulator R-837 on cytokine gene expression in the human epidermal carcinoma cell line COLO-16. Lymphokine Cytokine Res 1994; 13: 71–76.
13. Miller RL, Imbertson LM, Reiter MJ, et al. Inhibition of herpes simplex virus infection in a guinea pig model by S-26308. ASM Interscience Conference on Antimicrobial Agents and Chemotherapy 1985, 235.
14. Harrison CJ, Jenski L, Voychehovski T, Bernstein DI. Modification of immunological responses and clinical disease during topical R-837 treatment of genital HSV-2 infection. Antiviral Res 1988; 10: 209–224.

15. Bernstein DI, Harrison CJ. Effects of the immunomodulating agent R-837 on acute and latent herpes simplex virus type 2 infections. Antimicrob Agents Chemother 1989; 33: 1511–1515.

16. Harrison CJ, Stanberry LR, Bernstein DI. Effects of cytokines and R-837, a cytokine inducer, on UV-irradiation augmented recurrent genital herpes in guinea pigs. Antiviral Res 1991; 15: 315–322.

17. Bernstein DI, Miller RL, Harrison CJ. Effects of the immunomodulator (imiquimod, R-837) alone and with acyclovir on genital HSV-2 infection in guinea pigs when begun after lesion development. Antiviral Res 1993; 20: 45–55.

18. Chen M, Griffith BP, Lucia HL, Hsuing GD. Efficacy of S-26308 against guinea pig cytomegalovirus. Antimicrob Agents Chemother 1988; 32: 678–683.

19. Kende M, Lupton HW, Canonico PG. Treatment of experimental viral infections with immunomodulators. Adv Biosci 1988; 68: 51.

20. Sidky YA, Borden EC, Weeks CE, et al. Inhibition of murine tumor growth by an interferon inducing imidazoquinoline. Cancer Res 1992; 52: 3528–3533.

21. Sidky YA, Borden EC, Weeks CE. Inhibition of tumor-induced angiogenesis by the interferon inducer imiquimod. Proc Am Assoc Cancer Res 1992; 33: 77.

22. Sidky YA, Bryan GT, Weeks CE, et al. Effects of treatment with an oral interferon inducer, imidazoquinolinamine (R-837), on the growth of mouse bladder carcinoma FCB. J Interferon Res 1990; 10: S123.

33
Imiquimod in the Guinea Pig Model of Genital Herpes: An Antiviral and Adjuvant

David I. Bernstein
Children's Hospital Medical Center, Cincinnati, Ohio

Christopher J. Harrison
Creighton University and University of Nebraska Medical Center, Omaha, Nebraska

GUINEA PIG MODEL

The guinea pig model was chosen for these studies of genital herpes because it most closely mimics the human disease (reviewed in 1). After intravaginal inoculation of herpes simplex virus-2 (HSV-2), animals develop an acute vesiculoulcerative disease that begins 3 to 4 days after inoculation and lasts approximately 3 to 10 days. After recovery from the acute disease, the genital skin heals and animals develop spontaneous recurrences, which usually lasts 1 to 2 days (2). Recurrences are mild and consist of one to two vesicles or papules. Virus also can be isolated from the vaginal vault by swabbing for the first 10 days after HSV inoculation. Virus can be quantified and usually peaks 1 to 2 days after inoculation. As in humans, latent virus is detected in the lumbosacral ganglia and can be detected by cocultivation, as well as more sensitive techniques, such as polymerase chain reaction (PCR) (3). Stimuli, such as ultraviolet light exposure, can reactivate HSV and produce lesions in guinea pigs as it does in humans (4,5).

Thus, using the guinea pig model we can evaluate the effects of antivirals, immunomodulators, or vaccines on acute and recurrent HSV disease. We can quantitate the incidence and severity of disease, as well as the duration and magnitude of viral shedding. Using ultraviolet exposure, the effects of therapy on reactivatable lesions can be evaluated.

TREATMENT OF ACUTE GENITAL HSV-2

Our initial evaluation of imiquimod was performed using a topical (intra-vaginal) application of 1% suspension given twice a day for 5 days at a dose of 5 mg/kg beginning 12 hours after vaginal HSV-2 inoculation (6). As shown in Table 1, therapy completely prevented development of acute genital disease and significantly reduced both the peak viral titer and total viral shedding, as measured by the area under the $\log_{10}$ titer per day curve. Further, we were unable to detect latent virus in the dorsal root ganglia of treated animals by cocultivation. Significantly fewer treated animals developed recurrences, and the mean number of recurrent lesions days was also significantly reduced.

Because it appeared that therapy had reduced recurrent disease, we next determined whether virus had reached the neural tissue during the acute infection (7). Using the same treatment regimen, we sacrificed animals 3, 4, and 5 days after viral inoculation and determined the titer of HSV-2 in the lumbosacral dorsal root ganglia and spinal cord. As seen in Table 2, therapy decreased the number of animals with recoverable virus. In fact, virus was recovered from only one treated animal, and was present at the lowest detectable titer.

As discussed in previous chapters, high levels of circulating α-interferon were detected in treated animals whether or not they were inoculated with HSV-2. Levels peaked by days 2 to 3 and returned to baseline

Table 1 Effect of Imiquimod Therapy on Acute and Recurrent HSV-2 Disease

	Animals with acute disease (days 1–14)	Peak vaginal viral titer ($\log_{10}$)	Total viral shedding[a]	Number with recovered latent virus	Number with recurrence	Mean recurrent lesion days[b]
Placebo	12/12	6.8	35.5	5/6	9/9	6.8
Imiquimod	0/20[c]	4.9[c]	5.3[c]	0/8[d]	2/20[d]	0.4[c]

[a]Total viral shedding is measured by the area under the log10 viral titer per day curve.
[b]Mean number of days with recurrent lesions.
[c]$P < .001$
[d]$P < .02$

Table 2 Effect of Imiquimod on Acute Neural Infection

	Imiquimod (viral titer)[a]		Placebo (viral titer)	
	Ganglia	Spinal cord	Ganglia	Spinal cord
Day 3	0/5	0/5	1/5 (1.0)	2/5 (1.5)
Day 4	0/5	0/5	5/5 (1.4)	5/5 (2.6)
Day 5	0/6	1/6 (0.7)	4/5 (1.2)	4/4 (2.9)

[a]Viral titer log10

shortly after the drug was discontinued. Infection with HSV-2 also induced the production of lower levels of α-interferon, which peaked on days 4-8. Antibody titers to HSV were lower in treated animals, but lymphoproliferative responses to HSV and interleukin-2 (IL-2) production in response to HSV stimulation were detected earlier. Proliferative responses to PHA were also higher in noninfected imiquimod recipients compared to control animals.

In the initial experiments, virus was recovered from the vaginal vault for <36 hours in about one-third of treated animals (6). These animals did not develop an immune response and were susceptible to rechallenge. Thus, therapy was thought to be so effective that it had prevented the induction of protective immunity by decreasing viral replication to <36 hours. In our next experiments, therefore, the dose was decreased by applying drug once a day and delaying therapy until 36 hours after viral inoculation.

Using this regimen, treatment again reduced the peak lesion score of the acute disease from 3.7 in controls to 0.8 ($P < .001$) and the total acute lesion score (the sum of the daily scores for the first 14 days) from 14.1 to 0.6 ($P < .001$) (7). Viral titers were reduced by 24 hours after therapy and the duration of viral shedding was reduced from 6.9 to 3.2 days ($P < .001$). Recurrent disease was also reduced in treated animals from 5.1 to 2.0 recurrent episodes ($P < .001$). Further, latent virus was detected less frequently in treated animals with or without the addition of hexamethylenebisacetamide, a demethylating agent that increases the ability to detect latent virus by cocultivation (8).

Summary

In this model, imiquimod provided effective therapy for genital HSV-2 infection. Therapy markedly reduced the incidence and severity of acute disease and decreased viral shedding within 24 hours of initiating therapy. To our knowledge, this is the only therapy that has reduced subsequent recurrent disease when used to treat acute infection. Unlike acyclovir therapy in this model (9), imiquimod provided a significant reduction in recurrent lesions when used as late as 36 hours, but not when used at the onset of lesions (10).

TREATMENT OF RECURRENT GENITAL HSV-2

Because imiquimod appeared to have an effect against recurrent disease, we next evaluated its effectiveness as a suppressive therapy for recurrent HSV-2 disease in guinea pigs (11). In these trials, we compared 5 and 21 days of topical 1% cream given once a day. Treatment was initiated on day 15 after viral inoculation, a time when acute disease had resolved and the animals began to develop recurrent lesions.

Both the 5- and 21-day therapies significantly reduced recurrences while animals were receiving therapy (11). As opposed to 5 days of therapy, however, animals treated for 21 days continued to have a significant reduction in recurrence after drug therapy was stopped (Figure 1). This effect continued for at least 9 weeks after therapy was discontinued during the final week of observation. This resulted in an overall reduction (over the 8 to 10 weeks of treatment) of 16% for animals treated for 5 days and a 67% reduction when imiquimod was given for 21 days. Treatment did not appear to affect the ability to recover latent HSV.

Evaluation of cell-mediated immune responses revealed no significant increases in the 5-day treatment compared to control animals, but there were significant increases in the lymphoproliferative response to HSV and the amount of IL-2 produced by the mononuclear cells in response to HSV in the 21-day treatment group compared to control animals. Thus, it appeared that 21 days of imiquimod produced an up-regulation of the cell-mediated immune response. HSV antibody levels were depressed immediately after the 21-day treatment period, but were equivalent by day 60. Interferon was induced only during the period of treatment.

Summary

Treatment of recurrent HSV-2 disease with topical imiquimod decreased the number of recurrences during treatment. Prolonged therapy (21 days) up-regulated cell-mediated immunity and decreased recurrent disease for

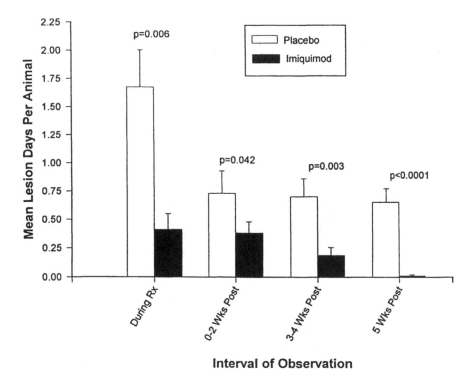

Figure 1 Effect of treatment with 21 days of imiquimod on genital HSV recurrences. Animals were treated topically (intravaginally) with imiquimod beginning on day 15 after HSV-2 inoculation. Animals were observed for recurrent HSV lesions during the 3 weeks of therapy and for 5 weeks after therapy was discontinued.

weeks after therapy was discontinued. Similar to the reduction of recurrent disease in acutely treated animals, this finding of prolonged activity appears to be unique for imiquimod.

ADJUVANT EFFECTS

Adjuvant for a Prophylactic HSV Vaccine

In our original studies (6), we noted that treated animals with >36 hours of viral replication developed accelerated cell-mediated immune (CMI) responses compared to placebo recipients, despite a markedly reduced level of viral replication. Antibody responses were not increased. Similarly, animals with a latent HSV-2 infection that were treated for 21 days developed enhanced CMI responses (11). Thus, it appeared that imiquimod might be acting as an adjuvant by accelerating the CMI responses when used to treat the initial infection and enhancing the responses to reactivated virus in latently infected animals. We believe that when treated animals reactivate virus during therapy, the virus serves as an antigen to boost the CMI response to HSV in the presence of imiquimod, even though the reactivated virus does not produce detectable lesions.

The potential of imiquimod to serve as an adjuvant, therefore, was evaluated. In the first experiments, we evaluated the adjuvant effects for a prophylactic vaccine (12). Animals received 35 μg of a lectin purified HSV-2 glycoprotein preparation with or without imiquimod at 14 and 35 days before intravaginal HSV-2 inoculation. Imiquimod was administered for 5 days with each dose of vaccine, either as a 1% cream intravaginally or subcutaneously in the back. Vaccine was given in the footpad. Imiquimod was begun either simultaneously with vaccine or delayed for 48 hours because it was unclear what effects the early presence of interferon would have on immune responses. These imiquimod-plus-vaccine groups were compared to a no vaccine/no imiquimod control group and groups receiving imiquimod alone, glycoprotein alone, or the glycoprotein mixed with complete Freund's adjuvant (CFA).

In the first experiment, immunization with the glycoprotein alone significantly reduced the severity of acute disease. The groups receiving adjuvants (imiquimod or CFA) had a further reduction in disease severity, but the differences were not significant because of the mild disease in the group receiving glycoprotein alone. Immunization with glycoprotein alone also reduced vaginal viral shedding, but this decrease was not significant unless an adjuvant was used. The addition of imiquimod to glycoprotein immunization reduced vaginal titers by about 2 logs, whereas CFA plus vaccine reduced titers by about 4 logs compared to control animals. Only the combination of glycoprotein immunization plus an adjuvant significantly reduced subsequent recurrent disease. The mean number of recurrent lesion days was reduced from 4.3 days in the glycoprotein immunized group to 0.8 in the group receiving imiquimod beginning 48 hours after immunization and 0.1 in the group receiving imiquimod simultaneously with immunization.

Similar results were observed in the second experiment (Table 3). None of the animals immunized with glycoprotein plus adjuvant developed

Table 3   Effect of Imiquimod as an Adjuvant for an HSV-2 Glycoprotein Vaccine

Group	Animals with acute disease	Peak vaginal viral titer (log_{10})	Number with recurrence	Mean recurrent lesion days
Control	11/11	6.1	10/10	5.7
gly alone	6/11	4.4	9/11	2.5
gly + imi (d)	0/10[a]	3.1a	4/10	0.4[b]
gly + imi (s)	0/10[a]	2.1[b]	3/10[a]	0.3[b]
gly + imi (sub q)	0/11[a]	1.3[b]	0/11[b]	0[b]
gly + CFA	0/9[a]	0[b]	0/9[b]	0[b]

gly = glycoprotein; imi = imiquimod; (d) = imiquimod delayed 48 hours after immunization; (s) = imiquimod given simultaneously with immunization; (sub q) = imiquimod given subcutaneously.
[a]$P < .05$ vs gly alone
[b]$P < .005$ vs gly alone

lesions acutely, producing a small but significant decrease from the group immunized with glycoprotein alone, where 6 of 11 animals developed genital lesions. The addition of imiquimod to glycoprotein immunization again decreased vaginal viral shedding. Compared to glycoprotein immunization alone, the groups also receiving imiquimod topically had decreases of 1 to 2 logs, whereas the group also receiving imiquimod subcutaneously had a 3-log reduction. Virus was not detected in animals receiving glycoprotein plus CFA. Recurrences were also significantly reduced in groups receiving imiquimod or CFA plus vaccine compared to vaccine alone. None of the animals immunized with glycoprotein and either imiquimod subcutaneously or CFA developed recurrent lesions.

Adjuvant for a Therapeutic HSV Vaccine

The concept of a therapeutic vaccine, that is, one given to patients with a history of recurrent HSV disease, dates back to the 1920s (see Chapter 26). The guinea pig model was recently used to test the concept that immunization could boost immune responses and thus reduce recurrences (13–15). Because cell-mediated immune responses, especially lymphoproliferative and IL-2 production, appear to be important for control of recurrent disease in this model (16), we next evaluated the potential of imiquimod to serve as an adjuvant for a therapeutic vaccine.

In these experiments, animals were immunized in the hind footpad with a similar mixture of HSV-2 glycoproteins given 14 and 35 days after HSV infection. During this period, animals have recovered from acute disease and are developing recurrent lesions. Animals received either nothing, glycoprotein immunization alone, or glycoprotein immunization plus imiquimod or CFA. Imiquimod was given at a dose of 3 mg/kg per day subcutaneously for either 1 or 5 days, beginning simultaneously with each immunization.

Similar results were obtained independently by the two investigators evaluating this therapy. The results of one experiment are shown in Figure 2. No significant reduction in recurrences was noted in animals immunized without adjuvants. The immunized groups that also received

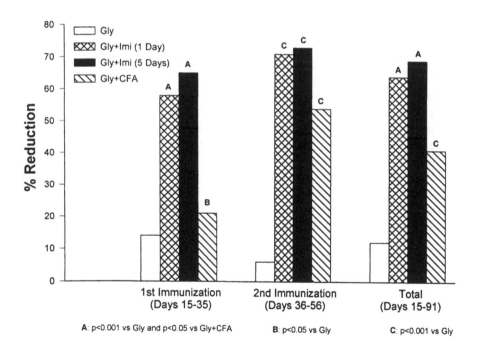

Figure 2 Effect of HSV-2 glycoprotein immunization with or without imiquimod on reducing recurrent HSV lesions in the guinea pig. Animals were immunized on days 14 and 35 after HSV infection along with either imiquimod given for 1 or 5 days, complete Freund's adjuvant (CFA), or nothing. Animals were observed for recurrent lesions for 11 weeks.

either 1 or 5 days of imiquimod, however, had significant reductions in recurrences ranging from 58% to 68% after the first vaccine dose and from 71% to 73% after the second vaccine dose compared to control animals. A total reduction of 64% to 69% was observed over the entire observation period (days 15 to 91). These reductions were significantly higher than the reduction observed in the animals immunized with vaccine plus CFA (41%). Antibody responses to HSV were slightly but significantly increased in imiquimod recipients compared to immunization alone, but this increase was less than in CFA recipients. Herpes simplex virus-specific MHC unrestricted cytolytic activity was increased only in the groups receiving imiquimod or CFA plus immunization.

Because both 21 days of imiquimod alone and vaccination with a short course of imiquimod as an adjuvant reduced recurrences, the combination of these approaches was evaluated (17). Animals received either placebo or 21 days of imiquimod alone (3 mg/kg subcutaneously) begun on day 15, or 21 days of imiquimod begun on day 15 plus immunization with HSV-2 glycoproteins on the first and last day of treatment. As discussed previously, imiquimod alone significantly reduced recurrences not only during therapy (89%), but also for each of the next 7 weeks of observation after therapy was discontinued (70%). Groups that received imiquimod plus vaccination had a reduction of 92% during the 3 weeks after the first immunization while receiving imiquimod and an 88% reduction during the next 7 weeks of observation. Further, this group continued to have a significant reduction in recurrent disease (56%) for an additional 4 weeks, which was not seen in the imiquimod alone group. Thus, 21 days of imiquimod reduced recurrence by 63% and imiquimod plus vaccination by 81% for the 15 weeks of observation.

In these experiments, imiquimod alone significantly increased the IL-2 production of mononuclear cells incubated with HSV-2, and imiquimod plus immunization produced an even greater increase. This response has been correlated to a reduction in recurrences in this model (16). Only immunization plus imiquimod increased the MHC unrestricted HSV cytolytic response or HSV antibody response to HSV.

Summary

Imiquimod appeared to act as an adjuvant for both prophylactic and therapeutic HSV vaccines. When used for prophylaxis, imiquimod plus glycoprotein immunization resulted in milder acute disease, decreased viral shedding, and especially a reduction in subsequent recurrences compared to glycoprotein immunization alone. When used therapeutically, it provided a significant reduction in recurrences compared to immunization alone. These clinical responses compared favorably to complete Freund's adjuvant, which is a potent but unacceptable adjuvant for clinical use. The best overall improvement was seen by the combination of 21 days of imiquimod and glycoprotein immunization.

CONCLUSION

Using the guinea pig model of genital HSV disease, the antiviral and adjuvant potential of imiquimod has been shown. Compared to acyclovir, imiquimod more effectively reduced acute disease and viral shedding in this model. Further, and more important, imiquimod therapy of the acute disease had an effect on subsequent recurrences that has not been demonstrated with acyclovir. When used to treat recurrent disease, imiquimod significantly suppressed recurrences, and unlike other antiviral therapies, imiquimod had a prolonged effect even after therapy was discontinued. This effect may be due to enhanced cell-mediated immune responses that develop in treated animals.

When used as an adjuvant for a prophylactic HSV-2 glycoprotein vaccine, imiquimod further enhances the protective effect so that acute disease and viral shedding are further reduced. The most profound effect, however, is a subsequent reduction in recurrent disease. Imiquimod also enhances the effectiveness of an HSV therapeutic vaccine, that is, a vaccine given to animals with recurrent disease to boost immune responses and reduce recurrences. When the two most effective antiviral and immunization schedules were combined, a greater than 80% reduction in recurrences was observed over an extended period. In the experiments evaluating imiquimod as an adjuvant, it appeared to produce effects at least equivalent to complete Freund's adjuvant, as well as other adjuvants, including monophosphoryl lipid A, Ribi triple mix, and muramyl dipeptide.

REFERENCES

1. Hsiung GD, Mayo DR, Lucia HL, Landry ML. Genital herpes: pathogenesis and chemotherapy in the guinea pig model. Rev Infect Dis 1984; 6: 33–50.

2. Stanberry LR, Kern ER, Richards JT, et al. Genital herpes in guinea pigs: pathogenesis of the primary infection and description of recurrent disease. J Infect Dis 1982; 146: 397–404.

3. Burke RL, Hartog K, Croen KD, Ostrove JM. Detection and characterization of latent HSV RNA by in situ and northern blot hybridization in guinea pigs. Virology 1991; 181: 793–797.

4. Spruance SL, Freeman DJ, Steward JCG, et al. The natural history of ultraviolet radiation-induced herpes simplex labialis and response to therapy with peroral and topical formulations of acyclovir. J Infect Dis 1991; 163: 728–734.

5. Harrison CJ, Stanberry LR, Bernstein DI. Effects of cytokines and R837, a cytokine inducer on UV irradiation augmented recurrent genital herpes in guinea pigs. Antiviral Res 1991; 15: 315–322.

6. Harrison CJ, Jenski L, Voychehovski T, Bernstein DI. Alterations in immunologic functions and clinical disease by topical treatment of genital HSV-2 infection with R837. Antiviral Res 1988; 10: 209–224.

7. Bernstein DI, Harrison CJ. Effects of the immunomodulating agent R837 on acute and latent herpes simplex virus type 2 infections. Antimicrob Agents Chemother 1989; 33: 1511–1515.

8. Bernstein DI, Kappes JC. Enhanced in vitro reactivation of latent herpes simplex virus from neural and extraneural tissues with hexamethylenebisacetamide. Arch Virol 1988; 99: 57–65.

9. Bernstein DI, Stanberry LR, Harrison CJ, et al. Antibody response, recurrence patterns and subsequent HSV-2 reinfection following initial HSV-2 infection of guinea pigs: effect of acyclovir. J Gen Virol 1986; 67: 1601–1612.

10. Bernstein DI, Miller RL, Harrison CJ. Effects of therapy with an immunomodulator (imiquimod, R-837) alone and with acyclovir on genital HSV-2 infection in guinea pigs when begun after lesion development. Antiviral Res 1993; 20: 45–55.

11. Harrison CJ, Miller RL, Bernstein DI. Posttherapy suppression of genital herpes simplex virus (HSV) recurrences and enhancement of HSV-specific T-cell memory by imiquimod in guinea pigs. Antimicrob Agents Chemother 1994; 38: 2059–2064.

12. Bernstein DI, Miller RL, Harrison CJ. Adjuvant effects of imiquimod on a herpes simplex virus type 2 glycoprotein vaccine in guinea pigs. J Infect Dis 1993; 167: 731–735.

13. Stanberry LR, Burke RL, Myers MG. Herpes simplex virus glycoprotein treatment of recurrent genital herpes. J Infect Dis 1988; 157: 156–163.

14. Stanberry LR, Harrison CJ, Bernstein DI, et al. Herpes simplex virus glycoprotein immunotherapy of recurrent genital herpes: factors influencing efficacy. Antiviral Res 1989; 11: 203–214.

15. Ho JR, Burke RL, Merigan TC. Antigen presenting liposomes are effective in treatment of recurrent herpes simplex virus genitalis in guinea pigs. J Virol 1989; 63: 2951–2958.

16. Bernstein DI, Harrison CJ, Jenski LJ, et al. Cell mediated immunological responses and recurrent genital herpes in the guinea pig: effects of glycoprotein immunotherapy. J Immunol 1991; 146: 3571–3577.
17. Harrison CJ, Miller RL, Bernstein DI. Adjuvant effect of imiquimod when combined with HSV glycoprotein vaccine in guinea pigs with recurrent HSV-2 genital herpes. Antiviral Res 1995; 26: 233.

34

Acute Pain Associated with Herpes Zoster and Its Impact on Quality of Life: Shingles Is a Pain

David U. Himmelberger
Health Outcomes Group, Palo Alto, California

Eva Lydick
Merck Research Laboratories, West Point, Pennsylvania

CLINICAL SYMPTOMS OF HERPES ZOSTER

Herpes zoster (shingles) is a painful condition in adults resulting from previous infection with varicella-zoster virus, the virus that causes chickenpox in children. The virus lies dormant in the nerve cells until the time when it reactivates, producing shingles.

Initially, the patient generally experiences fever, pain, and tenderness. The patient then usually develops a rash and small vesicles (blisters) on the skin or in the mouth. The skin rash, instead of covering large parts of the body as in chickenpox, usually appears only on a small area of skin in rows like shingles on a roof. A typical shingles rash follows the path of certain nerves on one side of the body only—generally in the trunk, buttocks, neck, face or scalp—usually stopping abruptly at the midline.

MAIN FEATURES OF HERPES ZOSTER

An episode of shingles typically begins with flu-like symptoms (chills, headache, upset stomach) and sometimes is accompanied by a prodromal itching or burning sensation. Pain may precede the rash by a few days (occasionally mistaken for a heart attack, lung infection, or back problem), but the discomfort is more commonly felt only during and/or

429

after the rash. The rash is usually confined to one side of the body. It starts as a series of raised red spots surrounded by a swollen area that turn into clear blisters. These blisters become cloudy, dry out, and crust over. The spots may bleed, then become very itchy and painful. In immuno-suppressed patients, attacks are severe, with the rash covering a wide area. In most cases, the rash takes several weeks to heal, and after healing may leave some whitish-silver or brown scars.

Shingles pain occasionally occurs alone, without any rash. The characteristic rash of herpes zoster generally disappears within 5 to 25 days of onset (1). However, many people, especially the elderly, continue to suffer pain long after the rash has healed. The severe pain that occurs along the affected nerve root is by far the worst aspect of herpes zoster. The severity and duration of the pain is highly variable (2), with some patients suffering severe pain for weeks while others have moderate pain for only a few days.

CAUSES OF HERPES ZOSTER

The herpes zoster virus is responsible for both chickenpox or varicella in children and shingles or zoster in adults. Shingles occurs most commonly in adults who had chickenpox as children, and have some, but not total immunity to the virus.

While chickenpox is highly contagious (caught by inhaling infected droplets), shingles is not generally transmitted from one person to another. However, children or adults who have not had the infection may catch chickenpox if they touch wet shingles blisters. Although childhood chickenpox almost always runs its course in a week or two (usually with full recovery), the virus is not fully eliminated from the body. It retreats to nerve cells, where it rests, silently hidden within nerve ganglia (centers near the spinal cord). Most people go through life without the virus ever becoming reactivated. If the virus is reactivated, it travels along affected nerve pathways, causing skin eruptions as it goes.

There is some evidence that shingles may be precipitated by excessive exposure to sunlight (ultraviolet radiation), stress (emotional), trauma (wounds, surgery, or inflammation), and other events that lower immune resistance. Shingles is a common problem for the elderly, and is rare among the young. The age-specific incidence rates vary from about 75 cases per 100,000 years of observation among individuals 15 to 24 years of age to more than 400 cases per 100,000 years of observation among individuals 74 years of age and older (3). The incidence rates are not appreciably different between males and females. It is most frequent among the immunosuppressed, such as those with Hodgkin's disease or leukemia, transplant, or AIDS patients, and people undergoing radiation treatment or taking immunosuppressants.

BACKGROUND ON NATURAL HISTORY STUDY

This chapter describes the results of a natural history study that was conducted to characterize the time course of pain and its impact on the quality of life of patients with herpes zoster. Pain is the single greatest cause of acute and chronic morbidity associated with herpes zoster and has devastating effects on a patient's quality of life. However, the magnitude of the negative impact of acute zoster pain on quality of life has not been well documented.

Brief Pain Inventory

Fifty patients, 55 years and older, were followed for a minimum of 8 weeks or until their pain disappeared. Patients were enrolled as soon after the onset of zoster rash and/or pain. Two-thirds of the patients were enrolled within 2 weeks (one-third within one week) of the onset of pain. Three-quarters were enrolled within 2 weeks of the onset of the rash. Those patients whose pain had not resolved by the end of 8 weeks were followed until they reported minimal pain. Pain was evaluated using the Wisconsin Brief Pain Inventory (4) (BPI) upon enrollment, daily during the first week and weekly thereafter. The BPI was developed to evaluate pain in cancer patients and has been shown to have good performance characteristics for evaluating pain in patients with different cancers.

In the BPI, pain is evaluated in the past 24 hours as one of 11 discrete levels ranging from 0 corresponding to NO PAIN AT ALL to 10 corresponding to PAIN AS BAD AS YOU CAN IMAGINE. The BPI evaluates four aspects of pain: worst pain, least pain, average pain, and pain right now. In addition to pain, the BPI includes questions about how pain interferes with seven activities of daily living: general activity, mood, walking ability, work (both inside and outside the home), relationships with others, sleep and enjoyment of life. The questions about interference with activities of daily living are scored from 0 to 10 with 0 corresponding to no interference and 10 corresponding to total interference. The BPI took only 3 to 5 minutes to complete and was well accepted by patients.

Pain is best characterized by examining not only its severity, but also its duration. "Area under the curve" (AUC) is a single numeric value that incorporates both the severity and duration of pain. A profile of one patient's "worst pain" and lesion area over 8 weeks is shown in Figure 1. The total area of lesions for this patient was largest at study week 0, 2 to 7 days after the rash first appeared. The lesions were large, but quickly decreased in size and were gone by the end of the third study week. In contrast to the rapid disappearance of the lesions, the severity of pain increased while the lesions were shrinking, and the pain persisted for 5 weeks after the lesions were totally healed. This patient had his maximum "worst pain" at level 10 during weeks 2 to 4. Although this patient's pain decreased to level 7 by week 5, the pain increased to level 9 at week 6 and was gone by week 8. The area under the pain curve is equal to 402.5 for this patient.

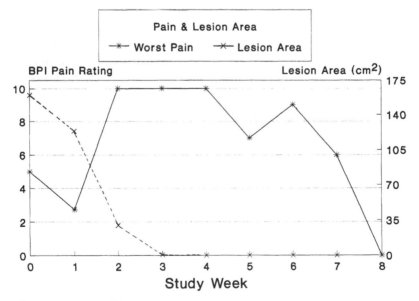

Figure 1 Pain and lesion area.

Quality of Life and Other Variables

A general quality of life questionnaire (MOS-36) comprised of 36 questions taken from the Medical Outcomes Study (5) was given every 2 weeks. There are eight domains in the MOS-36: physical functioning, role functioning-physical, bodily pain, general health perception, vitality, social functioning, role functioning-emotional, and mental health. Demographic data and comorbidity information were collected on each patient at enrollment. Demographic data and comorbidities were collected at baseline. Data on the extent and site of lesions were collected weekly. The extent of lesions was determined by placing a clear film over the patient's lesions and drawing the outline of the rash with a black pen. Photocopies of the film were retraced with a digitizing computer pad and the area of each lesion in cm^2 was computed. The area of each lesion was then summed to determine the lesion size for each patient.

RESULTS OF THE NATURAL HISTORY STUDY

This report focuses on the impact of herpes zoster on quality of life and responses to the question on "worst pain" since this question has previously been shown to have the greatest reliability (6). The BPI has been validated in patients with herpes zoster and has been shown to have good performance characteristics for evaluating pain in this patient population (7).

Worst Pain

The "worst pain" for most patients was day 0. The average "worst pain" at day zero was 6.4 compared to the maximum average "worst pain" which was 7.6. The maximum area under the curve for a single patient with two observations one week apart is 7 days times the maximum score of 10 or 70. Hence, each patient's AUC for pain is represented as a number between 0 and 560 for the 8 weeks of observation, although it could equal 840 for a few patients who were followed for 12 weeks.

As shown in Figure 2, the distribution of the "worst pain" is centered about the median AUC of 205, with a long trail ranging to 757. The mean AUC for "worst pain" is 215, with a standard deviation of 163.

AUC

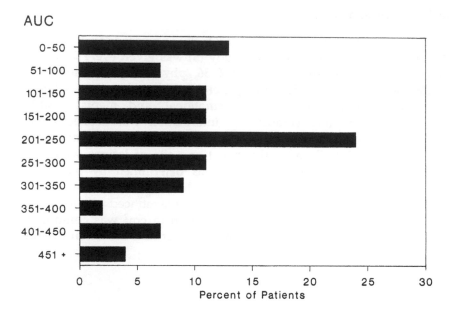

Figure 2   Area under the curve for worst pain.

Relationship Between Pain and Lesion Size

Although the characteristic lesions associated with herpes zoster are uncomfortable and disfiguring, as shown in Figure 3, patients experience significant levels of pain that persist well beyond the disappearance of lesions. By study week 4, more than 80% of the lesions have healed, and the remaining lesions have an average area of approximately 12 cm², an area slightly larger than the size of a silver dollar. In contrast, at week 4, more than 80% of the patients continue to experience pain at an average level of 3.6 on the BPI scale. A large proportion of patients continue to have pain through week 8.

Relationship Between Pain and Pain Medications

The patients with herpes zoster were taking a variety of medications for their pain. As shown in Table 1, although the mean "worst pain" was lower while patients were taking medication, none of the prescription medications was effective in alleviating the pain. Means rather than AUC were used to show the relationship between pain and treatment since

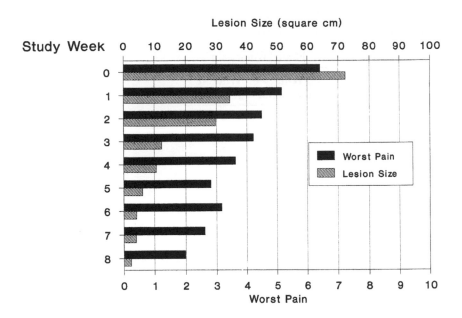

Figure 3 Relationship between worst pain and lesion size.

patients frequently changed the medication in search of anything that would receive their pain.

We also observed that the proportion of patients using opiates to relieve their pain was strongly related to the severity and duration of "worst pain" as expressed by the AUC. As the AUC increased, their physicians were more likely to prescribe opiates for the patient's pain. Opiates were usually reserved for extreme pain exceeding 7 on the 10 point BPI scale. However for this population of patients with herpes zoster, the opiates were no more effective than acetaminophen or NSAIDS in ultimately relieving pain.

The impact of the pain experienced by patients with herpes zoster is broad based, affecting many areas of their quality of life. The impact of the pain is directly related to the intensity and duration of the pain. As shown in Table 2, at week 2 when the pain was most intense, the proportion of patients reporting interference in their activities of daily living increases dramatically as the "worst pain" increases. In this table, a score of 3 or more represents interference with activities of daily living, and a score of 2 or less represents no interference. Even while patients were receiving

Table 1 Comparison of "Worst Pain" for Patients
Receiving and Not Receiving Pain Treatment

Treatment	Mean "worst pain"	
	With treatment	Without treatment
Acetaminophen	3.4	4.9
NSAIDs	3.9	4.6
Corticosteroids	3.6	5.5
Opiates	3.4	7.1
Other pain treatments (TENS, etc.)	3.8	7.5

medications for their pain as shown in Table 1, 10% to 30% of patients
reported interference in their activities of daily living. At pain levels of 9 to
10, all patients reported interference with some activities of daily living.
Pain interfered with sleep and general activity the most, while walking
ability and enjoyment of life were slightly less affected by pain.

Since the mean age of our population was 70, we used normative data
based on 442 patients within the ages 65 to 74 to help interpret the impact

Table 2 Association Between "Worst Pain" and Some Interference (Score of 3 or
More on a 10-Point Scale) with Individual Activities of Daily Living at Week 2

	% of patients reporting interference with activities of daily living						
Worst pain	General activity	Mood	Walking ability	Work[a]	Relationships with others	Sleep	Enjoyment of Life
0	0	0	0	0	0	0	0
1	0	0	0	2	0	7	0
2	1	4	1	4	4	2	4
3	5	5	5	11	6	11	10
4	32	27	17	29	22	30	27
5	43	29	22	25	18	41	29
6	57	43	35	59	49	78	57
7	71	61	40	55	51	65	67
8	76	65	54	58	53	84	64
9	93	73	58	78	51	83	66
10	80	77	77	80	74	86	74

[a]Includes both work outside the home and housework.

of herpes zoster on quality of life as measured by the MOS-36 (8). In Table 3 we show the differences in the mean quality of life score for each domain at selected study weeks compared with the age group norm. Negative numbers indicate that the quality of life of the herpes zoster patients is poorer than of age matched individuals without major health problems and positive numbers indicate better quality of life.

The physical and emotional aspects of the role functioning domain, and of course bodily pain, of the MOS-36 were most affected by pain. The social functioning and vitality domains were also significantly affected. There was a small impact on mental health, while physical functioning was practically unchanged. Interestingly, the general health perceptions domain was not affected by the episode of herpes zoster, and the domain scores were slightly above those for the general population.

The decrement in quality of life as measured by the MOS-36 appears, to a large extent, to be driven by pain. The correlations between domain scores on the MOS-36 and "worst pain" from the BPI at week 2 range from –0.32 to –0.63 for the eight domains, all statistically significantly different for zero with $P < 0.05$.

To help put the magnitude of the impact of herpes zoster into perspective, we have compared their quality of life with that of patients with five major medical conditions: hypertension, congestive heart failure (CHF), diabetes mellitus type II, recent acute myocardial infarction (acute MI), and clinical depression. In Figures 4 and 5 we have plotted the mean differences in quality of life for the herpes zoster patients at week 2 and the five other medical conditions compared to that of age matched individuals

Table 3 Differences in Quality of Life for the MOS-36 Domains and Age Group Norms by Study Week

Domain	Differences in quality of life from age group norms at indicated study week				
	0	2	4	6	8
Role functioning—physical	–24.9	–46.6	–32.2	–26.1	–20.3
Role functioning—emotional	–33.3	–35.8	–33.7	–23.7	–9.2
Bodily pain	–32.3	–34.2	–23.0	–12.9	–3.4
Social functioning	–16.8	–30.8	–24.6	–11.2	–3.4
Vitality	–15.5	–16.1	–14.7	–10.7	–0.5
Mental health	–8.9	–9.7	–8.7	–5.8	0.0
Physical functioning	–4.9	–5.5	–1.1	1.7	9.2
General health perception	10.3	9.4	5.4	7.0	7.3

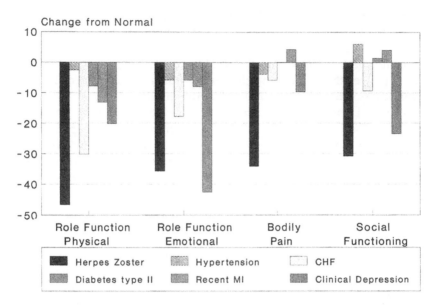

Figure 4 Impact of herpes zoster on quality of life relative to other medical conditions.

in the general U.S. population. Bars extending downward indicate quality of life worse than the general population and bars extending upward above the 0 norm line indicate quality of life better than the general population. As emphasized by the solid black bars, we observe that for almost all of the eight domains in the MOS-36, the quality of life of patients with herpes zoster is worse than for the other five medical conditions. Only patients with clinical depression have poorer quality of life in the vitality and role functioning-emotional domains.

DISCUSSION

The visible lesions that characterize herpes zoster, although uncomfortable and disfiguring, disappear in 3 to 4 weeks for most patients. However, the pain persists long after the lesions have disappeared. For most patients, the "worst pain" remains at a level of 2 or more out of 10 eight weeks after the onset of herpes zoster. These patients are taking virtually every type of analgesic for pain relief, including opiates, corticosteroids, nonsteroidal antiinflammatory drugs (NSAIDs), and acetaminophen.

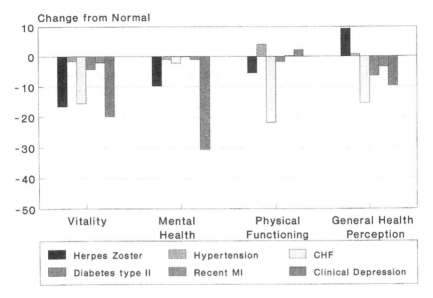

Figure 5 Impact of herpes zoster on quality of life relative to other medical conditions.

None of the analgesics was more effective than acetaminophen, and nothing was effective in providing complete relief from the pain.

Although the acute pain associated with herpes zoster resolves for the majority of patients, the impact of the pain is broad-based in terms of its impact on quality of life and persists for at least 8 weeks for more than 80% of patients. The disruption of quality of life is greatest in the areas of physical and emotional role functioning, social functioning, relationships with others, sleep, work, and vitality. The pain also had a negative effect on mood and interfered with patients' enjoyment of life.

The pain experienced by patients with herpes zoster is so severe that its impact on quality of life as measured by the MOS-36 is much greater than that experienced by patients with life-threatening diseases such as congestive heart failure or those with a recent acute myocardial infarction. Herpes zoster pain also has an impact on quality of life that is worse than or approximately equal to that experienced by patients with clinical depression.

Although the quality of life questions capture the effect that the zoster pain has on interference with work both inside and outside the home, they do not provide an estimate of the economic impact of the interference.

Based on our retrospective telephone interviews with the patients in the natural history study 1 year later, we found that 82% of the patients who were employed outside the home lost an average of 8 hours per week from their job during the 8 weeks of the study. Although not all patients could afford to pay for someone to help with the housework during their zoster episode, 8.5% of all patients did pay for someone. The average time for paid household work was 6 hours per week during the 8 weeks of the study.

Since the average age of the study population was 70, many were retired and not working for pay. We found that 13% of the patients engaged in volunteer work on a regular basis, and half of these patients were unable to perform their volunteer activities while they had zoster.

We found that the effects of zoster lingered on for a significant proportion of the patients. Six to twelve months after the onset of herpes zoster, 28% of the patients reported having pain at a level of 2.9 on the BPI scale. Some patients were permanently scared by their episode of herpes zoster. Virtually all the patients expressed a strong fear that the herpes zoster would recur.

With most adults at risk to have the dormant varicella virus reactivated, any treatment that can reduce the acute pain associated with herpes zoster will have a dramatic effect on improving quality of life and reducing the economic burden of this disease.

REFERENCES

1. Reuler JB, Chang MK. Herpes zoster: epidemiology, clinical features, and management. South Med J 1984; 77: 1148–1156.
2. Wood MJ. Herpes zoster and pain. Scand J Infect 1991; 78 (suppl): 53–61.
3. Rogozzino MW, Melton III LJ, Kurland LT, et al. Population-based study of herpes zoster and its sequelea. Medicine 1992; 61: 310–316.
4. Cleeland CS. Assessment of pain in cancer: measurement issues. Adv Pain Res Ther 1990; 16: 47–55.
5. Stewart AL, Hays RD, Ware JE Jr. The MOS short-form general health survey: reliability and validity in a patient population. Med Care 1988; 26: 724–735.
6. Daut RL, Cleeland CS, Flannery RS. Development of the Wisconsin brief pain questionnaire to assess pain in cancer and other diseases. Pain 1983; 17: 197–210.
7. Lydick E, Epstein RS, Himmelberger D, et al. Area under the curve: a metric for patient subjective responses in episodic diseases. Quality Life Res 1995; 4: 41–45.
8. Ware JE Jr, Snow KK, Kosinoski M, et al. SF-36 Health Survey: Manual and Interpretation Guide, Boston: The Health Institute, New England Medical Center, 1993.

35

Second Generation Antiherpes Drugs: Valaciclovir and Famciclovir

Komal Chopra, Angella Glidden, Patricia Lee, and Stephen K. Tyring

University of Texas Medical Branch, Galveston, Texas

INTRODUCTION

Although acyclovir has been the "gold standard" of antiherpes therapy for over a decade, its low bioavailability after oral administration and the necessity for frequent dosing stimulated the search for antiherpes agents with greater efficacy and efficiency than acyclovir. This search has led to various second-generation antiherpes drugs, two of which are now approved by the U.S Food and Drug Administration (FDA) for treatment of acute herpes zoster and herpes simplex genitalis: valaciclovir and famciclovir (Figure 1).

VALACICLOVIR

Valaciclovir Pharmacokinetics

Efforts aimed at improving the bioavailability of acyclovir have resulted in the synthesis of a variety of prodrugs, the most promising of which is valaciclovir (1). Valaciclovir is the L-valyl ester of acyclovir that demonstrates good oral absorption and extensive, nearly complete biotransformation to acyclovir. In both rat and monkey, the oral bioavailability of acyclovir derived from valaciclovir was approximately 65%, three to five times greater than oral acyclovir alone (2,3).

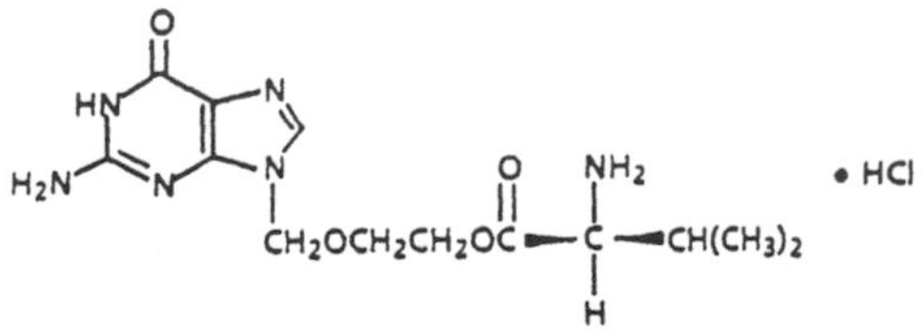

VALACICLOVIR

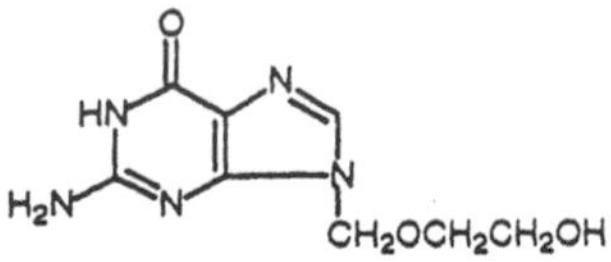

ACYCLOVIR

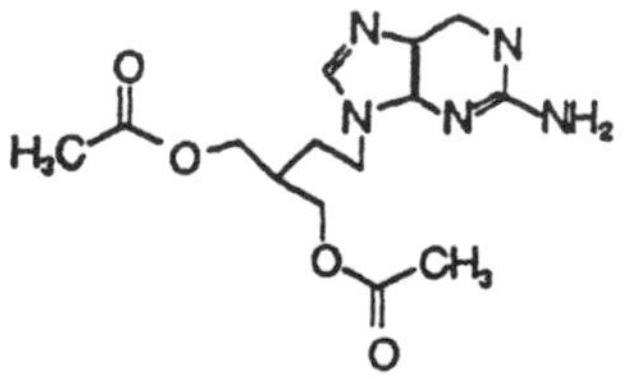

FAMCICLOVIR

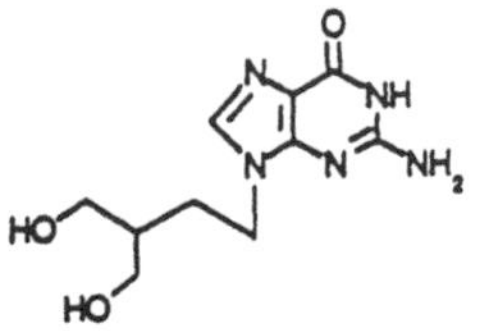

PENCICLOVIR

Figure 1 Second-generation antiherpes drugs.

Following oral administration of valaciclovir, a favorable pharmacokinetic profile was observed with maximum concentration (Cmax) and area under the curve (AUC) levels of acyclovir increasing proportionately with doses of 10 and 25 mg. Furthermore, while acyclovir was detected in plasma minutes after oral dosing, valaciclovir was essentially undetected. The half-life of acyclovir observed from oral valaciclovir was 1 hour compared with 7 minutes for the prodrug. The major urinary metabolite was acyclovir. With intravenous dosing, less extensive conversion was achieved, indicating first pass intestinal and/or hepatic metabolism (2,3).

Additional preclinical studies in humans indicate a similar pharmacokinetic profile. In normal human male volunteers, single valaciclovir doses of 100 to 1000 mg resulted in dose-proportionate increases in AUC levels of acyclovir (4). Similar steady state Cmax and AUC levels with multiple doses suggest the bioavailability does not decrease with increasing doses as it does with oral acyclovir alone (3). Administration of a single 1.0 g dose produced acyclovir peak plasma concentrations of 5 to 6 μg/ml. At a 2.0 g oral dose given four times daily to patients with advanced HIV disease, steady state acyclovir peak plasma levels are 8.4 μg/ml, and the AUC value approaches that of intravenous acyclovir. Because metabolism of valaciclovir produces only two derivatives, acyclovir itself and the amino acid L-valine, valaciclovir has not been found to be associated with any serious or unexpected adverse events or laboratory abnormalities (5). Nausea, vomiting, diarrhea, and abdominal pain were commonly reported in HIV-positive patients. However, in only one case was the adverse event, diarrhea, attributable to valaciclovir. No evidence of the nephropathy or neurotoxicity seen with high-dose intravenous acyclovir was observed with valaciclovir.

Valaciclovir for Therapy of Acute Herpes Zoster

In a large trial comparing the efficacy and safety of valaciclovir to acyclovir, 1141 immunocompetent patients aged 50 years and older (mean age 68 years) were randomized within 72 hours of their first vesicle of zoster to one of three treatment groups: valaciclovir 1 g orally three times a day for 7 days, valacyclovir 1 g three times a day for 14 days, or acyclovir 800 mg five times daily for 7 days (6). In terms of rash progression, valaciclovir was as effective as acyclovir in its effect on appearance of new lesions, time to crusting, and time to 50% healing. Analyses of subsets of patients between 50 and 60 years of age and over 60 years produced the same results. In evaluation of the effect on pain, valaciclovir conferred a slight benefit over acyclovir. Measuring times to cessation of pain, valaciclovir patients had a median of 40 days of pain after healing compared to 60 days for acyclovir recipients. At 6 months, 19% of valaciclovir patients had pain compared to 26% of acyclovir patients. Overall in terms of zoster-related discomfort, it is estimated that valaciclovir provided a 25% benefit over acyclovir (7). There were no substantial differences between 7 and 14 days of valaciclovir. The safety profile of valaciclovir was favorable as well, with nausea and headache being reported equally among treatment groups. The study concluded that valaciclovir is equal to acyclovir in terms of cutaneous resolution but provides a more convenient dosing schedule and significantly faster cessation of pain with valaciclovir. Therefore, valaciclovir was FDA approved for the treatment of shingles in July 1995.

Valaciclovir for Management of Herpes Simplex Genitalis

Various studies have now been completed with valaciclovir for treatment of first episode genital herpes, for episodic therapy of recurrent genital herpes, and for suppression of recurrent general herpes.

Valaciclovir for Treatment of First Episode Genital Herpes

Valaciclovir 1000 mg twice a day was compared to acyclovir 200 mg five times daily for 10 days in a randomized, double-blind, multicenter trial (8).

Therapy was initiated within 72 hours of lesion onset in 643 other-wise healthy patients. Median time to lesion healing was 9 days in both valaciclovir and acyclovir treatment groups. After 48 hours of therapy, development of new lesions was observed in 22% of valaciclovir recipients and in 24% of acyclovir recipients. Therefore, valaciclovir was demon-strated to be more convenient but not more effective than acyclovir for therapy of first episode genital herpes.

Valaciclovir for Episodic Treatment of Recurrent Genital Herpes

Valaciclovir has been evaluated in three randomized, double-blind, con-trolled trials for the episodic treatment of recurrent genital herpes:

1. Valaciclovir 1000 mg twice a day was compared to acyclovir 200 mg five times daily and to placebo (ratio 3:3:1)
2. Valaciclovir 1000 mg twice a day was compared to valaciclovir 500 mg twice a day and to placebo (ratio 3:3:2) (9); and
3. Valaciclovir 500 mg twice a day was compared to acyclovir 200 mg five times daily (ratio 1:1).

In all three studies patients self-initiated treatment within 24 hours of the first sign or symptom of recurrent genital herpes and continued therapy for 5 days. In total 2858 patients self-initiated treatment. Both valaciclovir regimens and acyclovir significantly accelerated resolution of all signs and symptoms compared with placebo ($P = 0.0001$), thus shortening the length of the episode. Hazard ratios for the valaciclovir regimens of 1.66 to 1.94 indicated that episode resolution occurred up to 94% faster with valaciclovir treatment compared with placebo. No differences were evi-dent between valaciclovir and acyclovir. Adverse events were rare, generally mild and similar in type across all treatment groups. Therefore, valaciclovir 1000 twice a day, valaciclovir 500 mg twice a day and acyclovir 200 mg five times daily were all equivalent for therapy of recur-rent genital herpes. The 500 mg twice a day regimen of valaciclovir was FDA approved for this purpose in December 1995 (9,10).

Valaciclovir for Suppression of Recurrent Genital Herpes

In a multicenter study of 382 patients comparing valaciclovir 500 mg once daily to placebo, valaciclovir recipients experienced an 85% reduction in recurrences of genital herpes (11). This reduction is similar to that seen with acyclovir 400 mg twice a day in other studies.

FAMCICLOVIR

Famciclovir Pharmacokinetics

Famciclovir is the diacetyl, 6 deoxyester of the guanosine analog, penciclovir, which exerts the antiviral effect. Oral penciclovir is poorly absorbed, but famciclovir is absorbed rapidly and converted to penciclovir in the intestinal wall and liver (12). Penciclovir has activity against herpes simplex virus (HSV-1), HSV-2, and Epstein-Barr virus (EBV) as well as varicella zoster virus (VZV). Like acyclovir, penciclovir must first be converted to its triphosphate form. The first phosphorylation is carried out by viral thymidine kinase and is then converted to penciclovir triphosphate by cellular enzymes. As with acyclovir triphosphate, penciclovir triphosphate inhibits viral DNA polymerase, blocking viral DNA synthesis and replication (13). The advantages of penciclovir over acyclovir include its enhanced bioavailability (77% following oral administration of famciclovir) and its persistent antiviral activity (14). Both the phosphorylation of acyclovir and penciclovir are efficient in VZV-infected cells, but the intracellular concentrations of acyclovir-triphosphate are 100 times less than penciclovir triphosphate (12). In VZV-infected cells, the half-life of penciclovir triphosphate is 7.2 to 11.0 hours compared to 0.8 hours for acyclovir triphosphate translating into prolonged antiviral activity for penciclovir triphosphate and less frequent losing for famciclovir. Inhibitory concentrations of penciclovir versus VZV are 3 to 4 µg/ml. Elimination of famciclovir is achieved by tubular secretion and glomerular filtration requiring dose adjustment in renal failure, similar to acyclovir. Penciclovir is eliminated unchanged in urine. There are no known drug interactions, but probenecid and other drugs eliminated by active renal tubular secretion may increase plasma levels of penciclovir. The drug may be removed during hemodialysis, but no overdosage has been reported (15). On the contrary, famciclovir has a very favorable safety profile, comparable to placebo and acyclovir when studied in over 1600 subjects including 816 herpes zoster patients (16). The most common adverse events were equal between famciclovir and placebo and included headache, nausea, and diarrhea. Compared to acyclovir, headache and nausea were equally reported as adverse events. No consistent laboratory abnormalities associated with famciclovir were found.

Famciclovir for Therapy of Acute Herpes Zoster

The efficacy and safety of famciclovir in herpes zoster were established in two large clinical trials (17,18). The first study of 419 adult patients with uncomplicated herpes zoster compared the efficacy of two different doses of famciclovir against placebo (17). Patients received either famciclovir 500 mg or 750 mg, versus placebo three times a day for 7 days. The 500 mg dose was equal to the 750 mg dose in efficacy, but there was a statistically significant reduction over placebo in the duration of viral shedding and time to cutaneous resolution both in the overall patient population and in the subsets of the elderly (> 50 years old) or those enrolled within 48 hours of rash onset. There was not a significant difference in acute pain among groups. In contrast, chronic pain both in the overall population and in the elderly subgroup was significantly reduced. Incidence of post herpetic neuralgia (PHN) was not affected by famciclovir, but medium time to loss of pain in the elderly patients was 63 days in the 500 mg treated patients and 163 days for patients in the placebo group, a reduction of 14 weeks in medium duration of pain. The second study, a multicenter trial of 545 immunocompetent adults, randomized patients to three different doses of famciclovir versus acyclovir (18). Like the first study, concomitant antiviral or immunomodifying treatments, topical or otherwise, were prohibited. Doses of famciclovir studied were 250 mg, 500 mg, and 750 mg three times a day versus acyclovir 800 mg five times daily for 1 week. Famciclovir was equal in efficacy to acyclovir at all doses tested for cutaneous lesion healing, but duration of acute pain was significantly reduced for all three doses of famciclovir in the subgroup of patients enrolled within 48 hours. For all patients treated, duration of acute pain was comparable between groups receiving 500 mg doses of famciclovir and 800 mg doses of acyclovir. Safety and tolerability were demonstrated in this study as well as in the placebo-controlled trial. In June 1995, the FDA approved famciclovir for uncomplicated herpes zoster at 500 mg three times a day for 7 days. Additional studies will elucidate the drug's effect and outline possible treatment for immunocompromised hosts, complications of zoster, ophthalmic zoster, and patients with renal and hepatic insufficiency.

Famciclovir for Management of Herpes Simplex Genitalis

Clinical trials have established the dosages and schedules for famciclovir in the therapy of first-episode genital herpes, for episodic treatment of recurrent genital herpes, and for suppression of recurrent genital herpes.

Famciclovir for Treatment of First Episode Genital Herpes

Studies conducted in the United States, Australia, and Canada compared famciclovir, 125 mg, 250 mg, 500 mg three times a day, with acyclovir

200 mg given five times daily for 10 days. These studies demonstrated that all three doses of famciclovir and acyclovir were effective in the treatment of first episode when considering cessation of viral shedding, complete healing, or loss of symptoms. A further study in Europe and Singapore compared famciclovir, 250 mg, 500 mg and 750 mg three times a day, with acyclovir 200 mg five times daily for 5 days and confirmed that all doses of famciclovir were effective and safe in treating first-episode genital herpes (19).

Famciclovir for Episodic Therapy of Acute Genital Herpes

Two double-blind, randomized, placebo-controlled, multicenter Canadian studies were conducted to evaluate the efficacy and safety of oral famciclovir in the treatment of recurrent genital herpes (20,21). Treatment was patient-initiated in one and clinic-initiated in the other. In both studies, patients received either 125 mg, 250 mg, or 500 mg of famciclovir or placebo twice daily for 5 days, with therapy initiated 6 hours or less after prodrome or lesion onset. Treatment was initiated in 467 (217 men; 250 women) patients in the patient-initiated study and 308 (162 men; 146 women) patients in the clinic-initiated study. Symptoms and lesions were assessed twice daily, and lesions were swabbed for viral culture twice daily for the first 5 days and then daily until complete healing. In the patient-initiated study, pretreatment viral cultures were positive in 74%, 79%, 67%, and 84% of the 125-mg, 250-mg, 500-mg famciclovir-treated and placebo-treated patients, respectively. In both studies, all famciclovir doses significantly reduced times to cessation of viral shedding and complete healing. In addition, time to loss of all symptoms was significantly reduced for all treatment groups when compared with placebo for both studies ($P < 0.05$).

Famciclovir for Suppression of Recurrent Genital Herpes

A multicenter, placebo-controlled trial was conducted to evaluate the efficacy of famciclovir in suppressing genital herpes recurrences in women with frequent episodes (≥ 6 per year) (22). A total of 375 women received oral famciclovir, at doses of 125 mg and 250 mg administered once or twice daily, 500 mg once daily, or placebo for 4 months. The median time to the first clinical recurrence was 3.8 months in the famciclovir treatment groups. This was in contrast to a median time to first clinical recurrence of 2.7 months for the placebo group. The time to first clinical recurrence was significantly prolonged in patients who received famciclovir 125 mg twice daily ($P = 0.031$) or 250 mg twice daily

Table 1 Current Recommendations for Valaciclovir and Famciclovir*

Indication	Valaciclovir	Famciclovir
Acute herpes zoster	1 g po TID for 7 days	500 mg po TID for 7 days
Recurrent genital herpes (episodic therapy)	500 mg po BID for 5 days	125 mg po BID for 5 days

*No official recommendations currently exist for either drug for therapy of first episode genital herpes nor for suppression of recurrent genital herpes.

($P = 0.0001$). The results for time to first virologically confirmed recurrence were similar to those noted for clinically confirmed recurrence, with statistical significance ($P < 0.05$) also achieved for the famciclovir 250 mg once daily group. Patients who were treated with famciclovir 250 mg twice daily had the most clinically significant prolongation in time to first recurrence. Oral famciclovir given twice daily for 4 months was well tolerated and appeared to effectively suppress recurrent genital herpes in this study population. The results from this trial highlight the potential future use of famciclovir for suppression of genital herpes.

CONCLUSION

These studies indicate that valaciclovir is preferable to acyclovir for oral therapy of recurrent genital herpes (in terms of convenience) as well as for acute treatment of herpes zoster (in terms of convenience and efficacy). No data, however, indicate a preference between valaciclovir and famciclovir for either of these indications. Both drugs are equally safe and equally convenient (Table 1). No study has yet compared their efficacies in the treatment of herpes simplex, but trials comparing valaciclovir to famciclovir for therapy of acute herpes zoster have been initiated. Approval of these two drugs for the therapy of first-episode genital herpes and for suppression of recurrent genital herpes, as well as recommendations for dosages and schedules, is expected in the near future.

REFERENCES

1. Jacobson MA. Valacyclovir (BW256U87): the 1-valyl ester of acyclovir. J Med Virol 1993; (suppl 1): 150–153.

2. Burnette TC, de Miranda P. Metabolic disposition of the acyclovir prodrug valacyclovir in the rat. Drug Metab Dispos 1994; 22: 60–64.
3. de Miranda P, Burnette TC. Metabolic fate and pharmacokinetics of the acyclovir prodrug valacyclovir in cynomolgus monkeys. Drug Metab Dispos 1994; 22: 55–59.
4. Weller S, Blum MR, Doucette M, et al. Pharmacokinetics of the acyclovir prodrug valacyclovir after escalating single- and multiple-dose administration to normal volunteers. Clin Pharmacol Ther 1993; 54: 595–605.
5. Darby G. Acyclovir- and beyond. J Int Med Res 1994; 22(suppl 1): 33A–42A.
6. Beutner KR, Friedman DJ, Forszpaniak C, et al. Valacyclovir compared with acyclovir for improved therapy for herpes zoster in immunocompetent adults. Antimicrob Agents Chemother 1995; 39: 1546–1553.
7. Beutner K. Antivirals in the treatment of pain. J Geriatr Dermatol 1994; 2(suppl A): 23A–28A.
8. Fife KH, International VHSVSG. Valaciclovir or acyclovir for the treatment of first episode genital herpes (abstr). In: 35th Interscience Conference on Antimicrobial Agents and Chemotherapy. 17 Sept 1995, San Francisco.
9. Spruance SL, Tyring SK, De Gregorio B, Miller C, Beutner K, International VHSVSG. A large-scale, placebo-controlled, dose-ranging trial of peroral valaciclovir for episodic treatment of recurrent herpes genitalis. Arch Intern Med 1996; 156: 1729–1735.
10. Tyring SK, International VHSVSG. Prevention of lesion development in recurrent genital herpes with oral valacyclovir HCl (abstr). In: 54th American Academy of Dermatology. 10–15 February 1996, Washington, DC.
11. Drucker JL et al. Once daily valaciclovir sustains the suppressive efficacy and safety record of acyclovir in recurrent genital herpes. The First European Congress of Chemotherapy. 14–17 May 1996. Glasgow, UK.
12. Bacon T. Famciclovir: potency, predictability, and persistence. 3rd Congress of the European Academy of Dermatology and Venereology, Copenhagen, Denmark, 1993 (abstract): 6–7.
13. Earnshaw DL, Vere Hodge RA. Effective inhibition of herpesvirus DNA synthesis by (S)-penciclovir-triphosphate. American Society for Microbiology, 32nd Interscience Conference on Antimicrobial Agents and Chemotherapy. Washington, DC: 1992: (Abstr 1707).
14. Pratt SK, Beerahee M, Pere MA, et al. The pharmacokinetics of penciclovir following oral administration of 500 mg famciclovir to patients with uncomplicated herpes zoster. 3rd Congress of the European Academy of Dermatology and Venereology, Copenhagen, Denmark, 1993.
15. Pratt SK, Fairless AJ, Peu MA, et al. The haemodialysis of penciclovir, Abstract 1286. 6th International Congress for Infectious Diseases, Prague, Czech Republic, April 26–30, 1994.
16. Saltzman R, Jurewicz R, Boon R. Safety of famciclovir in patients with herpes zoster and genital herpes. Antimicrob Agents Chemother 1994; 38: 2454–2457.

17. Tyring SK, Nahlik J, Cunningham A, et al. A double-blind, randomized, placebo-controlled, parallel group study of oral famciclovir for the treatment of uncomplicated herpes zoster. Ann Intern Med 1995; 123: 89–96.
18. Degreef H, Famciclovir Herpes Zoster Clinical Study Group. Famciclovir, a new oral antiherpes drug: results of the first controlled clinical study demonstrating its efficacy and safety in the treatment of uncomplicated herpes zoster in immunocompetent patients. Int J Antimicrob Agents 1994; 4: 241–246.
19. Loveless M, Harris W, Sacks S. Treatment of First Episode Genital Herpes with Famciclovir (abstr). In: 35th Interscience Conference on Antimicrobial Agents and Chemotherapy. 17–20 September 1995, San Francisco.
20. Sacks SL, Aoki F, Diaz-Mitoma F, Sellors J, Shafran S, for the Canadian Famciclovir Study Group. Patient-initiated, twice daily oral famciclovir for early recurrent genital herpes. JAMA 1996; 276: 44–49.
21. Sacks SL, Martel A, Aoki F, Shafran S, St-Pierre C, Lassondo M. Clinic-initiated treatment of recurrent genital herpes using famciclovir: results of a Canadian, multicenter study. Presented at the Int. Conf. Infectious Diseases. Apr. 1994. Prague, Czechoslovakia.
22. Mertz GJ, Loveless MO, Kraus SJ, Tyring SK, Fowler SL, Collaborative Famciclovir Genital Herpes Research Group. Famciclovir for suppression of recurrent genital herpes. Presented at 34th Interscience Conf. Antimicrobial Agents and Chemotherapy, Oct. 1994, Orlando, Fla.

36

Interferons for Treatment of Genital Warts

Angella Glidden, Komal Chopra, Patricia Lee, and Stephen K. Tyring
University of Texas Medical Branch, Galveston, Texas

INTRODUCTION

Interferons (IFN) have been available for the therapy of genital warts for over a decade. Interferons act via antiviral mechanisms as well as by a variety of nonantiviral actions. Interferon therapy is considered moderately effective and is associated with a low recurrence rate but has not become widely accepted as a therapy for genital warts. Major reasons for its limited acceptance include the need to administer IFN via an injection, its expense, its potential for systemic side effects, and its relatively slow rate of action. The future of wart therapy lies in induction of endogenous IFN at the local level.

THE NEED FOR ANTIVIRAL THERAPY FOR GENITAL WARTS

Traditional therapy for warts (including genital warts, condyloma acuminatum) has been cytodestructive or surgical intervention. Such treatments provide rapid relief of signs and symptoms (i.e., warts) but are usually associated with frequent recurrences as well as with possible pain, bleeding, secondary infection, and expense (when lasers are involved).

Genital warts can be associated with any of more than 20 of the greater than 70 recognized types of human papillomavirus (HPV). Recurrences of condyloma acuminatum following surgical removal of the warts are generally thought to be due to HPV lying latently (subclinically) in adjacent, clinically normal-appearing skin and mucous membranes (1).

Interferons are glycoproteins with broad-spectrum antiviral activity but do not directly inhibit viral replication. Instead IFNs induce cells to produce antiviral proteins that block subsequently infecting viruses at the stages of transcription, translation, and viral packaging. In addition, IFNs act against HPV-infected cells via a spectrum of nonantiviral mechanisms (e.g., immunomodulation, effects of cell differentiation, phenotypic reversion and regulation of oncogene and anti-oncogene expression) (Table 1). Therefore, IFNs have the potential to eradicate HPV in adjacent, normal-appearing tissue, thus reducing recurrences.

CLINICAL STUDIES OF IFNs FOR THERAPY OF CONDYLOMA ACUMINATUM

Of the three major classes of IFNs, most clinical trials for treatment of genital warts have involved IFNα, followed by IFNβ and IFNγ. Interferons have been administered topically, intralesionally, and systemically (i.e., either subcutaneously or intramuscularly). In addition, IFNs have been used as monotherapy and as part of combination treatment protocols.

Interferons as Monotherapy for Condyloma Acuminatum

Two IFNα subtypes are currently approved by the U.S. Food and Drug Administration (FDA) for intralesional (IL) therapy of condyloma acuminatum: IFNα2b (recombinant) (Intron, Schering Plough, Kennilworth, NJ) and IFNα3 (natural) (Alferon, Purdue Frederick, Norwalk, CT). Other IFNs and other routes of administration, however, have been extensively investigated. In addition, IFNs are approved for a number of other viral and non-viral diseases (Table 2). Although initial reports of topical IFN were promising (2,3), larger, well-controlled studies failed to support

Table 1 Mechanisms of Action of Interferons

1. Antiviral: regulation of viral transcription, translation and packaging.
2. Immunomodulatory: activation of lymphoid effector cells, regulation of antibody production, enhancement of surface antigens on target cells.
3. Differentiation: regulation.
4. Oncogene expression: down-regulation.
5. Tumor suppressor genes: up-regulation.

Table 2 Food and Drug Administration Approvals for Interferons

Interferonα	Hairy cell leukemia
	Kaposi's sarcoma (AIDS patients)
	Condyloma acuminatum
	Hepatitis B
	Hepatitis C
	Malignant melanoma (adjunct to surgery)
Interferonβ	Multiple sclerosis
Interferonγ	Chronic granulomatous
	Disease of children

the efficacy of topical IFN (4). Therefore, further discussion will be limited to IL and systemic routes of administration.

Therapy of Condyloma Acuminatum with Intralesional Interferons

Natural IFNα administered IL produced 50% (5/10 patients) complete responses (CR) of condyloma acuminatum with a 20% (1/5 patients) recurrence rate (RR) at 3 months (5). Although this trial involved no placebo group, a subsequent, larger study (6) yielded a 62% (41/66 patients) CR with natural IFNα compared to 21% (14/66 patients) CR with placebo. The RR at 4 months was 25% (9/36 patients) with IFNα; at 2 months the RR was 23% (3/13 patients) with placebo. In a third IL study (7) recombinant (r) IFNα2b, natural IFNα and IFNβ produced CRs of 48% (11/23 patients), 45% (7/15 patients) and 50% (10/20 patients), respectively, compared to 22% (4/18 patients) treated with placebo. Although none of the four placebo-treated patients who had cleared experienced a recurrence, 33% of the IFN-treated patients (all three groups) suffered a recurrence at a mean of 46 days. Other reports of IL rIFNα2b were associated with the following rates of CR: 36% (42/116 patients) with IFNα versus 17% (20/116 patients) with placebo; the RR with IFNα was 20% (5/25 patients) at 9 months (8); 28% (9/32 patients) with IFNα versus 16% (6/38 patients) with placebo (no RR given) (9); and 60% (6/10 patients) with IFNα; the RR was 17% (1/6 patients) at 2 months (10). The RR of placebo treated patients was not reported from these later three studies.

Therefore, IFN appears effective when administered IL for condyloma acuminatum, but IFN was injected two to three times per week for 3 to 8 weeks in these studies. Thus, IL use of IFN has limited practical value, especially for patients having numerous genital warts.

Systemic Therapy of Condyloma Acuminatum with Interferons

Use of systemic IFNs have been via subcutaneous (SQ) or intramuscular (IM) routes and have been given some distance from the genital warts (e.g., the arm). Complete responses with natural IFNα in one study were 43% (6/14 patients) with 1.0 mu (million units/treatment); 57% (17/30 patients) with 3.0 mu; and 69% (11/16 patients) with 5.0 mu (11). A subsequent investigation using IM or SQ natural IFNα produced 21% (6/28 patients) CR with 1.0 mu and 33% (21/63 patients) CR with 3.0 mu. Neither trial involved a placebo group or reported a RR. Reichman et al. (12) reported a 25% (19/77 patients) CR using 1.0 mu or 3.0 mu administered IM or SQ. At 4 months, an RR of 5% (1/19 patients) was observed. Olsen et al. (13) reported that natural IFNα (3.0 mu) administered IM produced 26% (9/34 patients) CR but with a 44% (4/9 patients) RR at 1 month. Subsequently, Reichman et al. (14) observed that natural IFNα, or IFNβ or IFNα2b given SQ (2.0 mu) produced a similar CR of 17% (22/133 patients) vs. 10% (4/42 patients) with placebo. At 176 days the RR was 23% (5/22 patients) with IFN; at 168 days the RR was 0% (0/4 patients) with placebo. Both 3.0 mu and 9.0 mu of rIFNα2a administered SQ yielded similar low rates of efficacy in a subsequent trial: 21% (11/53 patients and 12/56 patients, respectively) CR vs. 18% (10/57 patients) CR with placebo (15). At 9 months, a 36% (5/14 patients) RR was seen in the 9.0 mu group compared to a 9% RR in each of the other two groups. In contrast, Gross et al. (16) reported SQ administration of rIFNα2b in doses from 1.5 mu to 18 mu produced CRs from 43% (3/7 patients) to 71% (5/7 patients). The RR was 0% at 7 months in both groups. The same investigators later reported that rIFNα2c (5.0 mu) used SQ (17) produced a 71% (5/7 patients) CR. A 50% (12/24 patients) CR with IM use of rIFNα2a (3.0 mu) and a 36% (9/25 patients) CR with IM use of consensus IFN (2.5 mu or 5.0 mu) were reported by Gall et al. (18). Panici et al. (19) reported that rIFNα2b (3.0 mu) yielded a 20% CR whether IFN was administered IM (10/51 patients) or SQ (10/50 patients). The RR was 10% (1/10 patients) in both groups at 12 months.

Fewer reports exist with systemic use of IFNγ for condyloma acuminatum. When IFNγ was administered IM, the range of CRs was from 9% (1/11 patients) with 0.2 to 2.0 mu to 20% (3/15 patients) with 0.2 to 0.5 mu (20). In another report, only a 7% (2/28 patients) CR was seen with IFNγ (0.2 mu) given IM (21). Zouboulis et al. (22) observed no CRs (0/10 patients) when IFNγ (1.5 mu) was administered SQ. Fierlbeck (23), however, reported that IFNγ (1.5 to 3.0 mu) given SQ resulted in a CR of 29% (5/17 patients). Furthermore, Gross et al. (24) observed that IFNγ (0.75

to 6.0 mu) given SQ yielded a 56% (34/61 patients) CR; after 7 to 60 months the RR was 0%.

Therefore, systemic use of IFN appears less effective than IL administration for therapy of condyloma acuminatum but is better tolerated by many patients. Recurrence rates following CR with any route of administration of IFN are low in most studies but are difficult to compare to RR following CR with placebo therapy because the numbers of complete responders with placebo are very low in most reports.

Interferons as Adjunctive Therapy for Condyloma Acuminatum

Since the mechanisms of action of IFN differ from that of surgical/cytodestructive therapies, IFN would be expected to be additive, or even synergistic, when used in combination with nonantiviral treatments for condyloma acuminatum. A number of studies have been designed to test this hypothesis.

Since surgery/cytodestructive therapy can remove the genital warts caused by HPV, the primary criterion for determining the efficacy of combination therapy is the RR. Several reports (23,25–27) have documented the efficacy of surgery combined with IFN without providing the RR following surgery alone. In most reports in which laser surgery was followed by IFNα, however, the RR was less than for surgery without IFN. Vance et al. (28) noted a RR of 38% (18/47 patients) at 13 weeks with laser surgery in contrast to an RR of 19% (5/27 patients) with laser surgery followed by rIFNα2b. Likewise, Hohenleutner et al. (29) observed a 81% (13/16 patients) RR at 3 months following laser surgery compared to a 42% (8/19 patients) RR with laser surgery followed by rIFNα2b. A similar effect was noted by Petersen et al. (30) who noted a 77% (17/22 patients) RR at 3 months with laser alone compared to 48% (13/27 patients) RR with laser surgery followed by IFNα2b. At 11.5 months, the RR was 45% (9/20 patients) with laser alone in a study reported by Davis and Noble (31); at 9.5 months the RR following laser surgery with a single injection of rIFNα2b was 21% (3/14 patients). Reid et al. (32) reported that patients treated only with laser surgery suffered a 38% (3/8 patients) RR at 18 months compared to only a 4% (1/27 patients) RR in persons who received rIFNα2a after laser surgery. One study, however, demonstrated no benefit from laser surgery followed by rIFNα2a (i.e., 68% (48/71 patients) RR at 9 months versus 61% (39/64 patients) treated with laser alone) (33).

Less dramatic results were reported when electrocautery was combined with IFN in two small studies (34,35). Furthermore, no further benefit was observed with the addition of rIFNα2a to cryotherapy in two studies (36,37) or with the addition of rIFNα2b to podophyllin in another clinical trial (38).

IFN does appear to provide additive to synergistic benefits relative to nonantiviral therapy in terms of reduced RR if all visible warts are surgically removed and the patient is started immediately on a course of local (SQ) IFN. The dosage, schedule, and duration of IFN administration in these reports, however, vary widely. Although no specific recommendations exists for these parameters, the most effective use of exogenous IFN treatment appears to be as part of a combination regimen.

ADVERSE EVENTS ASSOCIATED WITH IFN THERAPY

Interferons are well tolerated by the majority of patients, particularly if doses less than 5.0 mu per treatment are given. Although doses above 1.0 mu per treatment can produce a flulike syndrome, the prevalence of this syndrome increases as the dose approaches 5.0 mu and usually only becomes problematic above 5.0 to 10 mu. Side effects are most frequently noted following the first in a series of injections; after the second and subsequent treatments the flulike syndrome usually is infrequent and/or mild. Premedication and/or treatment with acetaminophen decreases such adverse events. Slight lethargy may continue throughout a series of IFN injections but rarely has a major effect on the patients' activities.

Mild and transient changes in certain laboratory parameters have been reported with IFN doses from 1.0 to 5.0 mu but are usually rapidly reversible. These changes include mild to moderate leukopenia and thrombocytopenia as well as minor elevations in serum levels of certain liver enzymes.

Side effects associated with doses of IFN administered for treatment of condyloma acuminatum are a minor inconvenience, which are well tolerated by most patients, especially if they are forewarned of their possible occurrence.

FACTORS AFFECTING CLINICAL RESPONSES TO IFN THERAPY

Otherwise healthy persons with similar numbers and sizes of genital warts may vary widely in their response to exogenous IFN. Recent studies have demonstrated differences in the pretreatment status of responders to IFN compared to nonresponders. For example, responders to IFN demonstrate a higher pretherapy expression of the late HPV L1 gene in contrast to nonresponders who express mostly early HPV E7mRNA (39). Nonresponders (versus responders) were also characterized by condyloma acuminatum markedly depleted in Langerhans cells, which leads to decreases in major histocompatibility complex class II expression and to diminished attraction of CD_4+ T cells (40). In contrast to nonresponders, responders show a delayed-type hypersensitivity (DTH) reaction after IFN treatment, in which TH_1 cells and macrophages/natural killer cells predominate. Antigen presentation capability is also enhanced after IFN treatment in responders (41).

Response to exogenous IFN depends on a complex interaction of certain virological and immunological parameters. Optimalization of the effects of IFN on condyloma acuminatum would involve enhancement of both its antiviral and immunomodulatory activities.

THE FUTURE OF INTERFERON THERAPY FOR GENITAL WARTS

Whereas IFN is effective therapy for most cases of condyloma acuminatum, its acceptance for this indication has been limited by four factors: the need to administer IFN by injection, its expense, its potential for systemic side effects, and its slow rate of action. Although use of IFN as adjunctive therapy (e.g., following laser excision) for genital warts has several advantages over IFN monotherapy, the future of exogenous IFN for condyloma acuminatum is limited. Imiquimod is a topical inducer of endogenous IFN (as well as a spectrum of other cytokines) that has all the advantages of exogenous IFN with few (if any) disadvantages. Since imiquimod has been proven to be safe and effective therapy for condyloma acuminatum and is associated with low recurrence rates, it is destined to replace exogenous IFN, as well as most cytodestructive and surgical therapies for genital warts.

REFERENCES

1. Ferenczy A, Mitao M, Nagai N, et al. Latent papillomavirus and recurring genital warts. N Engl J Med 1985; 313: 784–788.
2. Ikic D, Bosnic N, Smerdel S, et al. Double blind clinical study with human leukocyte interferon in the therapy of condylomata acuminata. Proc Symposium Clin Use Interferon, Zagreb, Yugoslav: Acad Sci Arts, 1975: 229–233.

3. Ikic D, Orescanin M, Krusic J, Cestar Z. Preliminary study of the effect of human leukocyte interferon on condylomata acuminata in women. Proc Symposium Clin Use Interferon, Zagreb, Yugoslav: Acad Sci Arts, 1975: 223–225.

4. Keay S, Teng N, Eisenberg M, et al. Topical interferon for treating condyloma acuminata in women. J Infect Dis 1988; 158: 934–939.

5. Geffen JR, Klein RJ, Friedman-Kien AE. Intralesional administration of large doses of human leukocyte interferon for the treatment of condyloma acuminata. J Infect Dis 1984; 150: 612–615.

6. Friedman-Kien AE, Eron LJ, Conant M, et al. Natural interferon alfa for treatment of condylomata acuminata. JAMA 1988; 259: 533–538.

7. Reichman RC, Oakes D, Bonnez W et al. Treatment of condyloma acuminatum with three different interferons administered intralesionally: a double-blind, placebo-controlled trial. Ann Intern Med 1988; 108: 675–679.

8. Eron L, Judson F, Tucker S. et al. Interferon therapy for condylomata acuminata. N Engl J Med 1986; 315: 1059–1064.

9. Vance JC, Bart BJ, Hansen RC, et al. Intralesional recombinant alpha-2 interferon for the treatment of patients with condyloma acuminatum-verruca plantaris. Arch Dermatol 1986; 122: 272–277.

10. Boot JM, Blog B, Stolz E. Intralesional interferon alpha-2b treatment of condyloma acuminata previously resistant to podophyllin resin application. Genitourin Med 1989; 65: 50–53.

11. Gall SA, Hughes CE, Trofatter K. Interferon for the therapy of condyloma acuminata. Am J Obstet Gynecol 1985; 153: 157–163.

12. Reichman RC, Micha JP, Weck PK et al. Interferon alpha-nl (Wellferon) for refractory genital warts: efficacy and tolerance of low dose systemic therapy. Antiviral Res 1988; 10: 41–57.

13. Olsen EA, Trofatter KF, Gall SA, et al. Human lymphoblastoid alpha-interferon in the treatment of refractory condyloma acuminata. Clin Res 1985; 33: 673A.

14. Reichman RC, Oakes D, Bonnez W, et al. Treatment of condyloma acuminatum with three different interferon-α preparations administered parenterally: a double-blind, placebo-controlled trial. J Infect Dis 1990; 162: 1270–1276.

15. Condylomata International Collaborative Study Group. Recurrent condylomata acuminata treated with recombinant alfa-2a. JAMA 1991; 265: 2684–2687.

16. Gross G, Ikenberg H, Roussaki A, et al. Systemic treatment of condylomata acuminata with recombinant interferon-alpha-2a: low-dose superior to high-dose regimen. Chemotherapy 1986; 32: 537–541.

17. Gross G, Roussaki A, Schopf E, et al. Successful treatment of condyloma acuminata and bowenoid papulosis with subcutaneous injections of low-dosage recombinant interferon-α. Arch Dermatol 1986; 122: 749–750.

18. Gall SA, Constantine L, Koukol D. Therapy of persistent human papillomavirus disease with two different interferon species. Am J Obstet Gynecol 1991; 164: 130–134.

19. Panici PB, Scambia G, Baiocchi G, et al. Randomized clinical trial comparing systemic IFN with diathermocoagulation in primary multiple and widespread anogenital condyloma. Obstet Gynecol 1989; 74: 393–397.

20. Kirby P, Wells D, Kiviat N, Corey L. A phase I trial of intramuscular recombinant human gamma interferon for refractory genital warts. J Infect Dis 1986; 86: 485.

21. Kirby PK, Kiviat N, Beckman A, et al. Tolerance and efficacy of recombinant human interferon gamma in the treatment of refractory genital warts. Am J Med 1988; 85: 183–188.

22. Zouboulis C, Stadler R, Ikenberg H, Orfanos CE. Short-term systemic recombinant interferon-γ treatment is ineffective in recalcitrant condylomata acuminata. J Am Acad Dermatol 1991; 24: 302–303.

23. Fierlbeck G, Rassner G. Treatment of condylomata acuminata with systemically administered recombinant gamma interferon. Z. Hautkr 1987; 62: 1280–1287.

24. Gross G, Roussaki A, Brzoska J. Low doses of systemically administered recombinant interferon-gamma effective in the treatment of genital warts. J Invest Dermatol 1988; 90: 242.

25. Schneider A, Papendick U, Gissmann L, DeVilliers EM. Interferon treatment of human genital papillomavirus infection: Importance of viral type. Intl J Cancer 1987; 40: 610–614.

26. Weck PK, Buddin DA, Whisnant JK. Interferons in the treatment of genital human papillomavirus infections. Am J Med 1988; 85(suppl 2A): 159–164.

27. Erpenbach K, Derschum W, Vietsch HV. Adjuvant-systemische interferon-α2b-behandlung bei therapieresistenten anogenitalen condylomata acuminata. Urologe A 1990; 29: 43–45.

28. Vance JC, Davis D. Interferon alpha-2b injections used as an adjuvant therapy to carbon dioxide laser vaporization of recalcitrant ano-genital condylomata acuminata. J Invest Dermatol 1990; 95: 146S–148S.

29. Hohenleutner U, Landthaler M, Braun-Falco O. Post-operative adjuvante therapie mit interferon-alfa-2b nach laserchirurgie von condylomata acuminata. Hautarzt 1990; 41: 545–548.

30. Petersen CS, Bjerring P, Larsen J, et al. Systemic interferon alpha-2b increases the cure rate in laser treated patients with multiple persistent genital warts: a placebo-controlled study. Genitourin Med 1991; 67: 99–102.

31. Davis BE, Noble MJ. Initial experience with combined interferon alpha-2b and carbon dioxide laser for the treatment of condyloma acuminata. J Virol 1992; 147: 627–629.

32. Reid R, Greenberg MD, Pizzuti DJ, et al. Superficial laser vulvectomy V. surgical debulking is enhanced by adjuvant systemic interferon. Am J Obstet Gynecol 1992; 166: 815–820.

33. Condylomata International Collaborative Study Group. Randomized placebo-controlled double-blind combined therapy with laser surgery and systemic IFN-α2a in the treatment of anogenital condylomata acuminatum. J Infect Dis 1993; 167: 824–829.

34. Piccoli R, Santoro MG, Nappi C, et al. Vulvo-vaginal condylomatosis and relapse: combined treatment with electrocauterization and beta-interferon. Clin Exp Obstet Gynecol 1989; 16: 30–35.
35. Tiedemann KH, Ernst TM. Combination therapy of recurrent condylomata acuminata with electrocautery and alpha-2-interferon. Akt Dermatol 1988; 14: 200–204.
36. Handley JM, Horner T, Maw RD, et al. Subcutaneous interferon alpha 2a combined with cryotherapy vs cryotherapy alone in the treatment of primary anogenital warts: a randomized observer blind placebo controlled study. Genitourin Med 1991; 67: 297–302.
37. Eron LJ, Alder MB, O'Rourke JM, et al. Recurrence of condylomata acuminata following cryotherapy is not prevented by systemically administered interferon. Genitourin Med 1993; 69: 91–93.
38. Douglas Jr JM, Eron LJ, Judson FN, et al. A randomized trial of combination therapy with intralesional interferon alpha 2b and podophyllin versus podophyllin alone for the therapy of anogenital warts. J Infect Dis 1990; 162: 52–59.
39. Arany I, Goel A, Tyring SK. Interferon response depends on viral transcription in human papillomavirus containing lesions. Anticancer Res 1995; 15: 2865–2870.
40. Arany I, Tyring SK. Status of local cellular immunity in interferon-responsive and -nonresponsive human papillomavirus-associated lesions. Sex Trans Dis 1996; 23: 1–6.
41. Arany I, Tyring SK. Activation of local cell-mediated immunity in interferon-responsive patients with human papillomavirus-associated lesions. J IFN Cytokine Res 1996; 16: 453–460.

37
Genital Herpes Simplex Infection

Michael V. Reitano
*National Advice Centers, Sexual Health Magazine,
and New York University Hospital, New York, New York*

Jerry O. Stern
*National Advice Centers and
New York University Hospital, New York, New York*

Charles Ebel
*Sexual Health Magazine, Durham, and
Herpes Advice Center, Research Triangle Park, North Carolina*

OVERVIEW

While genital herpes remains a chronic infection that defies cure, the last decade has seen important advances in understanding the disease and refining its management.

A clinical entity characterized in the 1970s and 1980s as causing marked signs and symptoms and sometimes severe psychosocial morbidity, genital herpes today is known to be an extremely common viral infection that typically causes very mild symptoms and often goes unrecognized (1). Therapy with oral antiviral acyclovir has been shown to be safe and effective for treating the disease, and two newer compounds approved in 1995—valacyclovir and famciclovir—offer additional treatment options (2). Type-specific serological assays now available in research centers have shown that genital herpes is found in approximately one-quarter of U.S. adults, though many seropositive individuals are unaware of herpes's mild signs and symptoms and therefore, when interviewed, give no history (1,3,4).

While herpes was once considered contagious only during sympto-matic periods, more recent data show that the disease reactivates subclini-cally in the great majority of patients and can be transmitted at these times (5). The frequency of such reactivation and the lack of proven measures to stop transmission contribute to the continuing herpes epidemic and make patient counseling (and often partner counseling) an important aspect of disease management (6).

EPIDEMIOLOGY

Genital herpes is caused by herpes simplex type 2 (HSV-2) or, less fre-quently, herpes simplex virus type 1 (HSV-1), either of which can establish latency in the sacral ganglia (7). Still the more common type found in genital herpes infection, HSV-2 has been rising in prevalence since the early 1970s and is generally associated with the more severe manifesta-tions of the disease (3,8,9). While HSV-1 has long been appreciated as a near-ubiquitous infection associated with oral herpes symptoms, it now accounts for an increasing percentage of genital infection as well, with estimates ranging as high as 43% (10).

Between 1976 and 1980, the National Health and Nutrition Examina-tion Survey (NHANES) identified antibodies to HSV-2 in 16.4% of a cross-section of the U.S. population between the ages of 15 and 74 (11). A second NHANES study, however, reported that the seroprevalence of HSV-2 had reached 21.7% in 1991, a 32% increase (3). Extrapolating from the seroprevalence numbers, and allowing for a proportion of genital herpes caused by latent HSV-1 rather than HSV-2, the true prevalence of genital herpes in the United States is estimated to be in excess of 40 million.

Both the NHANES data and a number of smaller epidemiological studies have found significant demographic and behavioral correlates to seroprevalence. Rates of infection are higher in those of greater age, women, economically disadvantaged populations, and those with greater numbers of sexual partners (3,4,7,12).

The dramatic increase borne out by seroprevalence studies can be explained by the phenomena of frequently unrecognized or subclinical viral shedding and by the potential for transmission at such times (6).

Subclinical Reactivation

Studies using viral culture have shown that latent genital HSV-2 and geni-tal HSV-1 reactivate without causing clinical lesions in most seropositive individuals (9,13). Subclinical reactivation varies markedly from one individual to the next and changes over time (9). Rates of viral shedding as measured by culture have been shown to be higher in the first year after acquisition. One study found culture-proven viral shedding of 4.3% of days in the first year after primary HSV-2 versus rates of 2.3% and 2.1% in years 2 and 3 (14). More recent investigations using polymerase chain reaction (PCR) have detected viral shedding in culture-negative women (15). One investigator has found a median rate of viral shedding of 6.2% of days by culture and 23.9% of days by PCR (16).

While viral titer is generally lower in subclinical shedding, several investigators have shown that subclinical or unrecognized disease accounts for approximately 70% of genital herpes transmission (5). Patients thus must be counseled to consider themselves potentially infectious at times other than symptomatic outbreaks and to discuss risk and risk reduction measures with sexual partners.

CLINICAL DISEASE AND THE CLINICAL SPECTRUM

The most florid signs and symptoms of genital herpes have been characterized by Corey and others in patients acquiring infection for the time with one serotype in the absence of the other (for example, a first infection with HSV-2 in the absence of prior HSV-1 antibody) (17). Such patients, described as having *primary first episodes*, typically experience both systemic and local symptoms. These include lesions, pain, itching, dysuria, vaginal discharge, and inguinal adenopathy. In both men and women, pustular or ulcerative lesions are commonly found on the external genitalia. Lesions are often bilateral and may persist for two weeks or more. Inguinal adenopathy usually appears relatively later in the course of first-episode disease and may be the last symptom to resolve. Central nervous system complications such as stiff neck, headache, and photophobia are also common (17).

Patients acquiring genital herpes infection in the presence of prior infection with the alternate HSV type are described as having *nonprimary first episodes*. As with primary disease, bilateral lesions, pain, itching, and systemic symptoms commonly occur in these patients, though they are of shorter duration than in primary first episodes. Central nervous system complications also occur but are less frequent in nonprimary first episodes (17).

While first episodes can be acute, HSV symptoms in the first several weeks or months after infection may be minimal and may go unrecognized altogether. In one study, 25% of people presenting to a clinic for a supposed first attack were found to have antibody levels reflecting longstanding infection (18).

Symptomatic recurrences of genital herpes occur in 90% of patients with HSV-2—a frequency at least 1.5 times greater than that found in patients with HSV-1 (17,18). The classic herpes lesions often seen in first episodes may be present in recurrences as well, but lesions typically are smaller, less painful, and of shorter duration. Lesions are usually found on one side only, with an area of involvement one-tenth that of primary infection. Systemic symptoms such as inguinal adenopathy are less common. The mean duration of viral shedding in recurrences of HSV-2 is estimated at 4 days, as compared with 11 days in primary genital herpes (17).

Either first episodes or recurrences can be characterized by localized itching, tingling, burning, muscle aches, or other prodromal symptoms experienced by patients before the onset of frank lesions (18).

While many patients with first episode or recurrent disease will present with marked signs and symptoms, serological studies have demonstrated that the clinical spectrum is much broader than was previously understood (6). Koutsky and others have found that a variety of subtle or atypical genital fissures, cracks, and ulcerations are more common in HSV-2–positive subjects (1). In addition, when initially interviewed, seropositive individuals often do not give a history of genital herpes, but when educated about the full clinical spectrum of genital herpes, the majority learn to recognize the disease (1,19).

MANAGEMENT OF GENITAL HERPES

The antiviral agent acyclovir, a nucleoside analog that inhibits viral replication, provides an important therapy for patients with first-episode or recurrent genital herpes. Two newer antivirals, famciclovir and valacyclovir, also have been evaluated in the treatment of genital herpes; both are approved for recurrent disease and both have shown efficacy in first episodes as well. In a dose of 200 mg, 5 times a day for first episodes, oral acyclovir shortens the duration of viral shedding and speeds healing of lesions and other acute symptoms (2,20). Acyclovir has reduced duration of viral shedding in first episodes by 70% to 80% and duration of symptoms by 40% to 50% (21). The drug is well-tolerated, with minimal adverse effects and no long-term toxicity (2).

Topical acyclovir has seen clinical use in treatment of first episodes but has been shown to be less effective than oral acyclovir in reducing viral shedding and speeding healing of herpes lesions (21).

Oral therapy for primary and nonprimary first episodes can speed healing for patients by a week or more in some cases (22). Treatment is most effective when initiated early in the course of the disease but should be considered for first episodes even when patients present with florid symptoms.

Recurrent Herpes

Recurrent genital herpes can be treated either with episodic antiviral therapy or with a daily suppressive regimen.

Episodic Therapy

If initiated in the prodromal phase before the onset of lesions, treatment with acyclovir, valacyclovir, or famciclovir can reduce pain, speed healing, and reduce the duration of viral shedding (23,24). Given the importance of prompt administration, best results for episodic therapy are probably obtained with patient-initiated therapy (25). The three compounds have similar efficacy, and clinicians may weigh these therapeutic options on the basis of cost, convenience, and safety. Acyclovir, which has been available as an oral drug since 1985 in the United States, has the strongest safety profile by virtue of its long record. Famciclovir and valacyclovir, however, offer added convenience in the form of twice-daily dosing as opposed to the recommended five doses daily for acyclovir. In addition, patient-initiated valaciclovir has been shown to abort recurrences, preventing the progression of lesions to the vesicular or ulcerative stage in 31% of patients (23).

Suppressive Therapy

Antiviral drugs can be used alternately in a daily suppressive regimen to reduce the frequency of herpes symptoms or to stop recurrences altogether. Acyclovir in doses of 400 mg twice daily has been shown to bring about an 80% reduction in herpes recurrences overall, and in one five-year study 20% of participants had no recurrences for the entire duration of the study (26). Up to 15% of persons on suppressive therapy will develop a breakthrough recurrence in any given three-month period, but these are typified by a relatively short duration of viral shedding and mild symptoms (26,27). Six-year data on chronic acyclovir therapy also show no toxicity as measured by white blood cell count, serum creatinine, serum bilirubin, and other indicators (26).

Famciclovir and valacyclovir have been evaluated for use in suppressive therapy, and both have been shown effective. Famciclovir in a dose of 250 mg, twice daily effectively suppressed genital herpes in women, though a once-daily dose proved inadequate (28). Valacyclovir, meanwhile, has been trialed as a once-daily regimen and has provided results comparable to acyclovir in a six-month suppression study (29,30).

Viral Type and Recurrence Rates

A growing body of research has documented a substantial correlation between viral type, site of infection, and reactivation rates (8,9). Genital herpes caused by latent HSV-2 is more likely to reactivate both clinically and subclinically than genital HSV-1, and in one study HSV-2 was found to account for 98% of recurrent disease (8,9,31). Benedetti showed that those with HSV-2 have an average of 4 to 5 recurrences per year, while patients with HSV-1 have an average number of annual recurrences closer to 1 (8). The question of declining frequency of recurrences over time is still under study.

In addition, subclinical shedding is twice as frequent in those with HSV-2 as in those with HSV-1 (9). The leading correlates of frequent subclinical shedding are viral type and recent acquisition of HSV, with higher rates in the first year. Subclinical shedding also occurs at higher rates in those with frequent recurrences (9).

Assessing Patient Needs: Psychosexual Issues

Frequency and severity of herpes recurrences are often considered by clinicians in evaluating appropriate therapy. A number of management algorithms propose that patients with in excess of six or eight clinical recurrences per year are candidates for suppressive antiviral therapy. Clinicians, however, must also weigh the psychosocial impact of herpes and its effect on the patient's sex life. Numerous behavioral studies suggest that genital herpes causes emotional distress in the form of guilt, anxiety about recurrence, and fear of infecting a sexual partner (32,33). In addition, the social stigma that became attached to herpes in the early 1980s persists in the form of fear of discovery and in frequent communications barriers with clinicians and sexual partners. Some patients with few recurrences will benefit from suppressive therapy in gaining a sense of control and minimizing anxiety about recurrences (32).

Prevention Counseling

Because fear of infecting sexual partners ranks high among the concerns of herpes patients, many will appreciate guidance on the risks of transmission and ways to reduce this risk. Abstinence during symptomatic periods does not address the issue of subclinical shedding but is nonetheless a sound precaution. Condoms may be useful protection for some couples, but while they offer excellent sexually transmitted disease prevention in general, condoms are flawed with respect to HSV in that viral shedding may occur in places not covered or protected by condoms (5). Spermicides have shown some in vitro effectiveness against HSV but have not been tested in clinical settings (34). At least one study has shown that suppressive therapy reduces subclinical shedding by 95%, but follow-up studies on transmission rates have not been conducted (35). Patients may consider oral sex as a form of risk reduction, but they should be counseled about the possibility of oral-genital transmission and the prevalence of genital HSV-1, albeit a milder infection than genital HSV-2.

DIAGNOSIS

Numerous studies testify to the underdiagnosis of genital herpes, owing partly to the fact that the clinical spectrum of the disease has not been fully appreciated. The conventional diagnostic tools are also flawed. Viral culture, which remains the standard, offers the advantage of identifying viral type but is lacking in sensitivity, with a 50% false negative rate in recurrent herpes (1). Like viral culture, antigen detection tests require that samples be taken from active lesions and do not eliminate the problem of false negatives.

In an effort to identify genital herpes, physicians should take a detailed history and conduct a thorough examination, noting any type of recurring symptoms in the genital area. Recently formed lesions can be swabbed for viral isolation or antigen detection. Rapid methods such as cytologic exam or immunofluorescence also may be useful in conjunction with a history and visual examination (36).

Serologic Assays

Given the problem of false negatives with viral culture and antigen tests, serological assays have gained ground as a diagnostic tool. Most commercial serum tests for HSV reliably detect antibody but fail to distinguish accurately between HSV-1 and HSV-2 antibody (37). Because of the high background prevalence of HSV-1 from latent oral infection, the failure to make this distinction confounds interpretation. Newer HSV serum tests, however, such as the Western blot, are now in use at several research centers, and these may reach the commercial market in this decade (7,38). These truly type-specific assays allow clinicians to test a patient for HSV-2 antibody in the absence of lesions; a positive result, taken together with any history of genital symptoms, is highly suggestive of genital herpes (31).

SPECIAL CONSIDERATIONS

HSV in Pregnancy

Herpes simplex can be a devastating infection in newborns and continues to be seen in approximately 2000 births per year in the United States (39). Studies have suggested that protective HSV antibody is cross-placentally transferred to the fetus. Nonetheless, mothers with a history of recurrent herpes should be examined thoroughly during labor, and cesarean section remains the standard of care for those with herpes lesions or other signs of reactivation (40).

The highest risk of neonatal infection occurs in mothers who acquire herpes in pregnancy and experience a first episode at this time (41). As with sexual transmission, subclinical transmission accounts for the bulk of neonatal herpes cases, and viral shedding rates are higher in women who have recently acquired infection. Women who acquire herpes in late pregnancy lack time to establish a robust immune response to the infecting HSV type and therefore do not confer protective antibody cross-placentally, which further raises the risk of transmission (42).

Serological screening of all pregnant women and their partners may be useful in identifying those at maximum risk. Men with histories of recurrent HSV should be counseled about the risks of infecting sero-negative female partners during pregnancy and encouraged to reduce this risk through condom use or other appropriate measures, including abstinence (42).

HSV in the Immunocompromised Patient

Patients with weakened immune function, including those with HIV infection or recent kidney or bone marrow transplants, may experience more frequent recurrences of HSV (43). Therapeutic options in these cases include episodic or suppressive treatment with antiviral agents. Episodic therapy for recurrences may require doses from two to four times the typical regimen (18). Suppressive regimens have been successful in standard doses but may require adjustment in immunocompromised patients. In severely immunocompromised patients, a proportion of antiviral treatment failures may be due to acyclovir-resistant viral strains (18,44). While the majority of patients will respond to oral antiviral therapy, other options are available if lesions have not begun to clear in one week. Alternatives include intravenous acyclovir or foscarnet, or the topicals cidofovir and trifluorothymidine (45,46).

REFERENCES

1. Koutsky LA, Stevens CE, Holmes KK, Ashley RL, Kiviat NB, Critchlow CW, Corey L. Underdiagnosis of genital herpes by current clinical and viral-isolation procedures. N Engl J Med 1992; 326: 1533–1539.
2. Whitley RJ, Gnann JW Jr. Acyclovir: A decade later. N Engl J Med 1992; 327: 782–789.
3. Johnson R, Lee F, Hadgu A, McQuillan G, Aral S, Keesling S, Nahmias A. U.S. genital herpes trends during the first decade of AIDS: Prevalences increased in young whites and elevated in blacks. International Society of STD Research, Tenth Meeting. Helsinki, Finland, Aug. 29–Sept. 1, 1993, abstract 24.
4. Siegel D, Golden E, Washington AE, Morse SA, Fullilove ML, Catania JA, Marin B, Hulley SB. Prevalence and correlates of herpes simplex infections: the population-based AIDS in multiethnic neighborhoods study (AMEN study). JAMA 1992; 268: 1702–1707.
5. Mertz GJ, Benedetti J, Ashley R, Selke SA, Corey L. Risk factors for the sexual transmission of genital herpes. Ann Intern Med 1992; 116: 197–202.
6. Corey L. The current trend in genital herpes: Progress in prevention. Sexually Transmitted Diseases Supplement 1994; 21: S38–44.
7. Mertz GJ. Epidemiology of genital herpes infections. Infectious Disease Clinics of North America 1993; 7: 825–839.
8. Benedetti J, Corey L, Ashley R. Recurrence rates in genital herpes after symptomatic first-episode infections. Ann Intern Med 1994; 121: 847–854.
9. Wald A, Zeh J, Selke S, Ashley RL, Corey L. Virologic characteristics of subclinical and symptomatic genital herpes infections. N Engl J Med 1995; 333: 770–775.
10. Barton IG, Kinghorn GR, Najem S, Al-Omar LS, Potter CW. Incidence of herpes simplex virus types 1 and 2 isolated in patients with herpes genitalis in Sheffield. Br J Vener Dis 1982; 58: 44–47.

11. Johnson RE, Nahmias AJ, Magder LS, Lee FK, Brooks CA, Snowden CB. A seroepidemiologic survey of the prevalence of herpes simplex virus type 2 infection in the United States. N Engl J Med 1989; 321: 7–12.

12. Breinig MK, Kingsley LA, Armstrong JA, Freeman DJ, Ho M. Epidemiology of genital herpes in Pittsburgh: Serologic, sexual and racial correlates of apparent and inapparent herpes simplex infections. J Infect Dis 1990; 162(2): 306–312.

13. Brock VB, Selke S, Benedetti J, Douglas JM Jr., Corey L. Frequency of asymptomatic shedding of herpes simplex virus in women with genital herpes. JAMA 1990; 263: 418–420.

14. Koelle DM, Benedetti J, Langenberg A, Corey L. Asymptomatic reactivation of herpes simplex virus in women after the first episode of genital herpes. Ann Intern Med 1992; 116: 433–437.

15. Cone RW, Hobson AC, Brown Z, Ashley R, Berry S, Winter C, Corey L. Frequent detection of genital herpes simplex virus DNA by polymerase chain reaction among pregnant women. JAMA 1994; 272: 792–796.

16. Wald A, Cone R, Hobson A, Corey L. Frequent detection of herpes simplex virus DNA by polymerase chain reaction (PCR) in the genital tract. American Federation for Clinical Research. May 1995, abstract.

17. Corey, L. Genital Herpes. Sexually Transmitted Diseases. Holmes KK, Mardh P (eds.), McGraw-Hill, New York, 1990, 391–413.

18. Mertz GJ. Genital herpes simplex virus infections. Medical Clinics of North America 1990; 74: 1433–1454.

19. Langenberg A, Benedetti J, Ashley R, Selke SA, Corey L. Development of clinically recognizable genital lesions among women previously identified as having 'asymptomatic' herpes simplex type 2 infection. Annals of Int Med 1989; 110: 882–887.

20. Nilsen AE, Aasen T, Halsos AM, Kinge BR, Tjøtta, Wikström K, Fiddian AP. Efficacy of oral Acyclovir in the treatment of initial and recurrent genital herpes. Lancet 1982; 2: 571–573.

21. Kinghorn GR, Abeywickreme I, Jeavons M, Barton I, Potter CW, Jones D, Hickmott E. Efficacy of combined treatment with oral and topical Acyclovir in first episode genital herpes. Genitourin Med 1986; 62: 186–188.

22. Dorsky D, Crumpacker C. Drugs five years later: acyclovir. Annals of Internal Medicine 1987; 107: 859–874.

23. Spruance S, Tyring S, DeGragario B, Miller C, Beutner K. A large-scale, placebo-controlled trial of peroral valaciclovir for episodic treatment of recurrent genital herpes. Arch Intern Med 1996; 1729–1735.

24. Sacks S, et al. Famciclovir for the treatment of recurrent genital herpes. Proceedings of the 34th Interscience Conference on Antimicrobial Agents and Chemotherapy. Washington, DC: American Society for Microbiology; 1994, abstract.

25. Reichman, et al. Acyclovir in Genital Herpes. JAMA 1984; 251(16): 2107.

26. Goldberg LH, Kaufman R, Kurtz TO, Conant MA, Eron LJ, Batenhorst RL, Boone GS, the Acyclovir Study Group. Long-term suppression of recurrent genital herpes with Acyclovir. Arch Dermatol 1993; 129: 582–587.

27. Mindel A, Carney O, Freris M, Faherty A, Patou G, Williams P. Dosage and safety of long-term suppressive Acyclovir therapy for recurrent genital herpes. Lancet 1988; 1: 926–928.
28. Mertz GJ, Loveless MA, Kraus SJ, et al. Famciclovir for the suppression of recurrent genital herpes. Proceedings of the 34th Interscience Conference on Antimicrobial Agents and Chemotherapy. Washington, DC: American Society for Microbiology; 1994, abstract.
29. Drucker JL, Miller JM, and the International Valaciclovir Study Group. Once-daily valaciclovir sustains the suppressive efficacy and safety record of Acyclovir in recurrent genital herpes. The First European Congress of Chemotherapy. Glasgow, UK; 1996, abstract
30. Patel R, Crooks JR, Bell AR, and the International Valaciclovir Study Group. Once-daily valaciclovir for the suppression of recurrent genital herpes—the first placebo controlled clinical trial. The First European Congress of Chemotherapy. Glasgow, UK; 1996, abstract.
31. Reeves WC, Corey L, Adams HG, Vontver LA, Holmes KK. Risk of recurrence after first episodes of genital herpes: Relation to HSV type and antibody response. N Engl J Med 1981; 305: 315–319.
32. Catotti DN, Clarke P, Catoe KE. Herpes revisited: still a cause of concern. Sexually Transmitted Diseases 1993; 20: 77–80.
33. VanderPlate C, Aral SO. Psychosocial aspects of genital herpes virus infection. Health Psychology 1987; 6: 57–72.
34. Judson FN, Ehret JM, Bodin GF, Levin MJ, Rietmeijer CAM. In vitro evaluations of condoms with and without nonoxynol 9 as physical and chemical barriers against chlamydia trachomatis, herpes simplex virus type 2, and human immunodeficiency virus. Sexually Transmitted Diseases 1989; 16: 51–56.
35. Wald A, Zeh J, Barnum G, Davis LG, Corey L. Suppression of subclinical shedding of herpes simplex virus type 2 with acyclovir. Ann Intern Med 1996; 124: 8–15.
36. Ashley R. Laboratory techniques in the diagnosis of herpes simplex infection. Genitourinary Medicine 1993; 69: 174–183.
37. Ashley R, Cent A, Maggs V, Nahmias A, Corey L. Inability of enzyme immunoassays to discriminate between infections with herpes simplex virus types 1 and 2. Ann Intern Med 1991; 115: 520–526.
38. Safrin S, Arvin A, Mills J, Ashley R. Comparison of the Western immunoblot assay and a glycoprotein G enzyme immunoassay for detection of serum antibodies to herpes simplex virus type 2 in patients with AIDS. J Clin Micro 1992; 30: 1312–1314.
39. Whitley R, Arvin A, Prober C, Corey L. Predictors of morbidity and mortality in neonates with herpes simplex virus infections. N Engl J Med 1991; 324: 450–454.
40. Libman MD, Dascal A, Kramer MS, Mendelson J. Strategies for the prevention of neonatal infection with herpes simplex virus: A decision analysis. Reviews of Infectious Diseases 1991; 31: 1093–1104.

41. Brown ZA, Benedetti J, Ashley R, Burchett S, Selke S, Berry S, Vontver LA, Corey L. Neonatal herpes simplex virus infection in relation to asymptomatic maternal infection at the time of labor. N Engl J Med 1991; 324: 1247–1252.
42. Kulhanjian JA, Soroush V, Au DS, Bronzan RN, Yasukawa LL, Weylman LE, Arvin AM, Prober CG. Identification of women at unsuspected risk of primary infection with herpes simplex virus type 2 during pregnancy. N Engl J Med 1992; 326: 916–920.
43. Corey L, Spear P. Infections with herpes simplex viruses. N Engl J Med 1986; 314: 749–757.
44. Safrin S. Treatment of acyclovir-resistant herpes simplex virus infections in patients with AIDS. J AIDS 1992; 5(suppl 1): S29–S32.
45. Safrin S, Crumpacker C, Chatis P, Davis R, Hafner R, Rush J, Kessler HA, Landry B, Mills J, et al. A controlled trial comparing foscarnet with vidarabine for acyclovir-resistant mucocutaneous herpes simplex in the acquired immunodeficiency syndrome. N Engl J Med 1991; 325: 551–555.
46. Balfour H, Jr. Acyclovir-resistant herpesvirus infections: recognition and management. University of Alabama School of Medicine Division of Continuing Medical Education Dec 1995; 8.

Index

Abortion, spontaneous, genital herpes infection and, 279-280

Acetaminophen, 436

Acinetobacter, 29

Acrodermatitis chronica atrophicans (skin lesions of Lyme disease), 40, 41

Acute genital herpes, famciclovir for episodic therapy of, 447

Acute pain associated with herpes zoster, 335, 336, 429-440
  background on natural history study, 431-433
    brief pain inventory, 431-432
    quality of life and other variables, 433, 436, 437, 438
  causes of herpes zoster, 430-431
  clinical symptoms of herpes zoster, 429
  main features of herpes zoster, 429-430
  results of natural history study, 433-438
    relationship between pain and lesion size, 434, 435
    relationship between pain and pain medication, 434-438
    worst pain, 433, 434, 435, 436
  See Varicella zoster virus (VZV) neuralgia

Acute wounds, gram-negative microorganisms in, 101

Acyclovir (ACV), 270, 363, 441, 442
  acute zoster pain and, 336

[Acyclovir (ACV)]
  genital herpes and, 465
  herpes simplex labialis and, 357, 358-359
  HSV infection and, 271-273
  imiquimod compared to, 426
  neonatal herpes simplex and, 282, 283
  -resistant viral strain of HSV, 468-469
  valaciclovir as preferable to, 448
  See also Zovirax (acyclovir) capsules

African-American children, tinea capitis in, 170

Agar patch test, 56, 57-60

Age, effect on skin infections of, 53

AIDS epidemic, 217, 220-222

AIDS patients:
  antifungal drug resistance in, 233-243
  cidofovir and, 368-370

Alcohol, 1-minute alcohol cleansing, 7

Allodynia, 339

Allylamines, 145

Alopecia, 183

Alopecia areata, 170

"Alternative" herpes simplex treatment, 359

Aluminum chloride, 11

Amantadine, 267, 270

American Social Health Association (ASHA), 391
  public awareness survey of STDs by, 392-402

About the Editors

RAZA ALY is Professor of Dermatology and of Microbiology and Immunology at the University of California School of Medicine, San Francisco. The editor or coeditor of five books and the author or coauthor of over 120 professional papers, he is a member of the American Academy of Dermatology, the Society for Investigative Dermatology, the American Society of Microbiology, and the International Society for Human and Animal Mycology. Dr. Aly received the M.A. degree (1962) in biology and the M.P.H. degree (1965) from the University of Michigan, Ann Arbor, and the Ph.D. degree (1969) in medical microbiology from the University of Oklahoma, Oklahoma City.

KARL R. BEUTNER is Associate Clinical Professor of Dermatology at the University of California School of Medicine, San Francisco. A Fellow of the American Academy of Dermatology and a member of the Society for Pediatric Dermatology, the Society for Investigative Dermatology, and the American Society for Microbiology, among other organizations, he is the author or coauthor of over 50 key professional papers, book chapters, and abstracts focusing on new therapies for cutaneous viral infections. Dr. Beutner received the Ph.D. degree (1976) in microbiology and the M.D. degree (1979) from the State University of New York at Buffalo School of Medicine.

HOWARD MAIBACH is Professor of Dermatology, University of California School of Medicine, San Francisco. Dr. Maibach serves on the editorial boards of the *International Journal of Dermatology*, *Excerpta Medica*, and the *Journal of Toxicology: Clinical Toxicology* (Marcel Dekker, Inc.). His research includes work in dermatology, toxicology, and physiology, and he is the author of over 1400 papers in these and related fields, and coeditor of *Neonatal Skin* (with Edward K. Boisits), *Cutaneous Infestations and Insect Bites* (with Milton Orkin), *Percutaneous Absorption, Second Edition* (with Robert L. Bronaugh) and *Psoriasis, Second Edition* (with Henry H. Roenigk, Jr.) (all titles Marcel Dekker, Inc.). Dr. Maibach is a Fellow of the American College of Physicians and a member of the American Academy of Dermatology, the Society for Investigative Dermatology, the American Federation for Clinical Research, the American Medical Association, and the American Dermatologic Association. He received the M.D. degree (1955) from Tulane University, New Orleans, Louisiana.

Milton Keynes UK
Ingram Content Group UK Ltd.
UKHW031124141024
449569UK00006B/451